Urologic Issues for the Internist

Guest Editor

MICHAEL J. DROLLER, MD

MEDICAL CLINICS OF NORTH AMERICA

www.medical.theclinics.com

January 2011 • Volume 95 • Number 1

SAUNDERS an imprint of ELSEVIER, Inc.

W.B. SAUNDERS COMPANY
A Division of Elsevier Inc.

1600 John F. Kennedy Boulevard ● Suite 1800 ● Philadelphia, Pennsylvania 19103-2899

http://www.theclinics.com

MEDICAL CLINICS OF NORTH AMERICA Volume 95, Number 1
January 2011 ISSN 0025-7125, ISBN-13: 978-1-4377-2466-0

Editor: Rachel Glover
Developmental Editor: Donald Mumford

Medical Clinics of North America (ISSN 0025-7125) is published bimonthly by Elsevier Inc., 360 Park Avenue South, New York, NY 10010-1710. Months of issue are January, March, May, July, September, and November. Periodicals postage paid at New York, NY, and additional mailing offices. Subscription prices are USD 218 per year for US individuals, USD 404 per year for US institutions, USD 110 per year for US students, USD 277 per year for Canadian individuals, USD 525 per year for Canadian institutions, USD 173 per year for Canadian students, USD 336 per year for international individuals, USD 525 per year for international institutions and USD 173 per year for international students. To receive student/resident rate, orders must be accompanied by name of affiliated institution, date of term, and the *signature* of program/residency coordinator on institution letterhead. Orders will be billed at individual rate until proof of status is received. Foreign air speed delivery is included in all *Clinics* subscription prices. All prices are subject to change without notice. **POSTMASTER:** Send address changes to *Medical Clinics of North America*, Elsevier Health Sciences Division, Subscription Customer Service, 3251 Riverport Lane, Maryland Heights, MO 63043. **Customer Service: Telephone: 1-800-654-2452** (U.S. and Canada); **1-314-447-8871** (outside U.S. and Canada). **Fax: 1-314-447-8029. E-mail: journalscustomerservice-usa@elsevier.com** (for print support); **journalsonlinesupport-usa@ elsevier.com** (for online support).

Reprints. For copies of 100 or more of articles in this publication, please contact the Commercial Reprints Department, Elsevier Inc., 360 Park Avenue South, New York, NY 10010-1710. Tel.: 212-633-3812; Fax: 212-462-1935; E-mail: reprints@elsevier.com.

Medical Clinics of North America is also published in Spanish by McGraw-Hill Interamericana Editores S. A., P.O. Box 5-237, 06500 Mexico, D.F., Mexico.

Medical Clinics of North America is covered in *MEDLINE/PubMed (Index Medicus), Current Contents, ASCA, Excerpta Medica, Science Citation Index,* and *ISI/BIOMED.*

Printed in the United States of America.

GOAL STATEMENT

The goal of *Medical Clinics of North America* is to keep practicing physicians up to date with current clinical practice by providing timely articles reviewing the state of the art in patient care.

ACCREDITATION

The *Medical Clinics of North America* is planned and implemented in accordance with the Essential Areas and Policies of the Accreditation Council for Continuing Medical Education (ACCME) through the joint sponsorship of the University of Virginia School of Medicine and Elsevier. The University of Virginia School of Medicine is accredited by the ACCME to provide continuing medical education for physicians.

The University of Virginia School of Medicine designates this educational activity for a maximum of 15 *AMA PRA Category 1 Credits*™ for each issue, 90 credits per year. Physicians should only claim credit commensurate with the extent of their participation in the activity.

The American Medical Association has determined that physicians not licensed in the US who participate in this CME activity are eligible for a maximum of 15 *AMA PRA Category 1 Credits*™ for each issue, 90 credits per year.

Credit can be earned by reading the text material, taking the CME examination online at http://www.theclinics.com/home/cme, and completing the evaluation. After taking the test, you will be required to review any and all incorrect answers. Following completion of the test and evaluation, your credit will be awarded and you may print your certificate.

FACULTY DISCLOSURE/CONFLICT OF INTEREST

The University of Virginia School of Medicine, as an ACCME accredited provider, endorses and strives to comply with the Accreditation Council for Continuing Medical Education (ACCME) Standards of Commercial Support, Commonwealth of Virginia statutes, University of Virginia policies and procedures, and associated federal and private regulations and guidelines on the need for disclosure and monitoring of proprietary and financial interests that may affect the scientific integrity and balance of content delivered in continuing medical education activities under our auspices.

The University of Virginia School of Medicine requires that all CME activities accredited through this institution be developed independently and be scientifically rigorous, balanced and objective in the presentation/discussion of its content, theories and practices.

All authors/editors participating in an accredited CME activity are expected to disclose to the readers relevant financial relationships with commercial entities occurring within the past 12 months (such as grants or research support, employee, consultant, stock holder, member of speakers bureau, etc.). The University of Virginia School of Medicine will employ appropriate mechanisms to resolve potential conflicts of interest to maintain the standards of fair and balanced education to the reader. Questions about specific strategies can be directed to the Office of Continuing Medical Education, University of Virginia School of Medicine, Charlottesville, Virginia.
The faculty and staff of the University of Virginia Office of Continuing Medical Education have no financial affiliations to disclose.

The authors/editors listed below have identified no professional or financial affiliations for themselves or their spouse/partner:
Ardavan Akhavan, MD; Boback M. Berookhim, MD, MBA; David A. Bloom, MD; John W. Brock III, MD; David Y.T. Chen, MD; Donna Y. Deng, MD; Elodi J. Dielubanza, MD; George W. Drach, MD; Carl K. Gjertson, MD; Rachel Glover, (Acquisitions Editor); Thomas J. Guzzo, MD, MPH; Adam P. Klausner, MD; Vitaly Margulis, MD; W. Scott McDougal, MD; Jeffrey S. Montgomery, MD, MHSA; Kuwong B. Mwamukonda, MD; Craig S. Niederberger, MD; Jørgen Nordling, MD, DrMedSci, FEBU; Zamip P. Patel, MD; Mathew C. Raynor, MD; Mohummad Minhaj Siddiqui, MD; Jeffrey A. Stock, MD; Stacy T. Tanaka, MD; Britton E. Tisdale, MD; Jeremy B. Tonkin, MD; Naji J. Touma, MD, FRCS(C); Timothy Y. Tseng, MD; Robert G. Uzzo, MD; and Andrew Wolf, MD (Test Author).

The authors/editors listed below identified the following professional or financial affiliations for themselves or their spouse/partner:
Maaten Albersen, MD receives an unrestricted research grant from Bayer Healthcare Belgium.
Peter C. Albertsen, MD, MS is a consultant for Blue Cross Blue Shield and GSK, and is an investigator for Sanofi.
Natan Bar-Chama, MD is an industry funded research/investigatorAbbott pharmaceuticals and Vivus pharmaceuticals.
Culley C. Carson III, MD is a consultant and is on the Speakers' Bureau for AMS and GSK.
Michael J. Droller, MD (Guest Editor) is an industry funded research/investigator for GE/Photocure.
Magnus Fall, MD, PhD is a consultant and speaker, and has trial participation, with Pfizer and Astellas; is a consultant for Astra-tech and Sanofi-Aventis; is a consultant for and has trial participation with Medtronic and GSK.
Michael L. Guralnick, MD, FRCS(C) is on the Speakers' Bureau for Pfizer.
Philip Hanno, MD, MPH is on the Advisory Committee/Board for Pfizer, Astellas, and Trillium, and is on the Speakers' Bureau for Watson.
Gerald H. Jordan, MD is employed by Engineers and Doctors/Wallsten/PNN; is a industry funded research/investigator for Auxilium; and is a consultant for Auxilium, Cooke, and Coloplast.
Tom F. Lue, MD has a research grant from American Medical Systems, is a consultant for Pfizer, Lilly, Bayer, Medtronic, and Auxillium, and is a Board member for Genix.
J. Curtis Nickel, MD, FRCS(C) is an Industry funded research/investigator for GSK, Watson, Pfizer, J&J, Astellas, and Taris; is a consultant for GSK, Watson, Pfizer, J&J, Taris, Farr Labs, and Triton; and is an industry funded research/investigator for Astellas.
R. Corey O'Connor, MD is on the Speakers' Bureau for Astellas.
Claus G. Roehrborn, MD is on the Speakers' Bureau and the Advisory Committee/Board for GSK, Pfixer, Lilly, Sanofi, Neotract, AMS, and Watson; and is a consultant for Valeant.
Arthur I. Sagalowsky, MD is a consultant for Bioniche/Parexel.
Anthony J. Schaeffer, MD is the associate editor and a speaker for the American Urological Association; and is a consultant for Propagate Pharma, Hagen/Sinclair Research Recruiting, Inc., and SPD Development Company.
William A. See, MD is a consultant and is on the Advisory Committee/Board for AstraZeneca, and owns stock in Endocane.
Ira D. Sharlip, MD is a consultant, is on the Speakers' Bureau, and is on the Advisory Committee/Board for Lilly, Pfizer, Shionogi, and J&J.
Alan W. Shindel, MD is the Section Editor for Elsevier Inc, Yearbook of Urology.
William D. Steers, MD is an industry funded research/investigator for Allergan.
Marshall L. Stoller, MD owns stock in Ravine, is on the Advisory Committee/Board for EM Kinetics, and is a consultant and is on the Speakers' Bureau for Boston Scientific.

Disclosure of Discussion of Non-FDA Approved Uses for Pharmaceutical Products and/or Medical Devices.
The University of Virginia School of Medicine, as an ACCME provider, requires that all faculty presenters identify and disclose any off-label uses for pharmaceutical and medical device products. The University of Virginia School of Medicine recommends that each physician fully review all the available data on new products or procedures prior to clinical use.

TO ENROLL

To enroll in the Medical Clinics of North America Continuing Medical Education program, call customer service at 1-800-654-2452 or visit us online at http://www.theclinics.com/home/cme. The CME program is available to subscribers for an additional fee of USD 228.

FORTHCOMING ISSUES

March 2011
Prediabetes and Diabetes Prevention
Michael Bergman, MD,
Guest Editor

May 2011
Geriatric Medicine
John E. Morley, MB, BCh,
Guest Editor

July 2011
COPD
Stephen I. Rennard, MD, and
Bartolome R. Celli, MD,
Guest Editors

RECENT ISSUES

November 2010
Psychiatry for the Internist
Theodore A. Stern, MD,
Guest Editor

September 2010
Otolaryngology for the Internist
Matthew W. Ryan, MD, *Guest Editor*

July 2010
Drug Hypersensitivity
Werner J. Pichler, MD, *Guest Editor*

RELATED INTEREST

Urologic Clinics of North America, May 2011 (Volume 38, Issue 2)
Erectile Dysfunction
Culley C. Carson III, MD, *Guest Editor*

THE CLINICS ARE NOW AVAILABLE ONLINE!

Access your subscription at:
www.theclinics.com

Contributors

GUEST EDITOR

MICHAEL J. DROLLER, MD
Katherine and Clifford Goldsmith Professor of Urology, Professor of Oncology, Mount Sinai Medical Center, New York, New York

AUTHORS

MAARTEN ALBERSEN, MD
Research Fellow, Laboratory of Experimental Urology, Department of Urology, University Hospitals Leuven, Leuven, Belgium

PETER C. ALBERTSEN, MD, MS
Professor of Surgery (Urology), University of Connecticut Health Center, Farmington, Connecticut

ARDAVAN AKHAVAN, MD
Senior Resident, Department of Urology, Mount Sinai Medical Center, New York, New York

NATAN BAR-CHAMA, MD
Associate Professor, Departments of Urology and Obstetrics, Gynecology, and Reproductive Science, Mount Sinai Medical Center, Mount Sinai School of Medicine, New York, New York

BOBACK M. BEROOKHIM, MD, MBA
Resident, Department of Urology, Mount Sinai Medical Center, Mount Sinai School of Medicine, New York, New York

DAVID A. BLOOM, MD
Professor and Chief, Department of Urology, University of Michigan Health System, Ann Arbor, Michigan

JOHN W. BROCK III, MD
Surgeon-in-Chief and Professor, Division of Pediatric Urology, Monroe Carell Jr Children's Hospital at Vanderbilt, Nashville, Tennessee

CULLEY C. CARSON III, MD, FACS
Rhodes Distinguished Professor and Chief, Division of Urology, University of North Carolina School of Medicine, Chapel Hill, North Carolina

DAVID Y.T. CHEN, MD, FACS
Associate Professor of Surgery and Urologic Oncology Fellowship Director, Department of Surgery, Fox Chase Cancer Center, Temple University School of Medicine, Philadelphia, Pennsylvania

DONNA Y. DENG, MD
Assistant Professor of Urology, University of California, San Francisco, California

ELODI J. DIELUBANZA, MD
Department of Urology, Northwestern University, Feinberg School of Medicine, Chicago, Illinois

GEORGE W. DRACH, MD
Professor Emeritus of Urology, Division of Urology, Department of Surgery, Hospital of the University of Pennsylvania, Philadelphia, Pennsylvania

MAGNUS FALL, MD, PhD
Emeritus Professor of Urology, Institute of Clinical Sciences, Sahlgrenska Academy, University of Gothenburg, Sahlgrenska University Hospital, Gothenburg, Sweden

CARL K. GJERTSON, MD
Assistant Professor of Surgery (Urology), University of Connecticut Health Center, Farmington, Connecticut

MICHAEL L. GURALNICK, MD, FRCS(C)
Associate Professor, Department of Urology, Medical College of Wisconsin, Milwaukee, Wisconsin

THOMAS J. GUZZO, MD, MPH
Assistant Professor of Urology, Division of Urology, Department of Surgery, Hospital of the University of Pennsylvania, Philadelphia, Pennsylvania

PHILIP HANNO, MD, MPH
Professor of Surgery in Urology, Hospital of the University of Pennsylvania, Philadelphia, Pennsylvania

GERALD H. JORDAN, MD
Department of Urology, Eastern Virginia Medical School, Norfolk, Virginia

ADAM P. KLAUSNER, MD
Associate Professor and Warren W. Koontz Professor of Urologic Research, Division of Urology, Department of Surgery, Virginia Commonwealth University School of Medicine Richmond, Virginia

TOM F. LUE, MD
Professor and Vice Chair, Department of Urology, University of California at San Francisco, San Francisco, California

VITALY MARGULIS, MD
Assistant Professor, Department of Urology, University of Texas Southwestern Medical Center, Dallas, Texas

W. SCOTT MCDOUGAL, MD
Walter S. Kerr Jr Professor of Urology, Department of Urology, Massachusetts General Hospital, Harvard Medical School, Boston, Massachusetts

JEFFREY S. MONTGOMERY, MD, MHSA
Assistant Professor, Department of Urology, University of Michigan Health System, Ann Arbor, Michigan

KUWONG B. MWAMUKONDA, MD
Attending Physcian, SAUSHEC Urology Program, Brooke Army Medical Center, Houston, Texas

CRAIG S. NIEDERBERGER, MD
Professor and Head, Department of Urology, University of Illinois College of Medicine; Professor, Department of Bioengineering, College of Engineering, University of Illinois, Chicago, Illinois

J. CURTIS NICKEL, MD, FRCS(C)
Professor, Canada Research Chair in Urologic Pain and Inflammation, Department of Urology, Queen's University, Kingston General Hospital, Kingston, Ontario, Canada

JØRGEN NORDLING, MD, DrMedSci, FEBU
Professor of Urology, University of Copenhagen, Herlev Hospital, Denmark

R. COREY O'CONNOR, MD
Associate Professor, Department of Urology, Medical College of Wisconsin, Milwaukee, Wisconsin

ZAMIP P. PATEL, MD
Andrology Fellow, Department of Urology, University of Illinois College of Medicine, Chicago, Illinois

MATHEW C. RAYNOR, MD
Fellow, Division of Urology, University of North Carolina School of Medicine, Chapel Hill, North Carolina

CLAUS G. ROEHRBORN, MD
Professor and Chairman, Department of Urology, University of Texas Southwestern Medical Center, Dallas, Texas

ARTHUR I. SAGALOWSKY, MD
Professor, Department of Urology, University of Texas Southwestern Medical Center, Dallas, Texas

ANTHONY J. SCHAEFFER, MD
Professor and Chairman, Department of Urology, Northwestern University, Feinberg School of Medicine, Chicago, Illinois

WILLIAM A. SEE, MD
Professor and Chair, Department of Urology, Medical College of Wisconsin, Milwaukee, Wisconsin

IRA D. SHARLIP, MD
Clinical Professor, Department of Urology, University of California, San Francisco, California

ALAN W. SHINDEL, MD
Assistant Professor, Department of Urology, Lawrence J. Ellison Ambulatory Care Center, University of California at Davis, Sacramento, California

MOHUMMAD MINHAJ SIDDIQUI, MD
Clinical Fellow in Surgery, Department of Urology, Massachusetts General Hospital, Harvard Medical School, Boston, Massachusetts

WILLIAM D. STEERS, MD
Professor and Hovey Dabney Chair, Department of Urology, University of Virginia School of Medicine, Charlottesville, Virginia

JEFFREY A. STOCK, MD
Chief, Division of Pediatric Urology, Department of Urology, Mount Sinai Kravis Children's Hospital, New York, New York

MARSHALL L. STOLLER, MD
Department of Urology, University of California, San Francisco, California

STACY T. TANAKA, MD
Assistant Professor, Division of Pediatric Urology, Monroe Carell Jr Children's Hospital at Vanderbilt, Nashville, Tennessee

BRITTON E. TISDALE, MD
Department of Urology, Eastern Virginia Medical School, Norfolk, Virginia

JEREMY B. TONKIN, MD
Department of Urology, Eastern Virginia Medical School, Norfolk, Virginia

NAJI J. TOUMA, MD, FRCS(C)
Assistant Professor, Department of Urology, Queen's University, Kingston General Hospital, Kingston, Ontario

TIMOTHY Y. TSENG, MD
Department of Urology, University of Texas Health Science Center, San Antonio, Texas

ROBERT G. UZZO, MD, FACS
G. Willing "Wing" Pepper Chairman in Cancer Research, Professor and Chairman, Department of Surgery, Fox Chase Cancer Center, Temple University School of Medicine, Philadelphia, Pennsylvania

Contents

Preface: Urologic Issues for the Internist   xv

Michael J. Droller

Pediatric Urologic Conditions, Including Urinary Infections   1

Stacy T. Tanaka and John W. Brock III

Genitourinary complaints are common in children, and the busy primary care provider must determine initial treatment and assess need for specialty referral. Many complaints are self-limited, but some represent disorders that can threaten organ function. In this article, an initial approach in the primary care office and a guide to specialty referral for pediatric urologic conditions of the urinary tract, male genitalia, and female genitalia are suggested.

Long-term Follow-up and Late Complications Following Treatment of Pediatric Urologic Disorders   15

Ardavan Akhavan and Jeffrey A. Stock

Many pediatric urologic disorders have sequelae that may affect patients well into adulthood. Despite adequate treatment, many patients are at risk for progressive urologic deterioration years after surgical reconstruction. While many pediatric urologists follow their patients years after surgery, screening for late complications is a shared responsibility with primary care providers. This article discusses potential late complications and appropriate follow-up for patients who have a history of ureteral reimplantation, pyeloplasty, hypospadias repair, posterior urethral valve ablation, and intestinal interposition.

Urinary Tract Infections in Women   27

Elodi J. Dielubanza and Anthony J. Schaeffer

Urinary tract infection (UTI) is the most common extraintestinal infectious disease entity in women worldwide, and perhaps one of the most formidable challenges in clinical practice given its high prevalence, frequent recurrence, and myriad associated morbidities in the setting of rapidly evolving antimicrobial resistance. Achieving timely symptom relief and infection control and preventing morbidity, growth of resistant organisms, and recurrent infection are often difficult. This article reviews epidemiology and pathogenesis of urinary tract infection in women; characterizes common patterns of infection, clinical red flags, and appropriate laboratory testing and imaging; explores emerging patterns of antimicrobial resistance; and reviews the updated guidelines for the treatment of uncomplicated UTI in women.

Urinary Infections in Men   43

Mathew C. Raynor and Culley C. Carson III

Urinary tract infections are one of the most common bacterial infections and account for significant morbidity and mortality. This review of urinary infections in men provides an overview of the general presentation, diagnosis, and management of common genitourinary infections in men. The focus of this article is on clinical presentation, basic diagnostic evaluation strategies, treatment options, and when referral to a specialist is warranted.

Bladder Pain Syndrome 55

Philip Hanno, Jørgen Nordling, and Magnus Fall

Bladder pain syndrome is a deceptively intricate symptom complex that is diagnosed on the basis of chronic pelvic pain, pressure, or discomfort perceived to be related to the urinary bladder, accompanied by at least one other urinary symptom. It is a diagnosis of exclusion in a patient who has experienced the symptoms for at least 6 weeks in the absence of any confusable diseases that may give rise to the symptoms. Symptoms compatible with the diagnosis are now thought to affect up to 3% of the female population in the United States with a 5:1 female-to-male preponderance. Diagnosis and treatment can be challenging, and misdiagnosis as a psychological problem, overactive bladder, or chronic urinary infection has plagued patients with the problem.

Prostatitis and Chronic Pelvic Pain Syndrome in Men 75

Naji J. Touma and J. Curtis Nickel

Primary care physicians can and should diagnose, classify, and treat patients presenting with acute and chronic prostatitis syndromes. Although the chronic syndromes are a challenge to manage, this review article provides the necessary background to allow primary care physicians to take on this task. Patients who are unfortunate to be diagnosed with a prostatitis syndrome have the best chance for successful therapy at initial presentation. Those patients will ultimately benefit from an informed and educated physician.

Male Lower Urinary Tract Symptoms (LUTS) and Benign Prostatic Hyperplasia (BPH) 87

Claus G. Roehrborn

Male lower urinary tract symptoms, benign prostatic hyperplasia, enlargement of the prostate, and bladder outlet obstruction are common among aging men and will increase in socioeconomic and medical importance at a time of increased life expectancy and aging of the baby boomer generation. This article reviews the epidemiology, management, and therapeutic options for these conditions. In patients bothered by moderate to severe symptoms, providers can make educated and differential choices between several classes of drugs, alone or in combination, to treat effectively and improve the symptoms in most men. Despite the efficacy of medical therapy, there will be patients who require referral to a urologist either early, to rule out prostate cancer and other conditions, or later, after initial medical therapy and lifestyle management has failed. Perhaps as many as 30% of patients fail to achieve sufficient symptom improvement with medication, lifestyle adjustment, and fluid management, and may require more invasive or surgical treatment options.

Urinary Incontinence in Women 101

Donna Y. Deng

Urinary incontinence is a common and vexing problem that affects millions of adults. The main types of incontinence in women are stress, urge, and mixed. It is important to delineate the different types to target the treatment options better. Treatments include conservative or behavioral modifications, pharmacotherapy, and surgical interventions.

The Neurogenic Bladder: An Update with Management Strategies for Primary Care Physicians 111

Adam P. Klausner and William D. Steers

Patients with lesions of the central nervous system often have neurogenic bladder dysfunction. Lifelong bladder monitoring and management in these patients is necessary to prevent severe complications, including renal damage. The urodynamic test, performed by neurourologists or other specially trained providers, is the definitive test for diagnosis and management of neurogenic bladder dysfunction. This article describes the indications and technique of urodynamic testing and the interpretation of the results of such testing. The management of patients with neurogenic bladder dysfunction is also discussed.

Assessment and Management of Irritative Voiding Symptoms 121

Michael L. Guralnick, R. Corey O'Connor, and William A. See

Irritative voiding symptoms are to the urinary tract much as a cough is to the pulmonary system, that is, a nonspecific manifestation of multiple potential underlying causes. Key to the evaluation and management of patients with these symptoms is a clear understanding of the differential diagnosis, the diagnostic tests required for evaluation, and the role of specialists in diagnosis and treatment. This article outlines a general diagnostic approach for patients with irritative voiding symptoms. Treatment approaches for the diseases, as well as the initial management that may be performed in the primary care setting, are also discussed.

Urologic Aspects of HIV Infection 129

Alan W. Shindel, Ardavan Akhavan, and Ira D. Sharlip

Although lifespan has dramatically improved in the human immunodeficiency virus–positive (HIV+) population, HIV and its treatment continue to be a source of substantial morbidity in many organ systems, including the genitourinary tract. As the number of long-term survivors increases with advances in antiretroviral therapy, age-associated urologic symptoms are also becoming increasingly relevant considerations for people living with HIV. Primary care physicians have a major role to play in maintaining the genitourinary health of their HIV+ patients. This role is of great importance not just for the well-being of the individual patient but for the public health, as the genitourinary tract is a common vector for HIV transmission. In this article the authors review the management of the genitourinary system in patients with HIV infection. Particular consideration is given to urinary tract infections, lower urinary tract symptoms, renal insufficiency, sexual and fertility problems, and cancers of the genitourinary tract. Management algorithms are outlined and indications for referral to a urologist are emphasized.

Assessment of Hematuria 153

Vitaly Margulis and Arthur I. Sagalowsky

The most common causes of hematuria in adults include urinary tract infections, urolithiasis, benign prostatic enlargement, and urologic malignancy. Once hematuria is confirmed, its cause should be investigated through a comprehensive history, a focused physical examination, laboratory studies, an image-based assessment of the upper urinary tract, and a cystoscopic evaluation of the lower urinary system. Prompt evaluation and appropriate referral of patients with documented hematuria should be initiated in the primary care setting according to the proposed guidelines, and aimed at cost-effective and early detection of urologic abnormality.

Urologic Assessment of Decreasing Renal Function   161

Mohummad Minhaj Siddiqui and W. Scott McDougal

The discussion of renal failure as it relates to urology is largely a discussion of obstructive uropathy. Obstructive uropathy has been identified in multiple series to account for approximately 10% of all cases of renal failure. On a total population scale, autopsy series have shown the prevalence of hydronephrosis in 3% of men and women who are younger than 65 years and 6% of men older than 65 years. When benign prostatic hypertrophy and renal stone disease are considered, obstructive uropathy is also one of the most common indications for surgery. In this review, the different causes of obstructive renal insufficiency and management options available are discussed.

Medical and Medical/Urologic Approaches in Acute and Chronic Urologic Stone Disease   169

Timothy Y. Tseng and Marshall L. Stoller

Urinary stone disease is a condition with far-reaching implications. Patients with their initial instance of acute renal colic enter the health care system through 2 routes. Severe cases are generally seen in the emergency room, whereas more tolerable cases may be seen by primary care physicians. Patients with urinary stone disease are then managed in the long-term by a urologist. Timely and appropriate treatment of patients with urinary stone disease is essential to prevent the development of sepsis and progressive renal insufficiency. This article reviews the epidemiology, pathogenesis, presentation, and short- and long-term management of acute and chronic urinary stone disease.

Evaluation and Management of the Renal Mass   179

David Y.T. Chen and Robert G. Uzzo

The evaluation and management of renal cell carcinoma (RCC) has evolved in recent decades in response to the changing clinical presentation of the disease. Traditional teaching suggested that RCC usually presents with signs or symptoms. However, RCC discovered this way was usually locally advanced and often metastatic, requiring radical nephrectomy in most cases but often having a poor prognosis. As contemporary general medical practice began routinely using axial body imaging in the evaluation of many nonspecific abdominal complaints, today more than 70% of RCC cases identified are "screen-detected" as incidental findings having no attributable symptoms. This change has prompted a significant RCC stage migration over the past 20 years, with most kidney tumors seen in 2010 being smaller, organ-confined, and appropriate for nephron-sparing approaches with the anticipation of a favorable outcome. The approach to addressing patients with these incidentally detected, often localized, small renal masses raises different concerns than those for traditional patients presenting with symptomatic RCC. This article reviews the modern epidemiology of RCC, outlines the components of the evaluation of the incidental renal mass, details the current options of management, and discusses the long-term expectations for these patients.

Use and Assessment of PSA in Prostate Cancer   **191**

Carl K. Gjertson and Peter C. Albertsen

Since the introduction of prostate-specific antigen (PSA) screening in the late 1980s, more prostate cancers have been detected, and at an earlier stage. As a consequence, the majority of prostate cancers are now detected years before the emergence of clinically evident disease, which usually represents locally advanced or metastatic cancer. PSA screening has remained controversial, because many of the prostate cancers detected are low grade and slow growing. With this long natural history and a median survival without treatment that often approaches at least 15 to 20 years, many clinicians and researchers have questioned if prostate cancer screening and treatment actually improves survival, as many patients will die *with* prostate cancer rather than *of* prostate cancer. In this review, the authors discuss the rationale for prostate cancer screening and present the current guidelines for the use of PSA.

Evaluation and Treatment of Erectile Dysfunction   **201**

Maarten Albersen, Kuwong B. Mwamukonda, Alan W. Shindel, and Tom F. Lue

Erectile dysfunction (ED) is a prevalent and important disease that has been associated with various comorbidities. The evaluation of patients with ED should include a general health assessment followed by a discussion of reversible factors and lifestyle changes that might help preserve erectile capacity. Numerous effective treatment options are currently available. A frank discussion about use and side effects of these therapies is required to optimize success. Although oral pharmacologic treatments can be initiated and monitored by the primary care physician, patients who do not experience response to these treatments may be best served by referral to a sexual medicine specialist for further assessment and consideration of other treatment options. This article discusses the physiology and pathophysiology of erectile function in men, how the primary care physician may address the clinical problem of ED in practice, and when specialty referral is indicated.

Medical Implications of Erectile Dysfunction   **213**

Boback M. Berookhim and Natan Bar-Chama

Erectile dysfunction (ED) is a common condition in aging men, with a prevalence of 52% in men aged 40 to 70 years. It is frequently associated with several comorbid conditions, including cardiovascular disease, lower urinary tract symptoms, and testosterone deficiency. These conditions often have major consequences on the quality of life of patients and require adequate evaluation by the primary care practitioner. Complaints of ED, therefore, serve as a marker for these conditions and give the practitioner an opportunity to prevent the consequences of a delay in treatment. In this article, the evidence behind these associations is described.

Male Factor Assessment in Infertility   223

Zamip P. Patel and Craig S. Niederberger

> Male infertility assessment is more than a semen analysis. By interpreting
> a semen analysis, clinicians recognize its uses and limitations. Once
> understood, clinicians can then apply modern techniques of endocrine
> and radiologic evaluation to diagnosis of male reproductive dysfunction.
> It is important to identify patients with infertility not only to allow reproduc-
> tive potential but also to identify a population susceptible to future disease
> states.

The Diagnosis and Management of Scrotal Masses   235

Jeffrey S. Montgomery and David A. Bloom

> When evaluating a patient with a scrotal mass, a careful history and ingui-
> noscrotal examination are necessary. Malignant scrotal wall, paratesticu-
> lar, or spermatic cord tumors are rare. Scrotal ultrasound can confirm the
> precise location of a mass or rule out the presence of an inguinal hernia.
> Testicular masses deserve a formal workup, with serum tumor markers,
> a scrotal ultrasound as needed, and prompt consultation with a urologist
> for further staging and intervention. Scrotal masses in children are much
> rarer than in adults and should be evaluated by a urologist.

Assessment and Initial Management of Urologic Trauma   245

Jeremy B. Tonkin, Britton E. Tisdale, and Gerald H. Jordan

> This article discusses the appropriate assessment, initial management,
> timely referral to a urologist for abdominal, bladder, urogenital, and
> renal/renal collecting system injury. Appropriate laboratory and physical
> examinations, as well as radiologic imaging, are paramount to obtaining
> accurate diagnosis and to providing appropriate treatment.

Major Urologic Problems in Geriatrics: Assessment and Management   253

Thomas J. Guzzo and George W. Drach

> Elderly urologic patients require the same cautions as used in develop-
> ment of treatment programs for them in other disciplines. Because of
> potential interference with poor renal function or crossover effects with
> central or peripheral nervous system, however, many urologic drugs
> must be titrated appropriately. In treating cancer, erectile dysfunction,
> incontinence or urinary infection, patient quality of life and life span
> become dominant factors in making therapeutic decisions, by behavioral
> change, medication, or surgical intervention.

Index   265

Preface:
Urologic Issues for the Internist

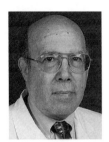

Michael J. Droller, MD
Guest Editor

When asked to edit this issue for *Medical Clinics of North America* on "Urologic Issues for the Internist," I had no hesitation in accepting. I had several reasons for this.

First was that an earlier issue of *The Clinics* on this topic had been edited by my colleague and close friend, Dr Martin I. Resnick (*Medical Clinics of North America*, volume 88, 2004). I considered editing this new updated issue a wonderful opportunity to honor my friend by providing a text that built upon and extended his important contribution.

Second was an appreciation that many conditions treated by urologists often represent problems that are to some extent, and often in large part, medically based. Thus, we as urologists (and our patients) might actually benefit from considering the medical perspectives offered by primary care physicians while they as our target audience in this issue of the *Medical Clinics in North America* (and their patients) might benefit from an understanding of these conditions from the urologist's point of view. I therefore envisioned this as an opportunity to provide our medical colleagues with a urologic perspective on the knowledge and approaches we considered important in what they could do for these patients, and when we considered it important for them to refer these patients to us for specialist attention.

Third was a perception that an updated presentation of urologic conditions from the urologist's perspective might more readily encourage primary care physicians to become true partners in assessing and initiating what we as urologists considered appropriate treatments for these patients. This might not only enhance overall urologic care through an improved understanding of these conditions from several perspectives but might also facilitate and enhance the application and efficacy of treatments when more specialist care might ultimately be needed.

Med Clin N Am 95 (2011) xv–xvi
doi:10.1016/j.mcna.2010.08.035
0025-7125/11/$ – see front matter © 2011 Elsevier Inc. All rights reserved.

medical.theclinics.com

Fourth was the potential opportunity I believed could be created in allowing leaders in our specialty to present their approaches and concepts on a variety of urologic conditions in a way that might prompt a general consideration of the issues involved, and that might encourage new thoughts on those issues that are still problematic.

In his preface to the earlier edition he edited, Dr Resnick commented that in his "review of the disorders managed by urologists, it became apparent that many applied to the general practice of medicine." He then suggested that although some "are potentially life-threatening, ... others tend to have significant impact on quality of life," and might favor a medical approach. On this basis, he described the contributions he compiled as intending to address "disorders that are common to urologic practice but also are common to all physicians practicing medicine. Some can be evaluated and treated by the primary care physician, (while, *sic*) others require referral to a urologic specialist." In sharing these thoughts and perspectives, I have attempted to apply this approach in presenting the various topics included in this issue of the *Medical Clinics of North America*.

The authors of the individual articles in this text have generously contributed their time and shared their knowledge in discussing the many issues comprising this text in which they are expert. In addition, they have selflessly adopted a highly informative and generalizeable approach in presenting state-of-the-art information that can be utilized by primary care physicians and urologists alike. Their amenability to accepting this approach has resulted in what I believe is a very understandable and practical text that can be utilized to excellent effect in the assessment and management of the variety of disorders and conditions presented. For this, I am profoundly appreciative. They merit full credit for their outstanding contributions.

It has been a pleasure to work with each of the contributors, with the editorial staff of *Medical Clinics of North America*, and with those who have made so many fine suggestions in the production of this text. I would also like to express my gratitude to Dr Datta Wagle for suggesting this project, and my appreciation in memoriam to Dr Martin Resnick for having initiated the concept and provided the foundation from which I could work with my urologic and our primary care colleagues in this effort.

Michael J. Droller, MD
Department of Urology
The Mount Sinai Medical Center
Box 1272
One Gustave L. Levy Place
New York, NY 10029, USA

E-mail address:
Michael.Droller@mountsinai.org

Pediatric Urologic Conditions, Including Urinary Infections

Stacy T. Tanaka, MD*, John W. Brock III, MD

KEYWORDS

- Pediatrics • Urologic diseases • Urinary tract
- Vesicoureteral reflux

Genitourinary complaints are common in children, and the busy primary care provider must determine initial treatment and assess need for specialty referral. Many complaints are self limited, but some represent disorders that can threaten organ function. Our goal is to suggest an initial approach in the primary care office and guide to specialty referral for pediatric urologic conditions of the urinary tract, male genitalia and female genitalia.

URINARY TRACT

Urinary Tract Infections, Febrile Urinary Tract Infections, and Vesicoureteral Reflux

Urinary tract infection (UTI) is frequent in children and can involve the bladder or kidney. Bladder infection typically presents with dysuria, urinary frequency, and/or new-onset incontinence. Kidney infection additionally presents with flank pain and high-grade fever. Kidney infections can also cause permanent renal injury. In infants, fever may be the only sign of a UTI. Kidney infections represent a significant health burden, accounting for 13,000 annual inpatient pediatric admissions at an estimated cost of $180 million in the United States.[1]

Because contaminated urine specimens can lead to unnecessary evaluation, the management of UTI begins with accurate diagnosis. Shaikh and colleagues[2] reviewed the accuracy of signs and symptoms associated with pediatric UTI and defined risk factors and clinical signs associated with increased likelihood of UTI. These risk factors are incorporated into the algorithm for UTI management in **Fig. 1**. In children with very low likelihood of UTI, urinalyses are not indicated. In children with higher likelihood, both urinalysis and urine culture should be sent. Hospitalization should be considered for children with the following characteristics: age less than 3 months, toxic appearance, dehydration, or inability to retain oral intake. Cefixime, a third generation cephalosporin, can be used for outpatient treatment (8 mg/kg/d in 2 divided

The authors have nothing to disclose.
Division of Pediatric Urology, Monroe Carell Jr Children's Hospital at Vanderbilt, 4102 Doctors' Office Tower, 2200 Children's Way, Nashville, TN 37232-9820, USA
* Corresponding author.
E-mail address: stacy.tanaka@vanderbilt.edu

Med Clin N Am 95 (2011) 1–13
doi:10.1016/j.mcna.2010.08.018
0025-7125/11/$ – see front matter © 2011 Elsevier Inc. All rights reserved.

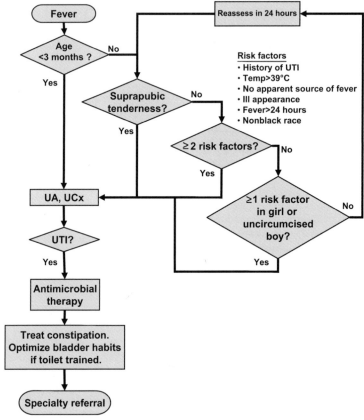

Fig. 1. Approach to UTI for children (*A*) younger than 24 months (*B*) older than 24 months. UA, urinalysis; UCx, urine culture. (*Adapted from* Shaikh N, Morone NE, Lopez J, et al. Does this child have a urinary tract infection? JAMA 2007;298:2895; with permission.)

doses). Children with febrile UTI should be treated for 7 to 14 days.[3] Duration of therapy can be shortened to 5 to 7 days for children older than 24 months without fever. Older children can also be treated with trimethoprim-sulfamethoxazole (6–12 mg/kd/d trimethoprim in 2 divided doses), but caution should be used in febrile UTIs because antibiotic resistance has been increasing in some communities.

Initial management after UTI treatment should focus on optimization of bladder and bowel habits. Infrequent voiding and constipation are common in children referred for UTIs.[4,5] Children should empty their bladders regularly every 2 hours during the day, allowing adequate time to empty completely. Constipation should be aggressively treated.[6] These learned behaviors are often frustrating and difficult for the parent and child to correct. Appropriate reassurance should be given rather than focusing on testing for an imagined underlying problem.

A history of high-grade fever with UTI suggests kidney involvement. There is no up-to-date consensus on the optimal workup of febrile UTI in children. In 1999, the American Academy of Pediatrics (AAP) recommended renal ultrasonography and voiding cystourethrogram (VCUG) to identify anatomic abnormalities with increased risk for

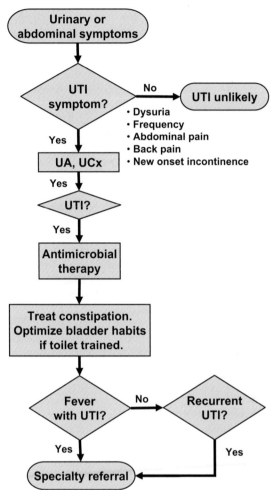

B Age>24 months

Fig. 1. (*continued*)

recurrence and kidney damage.[3] The renal ultrasonography is a noninvasive imaging technique that does not require radiation. Renal ultrasonography provides a gross assessment of urinary tract anatomy, including the size and shape of the kidneys and appearance of the bladder. The technique may also identify abnormalities such as hydronephrosis, ureteroceles, ectopic kidneys, solitary kidney, or renal dysplasia. However, with the prevalence of antenatal sonography, the likelihood of an abnormal ultrasonography after UTI is decreased. Furthermore, the sensitivity for renal ultrasonography to detect high grades of vesicoureteral reflux and renal scarring is low.[7]

Vesicoureteral reflux, the abnormal reflux of urine from the bladder to one or both kidneys, is the most commonly detected anatomic abnormality occurring in 30% to 40% of children presenting with febrile UTI.[8] VCUG primarily assesses for vesicoureteral reflux but can also identify bladder outlet obstruction from ureteroceles or posterior urethral valves. VCUG requires urethral catheterization and radiation exposure. Reflux severity is graded from 1 to 5 based on the associated dilatation of the ureter and collecting system on VCUG, and patients with high-grade reflux are more likely to have scarring than those with low-grade reflux.[3] However, even patients with grade 1 reflux can have problems with recurrent episodes of febrile UTI. The necessity of VCUG in the workup of febrile UTI has recently come into question. There is clearly a subset of patients with vesicoureteral reflux in whom medical treatment with antibiotic prophylaxis reduces neither the rate of infection nor the renal scarring.[9,10] As a result, some practitioners have argued that the diagnosis of vesicoureteral reflux and subsequent treatment is not beneficial for many children.

An alternative evaluation of the child with febrile UTI uses the "top-down" approach,[11] with initial dimercaptosuccinic acid (DMSA) renal scan and VCUG only for children with renal cortical defects, thereby avoiding urethral catheterization in many children. DMSA scan does not require urethral catheterization but requires intravenous access for administration of the radiotracer. Definitive data are not available to show the superiority of any of these imaging approaches. Because the renal ultrasonography is noninvasive and does not involve radiation, it is reasonable for the primary care provider to recommend an ultrasonography as an initial imaging technique for the child with a febrile UTI. The authors continue to recommend VCUG in all younger children with a history of febrile UTI. In younger children who are unable to verbally communicate lower urinary tract symptoms, delayed detection of recurrent pyelonephritis may be associated with significant morbidity. The detection of genitourinary abnormalities is especially important in younger infants in whom recurrent presentation with fever may necessitate an extensive medical workup.

The optimal management of children diagnosed with vesicoureteral reflux is controversial and evolving. Treatment options may include observation of antibiotics, continuous antibiotic prophylaxis, endoscopic surgical correction, or open surgical correction. Because of the variety of options available, specialty referral to discuss benefits and risks of these multiple approaches is warranted.

Antenatal Hydronephrosis

Antenatal hydronephrosis (ANH) affects 1% to 5% of all pregnancies. Most children with ANH have transient hydronephrosis that resolves without any intervention. Surgical intervention may be required for congenital obstructive processes, such as ureteropelvic junction obstruction, ureterovesical junction obstruction, ureterocele/ectopic ureter, and posterior urethral valves. These processes can cause varying degrees of hydronephrosis and renal damage. Vesicoureteral reflux, although not obstructive, can also cause dilation of the kidney collecting system.

The Society for Fetal Urology (SFU) recently published a consensus statement with recommendations for the postnatal evaluation of ANH.[12] The society recommended initial postnatal renal ultrasonography within the first week of life for unilateral ANH with a normal contralateral kidney and within the first 1 to 3 days of life for antenatal findings that suggested bladder outlet obstruction, including bilateral ANH, ANH in a solitary kidney, bladder or urethral abnormalities, or decreased amniotic fluid. In children with suspected bladder outlet obstruction, urologic consultation and potential surgical management optimally take place before hospital discharge of the newborn. In all other patients, specialty referral should be arranged by approximately 1 month of age. Because renal ultrasonography in the first week of life can underestimate hydronephrosis, a repeat ultrasonography should be performed at that time.

The efficacy of prophylactic antibiotics in the setting of ANH has not been proven by randomized controlled trial. The SFU has recommended initial antibiotic prophylaxis for children with moderate and severe hydronephrosis.[12] Because it may be difficult for the primary care provider to grade ANH severity, it is not unreasonable to start short-term antibiotic prophylaxis (amoxicillin, 10 mg/kg daily) for all neonates with ANH, pending further evaluation.

Additional studies may include VCUG and mercaptoacetyltriglycine (MAG3) diuretic renal scan. VCUG evaluates vesicoureteral reflux as well as lower urinary tract abnormalities, such as ureterocele and posterior urethral valves. MAG3 diuretic renal scan evaluates differential kidney function and severity of obstruction. Based on the results of the evaluation, specialty follow-up can range from serial ultrasonography to surgical intervention.

Multicystic dysplastic kidney (MCDK) can be confused with hydronephrosis. In contrast to hydronephrosis, the cysts in MCDK do not communicate, and there is no evidence of renal parenchyma. The contralateral solitary functioning kidney has a higher risk of urologic abnormalities, including vesicoureteral reflux, ureteropelvic junction obstruction, and ureterovesical junction obstruction. Varied, often contradictory, strategies for imaging evaluation and follow-up for MCDK have been published.[13] Specialty referral is warranted to discuss the benefits and risks of these strategies. **Fig. 2** presents an algorithm for the postnatal management of ANH.

Incontinence and Other Lower Urinary Tract Dysfunction

Urinary incontinence in the absence of UTI is a common concern in the pediatric population. Normal toilet training readiness occurs at different ages for different children. Nighttime bladder control frequently occurs years after daytime training is complete. Although most incontinence and lower urinary tract symptoms can be managed by the primary care provider, these symptoms may be the initial presentation of neurologic or other anatomic abnormalities in some children. Both neurogenic bladder and obstructive uropathy can threaten kidney function. A careful and directed initial evaluation by the primary care provider, as described later, is necessary to determine which children need immediate specialty referral.

The International Children's Continence Society has published recommendations for the evaluation of children with daytime incontinence.[14] Incontinence is the most apparent symptom of lower urinary tract dysfunction, but children and their families should also be questioned about increased urinary frequency; decreased urinary

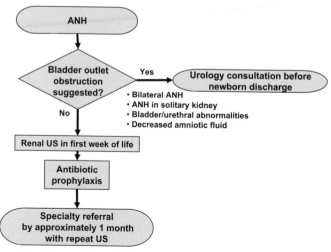

Fig. 2. Approach to history of ANH. US, ultrasonography.

frequency; urgency; holding maneuvers, such as pressing on the perineum or dancing with the urge to urinate; dysuria; interrupted stream during urination; straining during voiding; and weak stream. Because bladder dysfunction is commonly associated with bowel dysfunction, the frequency and consistency of bowel movements as well as fecal incontinence should be assessed.[6] The presence of polydipsia and type of fluid intake should be ascertained. Urine dipstick testing should be used in all children with urinary complaints to screen for UTI, diabetes mellitus, and proteinuria from kidney disease.

Immediate specialty referral is warranted in select children with lower urinary tract symptoms. Bladder dysfunction associated with suspected spinal cord disease should be addressed expediently. Clinical suspicion may arise from the history taking (eg, spinal cord injury, previous back surgery) or physical examination (eg, cutaneous manifestations of spinal dysraphism, such as sacral dimple, decreased strength or hypotrophy of lower extremities).[15] Bladder dysfunction associated with suspected nephrologic or urologic disease also warrants referral. Signs of kidney disease include hypertension, peripheral edema, and proteinuria. A history of febrile UTIs, prior urologic surgery, or continuous incontinence in a neurologically intact child raises the possibility of urologic anatomic abnormality.

The remaining children with daytime lower urinary tract symptoms do not necessarily need specialty referral. Most of them improve with optimization of bladder and bowel habits. In addition, for children with urinary frequency, urgency, and/or dysuria as the primary complaint, avoidance of bladder irritants, such as caffeine, chocolate, carbonated beverages, and citrus juices, may be helpful. Idiopathic hypercalciuria may also cause urinary frequency and dysuria. Anticholinergics should not be started without confirmation that the bladder is emptying well. Children with persistent symptoms benefit from specialty referral.

The International Children's Continence Society has also published recommendations for children who have monosymptomatic enuresis (bedwetting without any daytime lower urinary tract symptoms).[16] Families should be reassured that enuresis is a common condition, and active treatment should not be started before 6 years of age. Alarm therapy results in dryness in two-thirds of children when used correctly. It requires a highly motivated family to use the alarm every night for a minimum of 2 to 3 months and make sure the child awakens to the alarm to visit the toilet.[17] Desmopressin may also be used. The starting dose is 0.4 mg taken 30 to 60 minutes before sleep. The dose can be tapered down to 0.2 mg or up to a maximum of 0.6 mg. Only 30% of children are full responders, and the curative potential is low. In children with response, the desmopressin can be taken daily or only on important nights. If the medication is taken daily, regular drug holidays are essential to see if the medication is still needed. Children with persistent enuresis may benefit from specialty referral for additional evaluation.

Additional urologic workup for those children who are refractory to initial treatment may include ultrasound imaging and uroflowmetry consisting of noninvasive measurement of urine flow during voiding. Pelvic electromyography with patch electrodes during uroflowmetry assesses appropriate relaxation of the sphincter muscles necessary for coordinated voiding. A select number of patients may need cystourethroscopy to directly visualize the urethra and bladder and/or videourodynamics with urethral and rectal transducers to measure pressure in the bladder. Children with suspected neurogenic bladder disease should also be evaluated by lumbosacral magnetic resonance imaging (MRI) with subsequent neurosurgical evaluation, if necessary.

Fig. 3 presents an algorithm for the management of incontinence and other lower urinary tract symptoms.

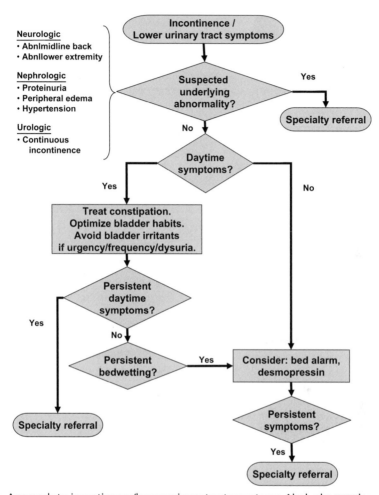

Fig. 3. Approach to incontinence/lower urinary tract symptoms. Abnl, abnormal.

Hematuria

There is no consensus on a standard approach to hematuria in children; however, several recent review articles present differential diagnoses and algorithms for management.[18–20] The evaluation of pediatric hematuria can be understandably intimidating for the primary care physician because of the extensive number of differential diagnoses. As a result, some children may have an overly extensive initial evaluation, whereas others have minimal, if any, evaluation before specialty referral. The goals for the primary care provider are: (1) to initiate a workup understanding that diagnosis may not be made before specialty referral, (2) to refer patients with suspected medical kidney disease expediently to a pediatric nephrologist, and (3) to refer patients with disorders that may need surgical management expediently to a pediatric urologist.

The evaluation of hematuria typically begins with abnormal urine dipstick analysis. Confirmation with microscopic analysis is essential before a true diagnosis of hematuria can be made because urine dipstick analysis can be falsely positive. The presence of more than 5 red blood cells per high-power field should be viewed as an indication for further testing.

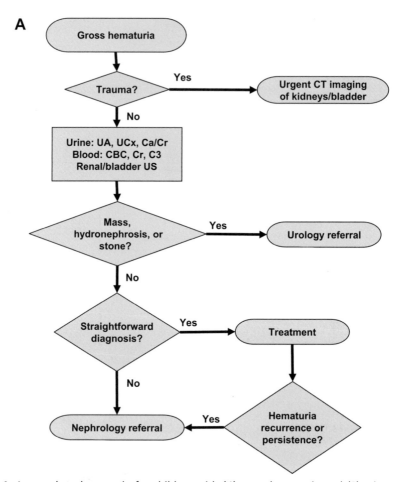

Fig. 4. Approach to hematuria for children with (*A*) gross hematuria and (*B*) microscopic hematuria. Ca/Cr, calcium/creatinine level; CBC, complete blood cell count; Cr, creatinine level; C3, complement level; CT, computed tomography; UA, urinalysis; UCx, urine culture; US, ultrasonography.

The causes of pediatric hematuria include glomerular diseases, interstitial and tubular diseases, infection, stones, tumors, and trauma. **Fig. 4** presents an algorithm for initial evaluation in the primary care setting and appropriate specialty referral based on recent review articles.[18–20]

MALE GENITALIA
Testicular Torsion and Other Causes Of Tender Scrotal Swelling

Testicular torsion is a truly urgent urologic problem. Surgical detorsion is required to salvage the testicle. Appropriate suspicion and timely referral should be based on careful history taking and physical examination. Acute onset of scrotal pain associated with nausea or vomiting in a pubertal boy is highly suspicious for torsion. On examination, the testicle may be lying transversely and may be higher riding than the contralateral testicle. The cremasteric reflex is absent so that stroking the inner thigh does

B

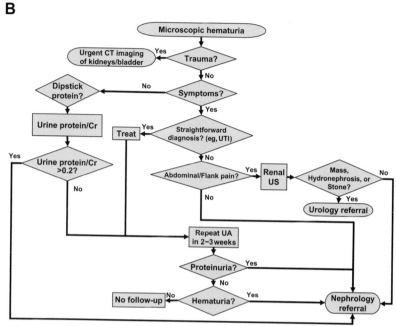

Fig. 4. (*continued*)

not cause further testicular ascent. As time progresses, the hemiscrotum becomes more indurated and erythematous. Although scrotal ultrasonography can confirm absence of vascular flow to the testicle, it can potentially delay definitive treatment. Patient presentation strongly suspicious for torsion warrants urologic consultation for scrotal exploration without additional imaging.

Other causes of tender scrotal swelling include incarcerated inguinal hernia, testicular trauma, torsion of an epididymal or testicular appendage, and epididymo-orchitis. With an incarcerated hernia, the swelling extends from the scrotum to the inguinal region. Manual reduction of the hernia should be attempted, but if the reduction is not successful, urgent referral to a surgical specialist is required. A direct blow to the scrotum can cause testicular rupture. If the testicle cannot be felt to be intact on examination, urgent urologic referral is required. Torsion of an appendage can be difficult to differentiate from testicular torsion, but it is usually not associated with nausea or vomiting. Occasionally, a blue dot sign and point tenderness can be localized to the upper pole of the testicle. Torsion of an appendage can be managed with ibuprofen and rest. Epididymo-orchitis presents with the gradual onset of pain and may be associated with urinary symptoms. Scrotal ultrasonography shows increased blood flow to the epididymis and testicle. If diagnosis is uncertain, consultation and/or scrotal ultrasonography is necessary.

Nontender Scrotal Swelling

Differential diagnoses of nontender scrotal swelling include intrascrotal tumor, hydrocele, and varicocele. Although testicular and paratesticular tumors are rare in children, a firm mass in the testicle or scrotum warrants prompt evaluation by a urologist because of the potential for malignancy. Scrotal ultrasonography is helpful to further define the mass.

Hydrocele is common in infants, and the hydrocele fluid transilluminates on examination. Hydroceles can be noncommunicating or communicating with the abdominal cavity through a patent processus vaginalis. Noncommunicating hydroceles typically do not require surgical correction. Persistent communicating hydroceles typically fluctuate in size and need surgical correction. In older children, hydrocele may also result secondary to testicular torsion, epididymo-orchitis, or tumor. Scrotal ultrasonography and/or urologic referral should be obtained if the hydrocele is tense enough to not allow adequate testicular examination.

Varicocele, or dilated veins around the spermatic cord, feels like a bag of worms that becomes more pronounced with standing or Valsalva. Varicocele is present in 15% to 20% of all men; some subset of those patients have problems with testicular growth and fertility. Because adolescent varicocele management is controversial, routine referral is warranted to discuss risks and benefits of intervention.

Undescended Testicle

The absence of a testicle from the scrotum occurs in 3% of full-term male newborns. Approximately, 75% of these boys have spontaneous testicular descent by 3 months of age.[21] The undescended testis is a well-established risk factor for testicular cancer.[22] Until recently, general consensus has been that surgical correction does not decrease malignancy risk. However, a recent cohort study showed that the relative risk of testicular cancer was decreased in those patients who underwent orchiopexy before 13 years of age.[23] Younger age at surgery is also associated with an increased adult sperm concentration in those patients who had appropriate germ cell development at the time of surgery.[24]

Examination of the pediatric patient for undescended testicle can be difficult. One hand should start at the hip at the superior-lateral aspect of the inguinal canal to sweep the testicle into the scrotum. The other hand is used to palpate the scrotal region. A retractile testicle can be easily brought down to the dependent scrotum without tension and does not need surgical intervention. If the presence of the testicle in the scrotum is not clear or if a retractile testicle cannot be differentiated from a true undescended testicle, urology referral is indicated. Imaging studies, such as ultrasonography, computed tomography, or MRI, are not indicated because they are neither specific nor sensitive enough to alter management. Previous recommendations by the AAP[25] recommended referral at 1 year of age; however, recent studies of germ cell development suggest that referral at 4 to 6 months of age is more appropriate.[26] Earlier referral for possible evaluation of disorders of sexual development is recommended if bilateral testicles are not palpable or if hypospadias is also present. Standard surgical treatment attempts to bring the testicle down to the dependent scrotum or confirms that a nonpalpable testicle is truly absent.

Hypospadias

Hypospadias is a common congenital defect of the male external genitalia in which the urethral meatus is located on the ventral underside of the penis instead of the tip. Hypospadias can also be associated with a ventral curvature of the penis (chordee) and an abnormal dorsal hood distribution of foreskin. Except in its mildest forms, hypospadias is usually apparent on newborn examination. Newborn circumcision, if desired by the parents, should be deferred until urologic consultation can be obtained if there is a question of hypospadias. Hypospadias is usually repaired at about 6 months of age as an outpatient procedure. Depending on the severity, the child may need androgen supplementation preoperatively for penile growth. Boys with more severe hypospadias may need several procedures. According to the AAP guidelines, the operation should be performed by a pediatric urologist.[27] If the hypospadias is associated with an undescended testicle, earlier referral is warranted for possible evaluation of disorders of sexual development.

Paraphimosis and Phimosis

Paraphimosis and phimosis are disorders of the foreskin in uncircumcised boys. Paraphimosis occurs when the retracted foreskin becomes trapped proximally behind the coronal sulcus, placing the glans at risk for ischemic injury. An attempt should be made to reduce the foreskin. Urologic consultation is required urgently if the foreskin cannot be reduced or routinely to discuss elective circumcision after the episode. With phimosis, the foreskin cannot be fully retracted over the head of the penis. Because of physiologic glanular adhesions, phimosis is normal in infants. As the child grows, the adhesions normally break down, allowing the foreskin to be retracted. Phimosis can be successfully treated with 0.1% betamethasone cream, 4 times daily, with a gentle stretch on the foreskin for 2 to 6 weeks. After the phimosis resolves, the foreskin should be retracted daily to prevent recurrence.

Circumcision Injury, Meatal Stenosis, and Redundant Foreskin

The most common circumcision injury is skin separation due to excessive foreskin removal. The injury typically heals well with topical antibiotic ointment, but specialty referral may be beneficial for parental reassurance. Meatal stenosis is a common condition acquired after neonatal circumcision that typically presents during toilet training with an upwardly deflected urinary stream. Lower urinary tract symptoms may also be present but are not usually attributable to the meatal stenosis and should be addressed separately as described earlier. Referral for meatotomy is indicated. Many parents are concerned about the appearance of excess skin after neonatal circumcision. Because of a prominent prepubic fat pad, the glans penis may often be covered in a circumcised infant. The appearance should improve as the child begins to walk. If the problem persists, elective specialty referral may be warranted.

FEMALE GENITALIA
Interlabial Masses

Multiple disorders present as interlabial masses during childhood. Masses may protrude from the urethral meatus (prolapsed ureterocele or prolapsed urethra), paraurethrally (paraurethral Skene cyst), or from the vaginal introitus (imperforate hymen with hydrocolpos, Gartner duct cyst, or sarcoma botryoides). Although intervention may not be required, specialty referral is warranted.

Labial Adhesions

Labial adhesions involve fusion of the labia minora. Labial adhesions should be treated when they divert the urinary stream or cause vaginal trapping of urine. Most labial adhesions resolve with the application of estrogen cream twice daily for up to 6 weeks with gentle separation of the labia. Parents should be warned that topical estrogen may be absorbed systemically with the possibility of minimal breast development. Rarely, manual separation of the adhesions using topical or general anesthetic may be necessary if estrogen therapy fails. Spread-leg voiding in toilet-trained girls helps to prevent recurrence.

Vulvitis

Prepubertal girls can present with vulvar discomfort and inflammation. Contact vulvitis may result from exposure to soaps and detergents as well as continuous exposure to a damp environment. General measures such as avoidance of harsh soaps and front-to-back wiping should be recommended. The vulvar area should be kept dry. Any urinary incontinence should be addressed. Spread-leg voiding should be encouraged to avoid vaginal trapping or urine. Tights, leotards, and wet bathing suits should not be worn all day. If symptoms are extremely bothersome, hydrocortisone 1% cream can be used to relieve the inflammation. Infectious organisms that can cause vulvitis include *Candida*, pinworms, and group A β-hemolytic streptococcus.[28] Because the child can learn to withhold bowel movements because of perineal pain, constipation should also be addressed.[29]

SUMMARY

Pediatric urologic conditions include a varied spectrum of disorders. A careful initial evaluation by the primary care provider lays the foundation for optimal management of these patients.

REFERENCES

1. Freedman AL. Urologic diseases in North America project: trends in resource utilization for urinary tract infections in children. J Urol 2005;173:949.
2. Shaikh N, Morone NE, Lopez J, et al. Does this child have a urinary tract infection? JAMA 2007;298:2895.
3. Practice parameter: the diagnosis, treatment, and evaluation of the initial urinary tract infection in febrile infants and young children. American Academy of Pediatrics. Committee on Quality Improvement. Subcommittee on Urinary Tract Infection. Pediatrics 1999;103:843.
4. Mazzola BL, von Vigier RO, Marchand S, et al. Behavioral and functional abnormalities linked with recurrent urinary tract infections in girls. J Nephrol 2003;16: 133.
5. Wan J, Kaplinsky R, Greenfield S. Toilet habits of children evaluated for urinary tract infection. J Urol 1995;154:797.
6. Evaluation and treatment of constipation in infants and children: recommendations of the North American Society for Pediatric Gastroenterology, Hepatology and Nutrition. J Pediatr Gastroenterol Nutr 2006;43:e1–13.
7. Calisti A, Perrotta ML, Oriolo L, et al. Diagnostic workup of urinary tract infections within the first 24 months of life, in the era of prenatal diagnosis. The contribution of different imaging techniques to clinical management. Minerva Pediatr 2005;57: 269.
8. Downs SM. Technical report: urinary tract infections in febrile infants and young children. The Urinary Tract Subcommittee of the American Academy of Pediatrics Committee on Quality Improvement. Pediatrics 1999;103:e54.
9. Pennesi M, Travan L, Peratoner L, et al. Is antibiotic prophylaxis in children with vesicoureteral reflux effective in preventing pyelonephritis and renal scars? A randomized, controlled trial. Pediatrics 2008;121:e1489.
10. Roussey-Kesler G, Gadjos V, Idres N, et al. Antibiotic prophylaxis for the prevention of recurrent urinary tract infection in children with low grade vesicoureteral reflux: results from a prospective randomized study. J Urol 2008;179:674.
11. Pohl HG, Belman AB. The "top-down" approach to the evaluation of children with febrile urinary tract infection. Adv Urol 2009:783409.
12. Nguyen HT, Herndon CD, Cooper C, et al. The Society for Fetal Urology consensus statement on the evaluation and management of antenatal hydronephrosis. J Pediatr Urol 2010;6(3):212–31.

13. Hains DS, Bates CM, Ingraham S, et al. Management and etiology of the unilateral multicystic dysplastic kidney: a review. Pediatr Nephrol 2009;24:233.
14. Hoebeke P, Bower W, Combs A, et al. Diagnostic evaluation of children with daytime incontinence. J Urol 2010;183:699.
15. Bauer SB. Neurogenic bladder: etiology and assessment. Pediatr Nephrol 2008; 23:541.
16. Neveus T, Eggert P, Evans J, et al. Evaluation of and treatment for monosymptomatic enuresis: a standardization document from the International Children's Continence Society. J Urol 2010;183:441.
17. Glazener CM, Evans JH, Peto RE. Alarm interventions for nocturnal enuresis in children. Cochrane Database Syst Rev 2005;2:CD002911.
18. Diven SC, Travis LB. A practical primary care approach to hematuria in children. Pediatr Nephrol 2000;14:65.
19. Meyers KE. Evaluation of hematuria in children. Urol Clin North Am 2004;31:559.
20. Pan CG. Evaluation of gross hematuria. Pediatr Clin North Am 2006;53:401.
21. Berkowitz GS, Lapinski RH, Dolgin SE, et al. Prevalence and natural history of cryptorchidism. Pediatrics 1993;92:44.
22. Dieckmann KP, Pichlmeier U. Clinical epidemiology of testicular germ cell tumors. World J Urol 2004;22:2.
23. Pettersson A, Richiardi L, Nordenskjold A, et al. Age at surgery for undescended testis and risk of testicular cancer. N Engl J Med 1835;356:2007.
24. Hadziselimovic F, Hocht B, Herzog B, et al. Infertility in cryptorchidism is linked to the stage of germ cell development at orchidopexy. Horm Res 2007;68:46.
25. Timing of elective surgery on the genitalia of male children with particular reference to the risks, benefits, and psychological effects of surgery and anesthesia. American Academy of Pediatrics. Pediatrics 1996;97:590.
26. Tasian GE, Hittelman AB, Kim GE, et al. Age at orchiopexy and testis palpability predict germ and Leydig cell loss: clinical predictors of adverse histological features of cryptorchidism. J Urol 2009;182:704.
27. Guidelines for referral to pediatric surgical specialists. Pediatrics 2002;110:187.
28. Kass-Wolff JH, Wilson EE. Pediatric gynecology: assessment strategies and common problems. Semin Reprod Med 2003;21:329.
29. Yerkes EB. Urologic issues in the pediatric and adolescent gynecology patient. Obstet Gynecol Clin North Am 2009;36:69.

Long-term Follow-up and Late Complications Following Treatment of Pediatric Urologic Disorders

Ardavan Akhavan, MD[a], Jeffrey A. Stock, MD[b],*

KEYWORDS

• Ureteral reimplantation • Ureteral pelvic junction obstruction
• Pyeloplasty • Hypospadias • Intestinal reconstruction

Long-term sequelae of reconstructive urologic surgery can affect children for years and even decades after surgery. The need for life-long surveillance is critical in ensuring effective identification and management of late complications. However, as children mature into adolescence and adulthood, follow-up with the treating urologist becomes poor, and the responsibility for identifying late complications often rests upon the primary care provider. This article's reviews the potential issues following various reconstructive urologic surgeries to help define guidelines for appropriate long-term surveillance of common pediatric urologic conditions for primary care providers.

VESICOURETERAL REFLUX AND URETERAL REIMPLANTATION

Primary vesicoureteral reflux (VUR) is present in 30% to 50% of all children who have urinary tract infections (UTI).[1,2] Given that the incidence of UTI in children is 5% to 10%,[3] VUR is the most common urologic abnormality in the pediatric population.[4] This is especially significant given that reflux nephropathy is the cause of end-stage renal failure (ESRD) in 3% to 25% of children and 10% to 15% of adults on dialysis.[4]

 With widespread use of fetal imaging, VUR is now most commonly diagnosed after the finding of hydronephrosis on prenatal ultrasound screening. Otherwise, it is detected upon evaluation of children presenting with UTI. Potentially-associated

[a] Department of Urology, Mount Sinai Medical Center, One Gustave L. Levy Place, New York, NY 10029, USA
[b] Division of Pediatric Urology, Department of Urology, The Mount Sinai Kravis Children's Hospital, One Gustave L. Levy Place, New York, NY 10029, USA
* Corresponding author.
E-mail address: jeffrey.stock@mountsinai.org

Med Clin N Am 95 (2011) 15–25
doi:10.1016/j.mcna.2010.08.032
0025-7125/11/$ – see front matter © 2011 Elsevier Inc. All rights reserved.

conditions include posterior urethral valves (PUV), prune-belly syndrome, and spinal dysraphism.

Whereas all children are treated initially with antibiotics, definitive treatment is reserved for children with severe or refractory disease. Factors affecting treatment include age of the child, failure of prior treatments, degree of reflux, presence of bilateral disease, medical comorbidities, and surgeon preference. If definitive treatment is elected over observation, multiple surgical methods have been described, and include intravesical and extravesical approaches to ureteral reimplantation, with or without tapering of the distal ureter.[5] Alternatively, endoscopic treatment with injection of a bulking agent is also a treatment option.[4]

When evaluating patients with a history of ureteral reimplantation, it is important for primary care providers to recognize that UTI is the most common long-term complication. The rate of cystitis up to 25 years following reimplantation is up to 43% in women and 24% in men; pyelonephritis affects 27% of women and 9.5% of men.[6–8] This compares with an overall 6% incidence of UTI in normal young healthy females.[6] Of the women who experience UTI, 54% have recurrent, frequent, complicated infections.[6] Interestingly, Duckett and colleagues[9] reported that at 5 years, patients managed nonsurgically had similarly elevated rates of lower tract infection compared to those of children managed surgically; however, surgical patients had half the long-term rate of pyelonephritis than those who were managed with antibiotics and observation.

This last finding suggests that patients with history of reflux may have underlying bladder or voiding abnormalities that predispose them to infection. Whereas this may be the case in patients with secondary VUR, the incidence of voiding dysfunction in patients with primary VUR is not known. Upadhyay and colleagues[10] reported on uroflowmetry, postvoid residuals, and voiding questionnaires from 14 girls and 7 boys, 5 to 13 years after surgery and determined that only one patient had elevated postvoid residual urine (PVR) and eight (38%) reported infrequent voiding. Otherwise, voiding patterns were normal. To the authors' knowledge, no study has reported urodynamics findings of patients following ureteral reimplantation for primary VUR to help explain the elevated incidence of lower tract UTI.

Regardless, the authors advocate that all children who are status-post surgical correction of VUR with breakthrough febrile UTI be referred for urologic evaluation for screening of recurrence. In addition, patients with a history of reflux secondary to outlet obstruction, spinal dysraphism, or prune-belly syndrome should be screened regularly for voiding dysfunction and evaluated routinely with urodynamics as they are at lifelong risk of dysfunctional voiding and recurrent secondary reflux.

The increased incidence of upper tract UTI predisposes patients to scarring and chronic pyelonephritis. In general, the reported incidence of renal scarring in patients with primary VUR ranges from 23% to 80%, with greater scarring occurring in patients with higher grades of reflux.[11,12] Various studies have demonstrated progressive scarring in 3% to 22% of patients followed from 3 to 20 years postoperatively.[6,8,11,13,14] Up to 85% of patients with new scars were female.[6] Other associated risk factors for progressive scarring included degree of reflux, bilateral disease, and the presence of already severely-scarred kidneys. Multiple studies have also demonstrated that patients with severe scarring also experienced poor long-term growth of the affected kidney.[6,15] It is important to note that only "high risk" and symptomatic patients were screened for renal scars; the reported incidence of renal scarring is likely an underestimate as all patients were not screened.

The test of choice to evaluate for scarring is the dimercaptosuccinic acid (DMSA) scan as it is not only sensitive for detection of scarring, but also evaluates differential kidney function.[14] The authors do not advocate routine screening for all patients for scarring or function; rather, such imaging should be reserved for patients with recurrent UTI, progressive renal failure, or severe scarring preoperatively.

Whereas renal scarring can be common in patients with reflux, renal failure is typically only found when the scarring is bilateral and severe.[6] Given the lack of comprehensive, prospective, long-term studies of patients with reflux, the true incidence of end-stage renal disease in patients with reflux is unknown. In 2006, reflux was noted to be the cause of renal failure in 3.5% of patients on dialysis and 5.2% of patients undergoing transplant, making it the fourth most common cause of renal insufficiency or failure.[16] Furthermore, despite advances in screening and management of reflux, there has been no significant change in this incidence of reflux-associated renal failure over the past 40 years, which suggests that patients destined for renal failure may have an intrinsic parenchymal defect or that the process, once begun, is inexorable.[17] In addition to the pattern of renal scarring, progression to end-stage renal disease is typically predicted by proteinuria, severity of reflux, age at diagnosis, and blood pressure.[6,16] Whereas progression to end-stage renal disease overall is uncommon in these patients, when it does occur the results are devastating. As such, primary care providers should consider more aggressive screening in patients with a history of high-grade reflux. Otherwise, annual blood pressure screening and urinalysis with protein determination should be sufficient in the majority of patients. If renal function is impaired, DMSA scan should be the next test of choice, followed by voiding cystourethrography (VCUG).

Renal scarring is also associated with the development of early hypertension. The mechanism for this is believed to be mediated by activation of the renin-angiotensin system.[16] Beetz and colleagues[8] reported follow up results of 189 children treated surgically for primary VUR and found that, at 11 years, 11.5% of the 61 patients with renal scarring had hypertension, whereas only 2.3% of those without renal lesions had problems with blood pressure. Similarly, Smellie and colleagues[18] reported a 7.5% incidence of hypertension in 226 patients followed for 18 to 35 years; 88% of hypertensive patients had evidence of renal scarring. Additionally, Wallace and colleagues[19] reported an 18.5% incidence of hypertension among children with reflux and bilateral scarring compared with an incidence of 11.3% in patients with only unilateral scars after an average of 12 years following surgical correction. In a study of 55 patients followed prospectively for 15 years, Goonasekera and colleagues[20] reported an 18% incidence of hypertension, with peak incidence in patients between 15 to 30 years of age.

The overall rate of hypertension in these patients varies with duration of follow-up, age of patient, extent and laterality of scarring, and degree of reflux. Most intermediate follow-up studies demonstrate a 15% to 20% incidence of hypertension in older children and young adults, whereas longer term studies following patients into adulthood reveal a 30% to 40% incidence.[16] Patients with a history of reflux, particularly those with bilateral disease or extensive scarring, should be aggressively screened throughout life for hypertension, and treated aggressively with ACE inhibitors or angiotensin receptor blockers.

Women with a history of VUR are also at increased risk for gestational complications during pregnancy. The incidence of UTI in normal women during pregnancy ranges from 4% to 7%.[6] In comparison, the risk of UTI among women with a history of reflux ranges from 17% to 65%.[21] Furthermore, these women are at increased risk of gestational renal failure, spontaneous abortion, early labor, and preeclampsia.[6,21] Studies have demonstrated that women status-post surgical correction of reflux have increased risk of these gestational complications over women who were managed conservatively (65% vs 15%).[18,22] However, this may be secondary to selection bias in that women with more severe reflux and scarring would have been more likely to have undergone surgical intervention than those managed conservatively. Primary care providers should also be familiar with the increased risk of ureteral obstruction in pregnant women who have undergone open ureteral reimplantation, necessitating emergent percutaneous nephrostomy drainage. Complaints of flank pain should warrant regular screening with blood pressure measurement, serum creatinine assessment, and renal ultrasound.[23]

URETEROPELVIC JUNCTION OBSTRUCTION AND PYELOPLASTY

Ureteropelvic junction (UPJ) obstruction is a form of obstructive uropathy found in both adults and children. UPJ obstructions can be acquired, secondary to trauma from instrumentation, calculus, or ischemia; or they can be primary, arising from a congenital intrinsic defect of the renal pelvis or extrinsic crossing vessel. Patients are typically diagnosed by prenatal ultrasound, whereas older children may present with complaints of flank pain, recurrent UTI, or nausea. Findings can include palpable mass or even hypertension. Hypertension is believed to be renin-mediated secondary to the enlarged collecting system obstructing blood flow to the kidney. Initial imaging comprises renal ultrasound, which will reveal hydronephrosis, followed by a functional mercaptoacetyltriglycine (MAG3) diuretic renal scan, which will demonstrate delayed washout of radiotracer in the affected kidney. Standard treatment is to perform an open, laparoscopic, or robotic-assisted pyeloplasty.

Postoperatively, hydronephrosis (which only indicates renal pelvis dilation and not necessarily obstruction) may not resolve immediately. Amling and colleagues[24] reported that hydronephrosis improved in only 8% of patients one month following pyeloplasty. This value increased to 36% by six months, 60% by one year, 81% by two years, and 91% at eight years. As such, serial ultrasounds may be necessary until hydronephrosis is resolved to document baseline status of the renal pelvis to interpret future imaging studies if symptoms suggest recurrent obstruction. If such baseline imaging is not available and obstruction is suspected, MAG3 diuretic renal scan is warranted.

There are no guidelines for the follow-up of patients after pyeloplasty. Late complications include recurrent UPJ stricture, stone formation, UTI, and hypertension. Symptoms that should alert the primary care provider include flank pain, dysuria, fever, signs of poorly controlled hypertension, and tenderness at the surgical site. Psooy and colleagues[25] evaluated the late complications in their cohort of 118 patients followed for a median of 5.5 years. The investigators noted that 13% of patients had continued prolonged or incomplete drainage on MAG3 diuretic renal scan at one year, one of whom developed a symptomatic recurrence at eight years, necessitating repeat pyeloplasty. Of those patients with normal renal scans at one year, none had late obstruction. Similarly findings were reported by Pohl and colleagues[26] who reported on 117 patients following pyeloplasty and determined that the results of the three-month postoperative renal scan was predictive of late obstruction. These investigators suggested that follow-up and repeat imaging should be reserved for patients with renal units whose half times of isotopic clearance were greater than 20 min.

Other late complications in the Psooy and colleagues[25] study included hypertension in two, and wound complications in seven. The investigators reported that 18% of patients presented to their providers with a total of 30 complaints suggestive of repeat UPJ obstruction, but only one represented a true recurrent obstruction.[25] The majority of these patients presented within the first year postoperatively. The investigators recommended performing a renal scan between three and four months postoperatively, and then following the patients clinically for one year before having patients followed by their primary care providers for annual blood pressure screening. Patients should be immediately referred back to their urologists if any complaints are suggestive of recurrent obstruction.

HYPOSPADIAS REPAIR

Hypospadias affects 1:200 to 1:300 of male births, making it one of the most common congenital defects.[27] Failure of closure of the ventral urethra leads to a proximal, ventral displacement of the urethral meatus, which may be located anywhere from the glans to the perineum. Referral for repair should be done once the hypospadias is identified, and repair should be performed before 18 months of age. The goals of surgical correction include reconstruction of a normal-appearing phallus that allows the male to void straight in the standing position, have a straight erection, and allow for intravaginal deposition of semen during coitus. Many children have a concomitant penile chordee that must be corrected at the time of surgery as well. Chordee is defined as a congenital ventral curvature of the penis that can range from a slight angle to a tethering of the entire phallus to the scrotum. Surgical correction depends on the location of the hypospadias; over 200 types of repairs have been described,[27] and can range in complexity from a simple primary closure of the distal urethra to a staged interposition of a harvested buccal graft or foreskin flap.

Comprehensive follow-up studies of these children is lacking owing to, in part, the logistical problems associated with tracking patients decades after they underwent surgery as infants. There are a handful of questionnaire studies on small numbers of patients who were able to be located. The majority of late complications may present as voiding dysfunction. Hoag and colleagues[28] cited a 10% incidence of urethral stricture and 11% rate of urethrocutaneous fistula in their follow-up of 28 patients questioned an average of 13.7 years after hypospadias repair. Similarly, Nelson and colleagues,[29] reporting on 43 patients at a mean of 6.9 years after surgery (using oral mucosal graft to repair proximal hypospadias), found meatal stenosis in 12%, with urethral strictures in 14%, and urethrocutaneous fistulae in 12%.

Voiding dysfunction has also been examined in these patients postoperatively. In the Hoag and colleagues[28] study, 18% to 81% of patients reported dissatisfaction with voiding.[28,30] Complaints included difficulty initiating micturition in 26% to 52%, and spraying in 28% to 52%.[28,29] Furthermore, Rynja and colleagues[27] evaluated 33 patients years after hypospadias repair and found that 43% had elevated PVR on bladder scan; average residual urine in those with elevated levels was 124mL. In all the above studies, patients with more proximal hypospadias repairs were more likely to have voiding dysfunction and late complications. Primary care providers should be aware of the potential for urethral pathology and should screen for and refer all complaints of voiding dysfunction, especially spraying and hesitancy, for formal urologic evaluation.

Former hypospadiacs may also present to their primary care physicians with concerns of sexual functional development. Studies have demonstrated that patients may be more apprehensive of the appearance of their genitals, leading to later realization of sexual milestones, including onset of intercourse, masturbation, and emotional intimacy.[28,31–35] However, once these milestones were met, follow-up studies have determined no difference in marriage rates, number of sexual partners, frequency of intercourse, or differences in psychosocial development.[27,30,32] Many studies have reported self-perceived concern with penile length as the predominant sexual complaint of most men following hypospadias repair.[27,30,32] Primary care doctors should be sensitive to the concerns of adolescent males over the appearance of their phallus, and reassure them that outcomes for erectile and sexual function and development are generally excellent.

Patients may also present to their primary care physician with complaints of sexual dysfunction. Rynja and colleagues,[27] using an International Index of Erectile Function-15 sexual inventory questionnaire on hypospadias patients, found that hypospadiac men had decreased frequency of ejaculation and sensation of orgasm following stimulation. In the Hoag and colleagues[28] study, 13% of patients reported pain with intercourse, likely secondary to persistent curvature of the penis. Moriya and colleagues[32] determined that 14% had ejaculatory dysfunction, including dribbling and an inability to ejaculate without milking. Similar complaints were present in 12% of the patients in the Aho and colleagues[30] study. Such findings are most commonly associated with more proximal hypospadias repairs, where the contractile tissue of the urethra is replaced by more rigid grafts, thereby compromising the expulsion properties of the native urethra necessary for proper ejaculation.

POSTERIOR URETHRAL VALVES

PUV occur in 1:8000 to 1:25,000 live births, and is the most common cause of obstructive uropathy in male newborns.[36] Associated conditions include upper tract dysplasia, bladder dysfunction, VUR, and prune-belly syndrome. Diagnosis is typically by prenatal or postnatal ultrasound and VCUG demonstrating a pathognomonic "keyhole sign" at the bladder neck. Treatment is directed at alleviating the obstruction as early as possible. Modalities include vesicostomy, upper urinary tract diversion, and primary valve ablation. Whereas no treatment option is superior at preserving renal function, patients with histories of upper tract diversion are at increased risk for bladder dysfunction and ureteral stricture disease, and are at much higher likelihood for subsequent procedures, including ureteral reimplantation and bladder augmentation.[37]

Despite early alleviation of obstruction, these patients are always at risk for renal insufficiency. Smith and colleagues[37] evaluated long-term outcomes of 100 patients treated for PUV and found that 10% had ESRD by age 10, and 38% required dialysis by age 20. Chronic renal failure was present in 34% and 51% at 10 and 20 years of age, respectively. Whereas renal failure in the newborn setting is frequently secondary to renal dysplasia, renal insufficiency that develops over years following treatment of PUV is often secondary to associated hyperfiltration injury and bladder dysfunction.[38] Up to 75% of patients have persistent polyuria secondary to a defect in the kidney's concentrating ability.

Ansari and colleagues[39] reported on 260 children with PUV and determined that bladder dysfunction was an early independent risk factor for the eventual development of ESRD. In the setting of a dysfunctional bladder, increased hydrostatic pressures of the bladder can be transmitted to the upper tracts, predisposing the patient to further renal deterioration.[40] As the child grows, the increasing demands for renal clearance are met with hyperfiltration in the remaining functional nephrons to help preserve renal function; the resultant proteinuria and focal segmental glomerulosclerosis lead to kidney failure. Proteinuria is present in up to 79% of PUV patients with chronic renal failure, compared with 17% of patients with normal renal function.[41] All patients with a history of valves should be screened throughout life for proteinuria. Any patient with this finding should be started on ACE inhibitors to prevent progressive renal deterioration.

The rate of urinary incontinence in these patients ranges from 19% to 81%.[38] Whereas not all patients with dysfunctional bladders have incontinence, all patients with incontinence have dysfunctional bladders, which are found in up to 75% of all patients following valve ablation.[38] Prolonged incontinence is expected in children and adolescents with posterior valves, with almost half of patients still wetting by age 10. However, parents should be reassured that 99% of patients obtain full continence by age 20.[37] Any patient with a complaint of irregular voiding habits, or those being considered for kidney transplantation should be referred to a urologist for formal urodynamics testing. The most common findings on urodynamics are bladder instability, myogenic failure, and poor compliance, with the latter being most dangerous for potential deterioration of kidney function.[42] Whereas patients tend to grow out of unstable and poorly compliant bladders, myogenic failure typically persists into adulthood.[38]

Studies have reported that 26% to 72% of cases are associated with unilateral or bilateral VUR.[43] The cause is most commonly secondary to upper tract transmission of bladder pressures from bladder outlet obstruction, although primary reflux from an incompetent ureteral orifice is also possible. Following treatment of the valves, the rate of spontaneous resolution of reflux ranges from 27% to 64%. Persistent reflux is associated with progressive renal deterioration. Therefore, long-term screening of symptomatic children may help preserve renal function.[43] All complaints of febrile urinary tract infection should be worked up with renal ultrasound or VCUG.

BLADDER DYSFUNCTION AND INTESTINAL RECONSTRUCTION AND DIVERSION

Bladder dysfunction can be one of the most disabling complications of both acquired and congenital nervous system and pelvic disorders in children. The goal of treatment for the neurogenic bladder is a continent, highly compliant, normal capacity bladder with low filling and voiding pressures and emptying to completion. When conservative measures fail to meet this objective, patients can be managed with bladder augmentation using either ureter, stomach, intestine, or colon. Alternatively, patients may also undergo upper tract urinary diversion with either a continent intestinal pouch or an incontinent conduit, depending on the severity of bladder dysfunction, response to prior treatment, degree of physical impairment, and renal function.

Metabolic derangements can occur secondary to both the functional loss of intestine from the digestive tract, as well as from the intestinal absorption of electrolytes from and secretion of solutes into the urine. Patients with terminal ileum substitutions are at risk for pernicious anemia; if clinically indicated, physicians should screen these patients for B12 deficiency and supplement as necessary.

The nature of the metabolic defect depends on the segment of viscera used, and the severity is a function of its length. **Table 1** is a simple chart of the metabolic derangements seen with the various intestinal segments used in urinary tract substitution. The causes of metabolic disturbances in diverted patients is described in detail

Table 1
Serum electrolyte disturbances following intestinal urinary diversion by segment

	pH	Potassium	Chloride
Stomach	↑	↓	↓
Jejunum	↓	↑	↓
Ileum or Colon	↓	↓	↑

elsewhere.[44] The most relevant complication, though, is metabolic alkalosis caused by aciduria in patients with gastric-based reconstructions. If severe, aciduria may cause hematuria-dysuria syndrome, known to occur in up to 36% of patients, where acidification of the urine from the stomach leads to hematuria and abdominal, penile, or urethral pain in the absence of infection.[45]

Overall, the rates of metabolic disturbances in long-term follow-up of children reconstructed for benign disease are poorly documented. DeFoor and colleagues[46] reported a 23% incidence of metabolic acidosis in children undergoing enteric-only neobladders, all necessitating bicarbonate treatment. Typically, patients with a glomerular filtration rate (GFR) of 55 mL/min/1.73 m^3 have enough renal function to compensate for any resultant acid and electrolyte loads or losses.[47] Patients with augmented or diverted urinary tracts require lifelong electrolyte monitoring.

Both the main purpose and requirement for urinary reconstruction with intestine is preservation of renal function. In the adult literature, many studies have demonstrated that in compliant patients with functioning urinary diversions, the rate of decline in GFR was no different than that associated with normal aging.[48] Fontaine and colleagues[49] reported results in 53 patients with reconstructed urinary reservoirs performed for bladder exstrophy and followed for at least 10 years. Unlike patients with PUV, any renal failure in this population could be directly attributable to the reconstruction and not an intrinsic defect in the kidney itself. The investigators found that 19% had a decline in GFR by at least 20%. In all cases, renal failure was secondary to chronic retention or chronic urinary tract infections secondary to ileoureteral stenosis, poorly compliant reservoirs, or poor compliance.[49] The authors recommend that all patients be screened for renal function regularly. If GFR is compromised, aggressive investigation is warranted, including voiding history, imaging for hydronephrosis and PVR, urine culture, and urodynamics.

Patients having undergone bowel reconstruction of the urinary tract are at lifelong risk of UTI and urolithiasis. Bacterial colonization is the rule, so treatment should be reserved only for patients who are symptomatic, as evidenced by fever, leukocytosis, and dysuria in the setting of a positive urine culture without another possible source of infection.[50] Additionally, patients colonized with urease-splitting organisms should be treated to minimize the risk of stone formation. Recurrent upper tract infections may cause scarring if severe, so prompt treatment is important. In the setting of incomplete voiding, colonization with urease-splitting bacteria, or noncompliance with self-catheterization or irrigation regimens, bladder stones can develop over mucous clots or exposed staples over a period of 24 to 45 months.[48] Such patients should be referred back to the urologist for treatment, and should also be evaluated for bladder function and catheterization and irrigation habits. Excessive mucous secretion can also lead to false-positive urine-based pregnancy tests in both men and women in up to 57% of patients.[51]

The risk of cancer development following intestinal urinary diversion is controversial. Ureterosigmoidostomy is now only used as a last option for patients with severe urologic and bowel deformities such that no other diversion is possible. The ureters, connected directly into the sigmoid colon, carry urine into the digestive tract. For reasons not clear, the mixture of urine and feces is carcinogenic to the lining of the digestive tract. The overall incidence of colon cancer in this population ranges from 3.5% to 19% at 15 to 25 years following diversion. Pathology typically shows adenocarcinoma.[48] Fortunately, patients with ureterosigmoidostomy are rare.

In contrast, patients diverted with cutaneous diversion or augmented with bowel, where feces and urine do not mix, do not have as pronounced an increase in cancer risk. Whereas there are case reports of transitional cell carcinomas and sarcomas developing, the vast majority of tumors are adenocarcinomas. Such tumors were discovered an average of 22 years following reconstruction for benign disease.[48]

The actual rate of cancer is unknown given poor rates of follow-up and confounding factors in the studies. Various investigators have suggested routine cystoscopy for patients starting 10 years following surgery; however, this is controversial. Hamid and colleagues[52] followed 92 patients with intestinal bladder augmentation for benign disease over 10 years and found only one cancer that was discovered upon workup for symptomatic hematuria.

SUMMARY

Many pediatric urologic disorders have sequelae that may affect patients well into adulthood. Lifelong monitoring of renal and voiding function is necessary. Primary care physicians caring should have a low threshold for early urologic referral in these patients to minimize potential complications.

REFERENCES

1. Matouschek E. [Treatment of vesicorenal reflux by transurethral teflon-injection (author's transl)]. Urologe A 1981;20:263–4 [in German].
2. Bisignani G, Decter RM. Voiding cystourethrography after uncomplicated ureteral reimplantation in children: is it necessary? J Urol 1997;158:1229–31.
3. Rushton HG. Urinary tract infections in children. Epidemiology, evaluation, and management. Pediatr Clin North Am 1997;44:1133–69.
4. Chertin B, Colhoun E, Velayudham M, et al. Endoscopic treatment of vesicoureteral reflux: 11 to 17 years of followup. J Urol 2002;167:1443–5 [discussion: 1445–6].
5. Elder JS. Guidelines for consideration for surgical repair of vesicoureteral reflux. Curr Opin Urol 2000;10:579–85.
6. Mor Y, Leibovitch I, Zalts R, et al. Analysis of the long-term outcome of surgically corrected vesico-ureteric reflux. BJU Int 2003;92:97–100.
7. Cooper A, Atwell J. A long-term follow-up of surgically treated vesicoureteric reflux in girls. J Pediatr Surg 1993;28:1034–6.
8. Beetz R, Schulte-Wissermann H, Troger J, et al. Long-term follow-up of children with surgically treated vesicorenal reflux: postoperative incidence of urinary tract infections, renal scars and arterial hypertension. Eur Urol 1989;16:366–71.
9. Duckett JW, Walker RD, Weiss R. Surgical results: International Reflux Study in Children—United States branch. J Urol 1992;148:1674–5.
10. Upadhyay J, Shekarriz B, Fleming P, et al. Ureteral reimplantation in infancy: evaluation of long-term voiding function. J Urol 1999;162:1209–12.
11. Piepsz A, Tamminen-Mobius T, Reiners C, et al. Five-year study of medical or surgical treatment in children with severe vesico-ureteral reflux dimercaptosuccinic acid findings. International Reflux Study Group in Europe. Eur J Pediatr 1998;157:753–8.
12. Macedo CS, Riyuzo MC, Bastos HD. [Renal scars in children with primary vesicoureteral reflux]. J Pediatr (Rio J) 2003;79:355–62 [in Portuguese].
13. Belloli G, Bedogni L, Salano F, et al. [Long- term evaluation of renal damage in primary vesico-renal reflux after corrective surgery]. Pediatr Med Chir 1985;7: 643–52 [in Italian].
14. Webster RI, Smith G, Farnsworth RH, et al. Low incidence of new renal scars after ureteral reimplantation for vesicoureteral reflux in children: a prospective study. J Urol 2000;163:1915–8.

15. Beetz R, Hohenfellner R, Schofer O, et al. Long-term follow-up of children with surgically treated vesicorenal reflux: renal growth. Eur Urol 1991;19:39–44.
16. Cendron M. Reflux nephropathy. J Pediatr Urol 2008;4:414–21.
17. Craig JC, Irwig LM, Knight JF, et al. Does treatment of vesicoureteric reflux in childhood prevent end-stage renal disease attributable to reflux nephropathy? Pediatrics 2000;105:1236–41.
18. Smellie JM, Prescod NP, Shaw PJ, et al. Childhood reflux and urinary infection: a follow-up of 10–41 years in 226 adults. Pediatr Nephrol 1998;12:727–36.
19. Wallace DM, Rothwell DL, Williams DI. The long-term follow-up of surgically treated vesicoureteric reflux. Br J Urol 1978;50:479–84.
20. Goonasekera CD, Shah V, Wade AM, et al. 15-year follow-up of renin and blood pressure in reflux nephropathy. Lancet 1996;347:640–3.
21. Hollowell JG. Outcome of pregnancy in women with a history of vesico-ureteric reflux. BJU Int 2008;102:780–4.
22. Mansfield JT, Snow BW, Cartwright PC, et al. Complications of pregnancy in women after childhood reimplantation for vesicoureteral reflux: an update with 25 years of followup. J Urol 1995;154:787–90.
23. Austenfeld MS, Snow BW. Complications of pregnancy in women after reimplantation for vesicoureteral reflux. J Urol 1988;140:1103–6.
24. Amling CL, O'Hara SM, Wiener JS, et al. Renal ultrasound changes after pyeloplasty in children with ureteropelvic junction obstruction: long-term outcome in 47 renal units. J Urol 1996;156:2020–4.
25. Psooy K, Pike JG, Leonard MP. Long-term followup of pediatric dismembered pyeloplasty: how long is long enough? J Urol 2003;169:1809–12 [discussion: 1812; author reply: 1812].
26. Pohl HG, Rushton HG, Park JS, et al. Early diuresis renogram findings predict success following pyeloplasty. J Urol 2001;165:2311–5.
27. Rynja SP, Wouters GA, Van Schaijk M, et al. Long-term followup of hypospadias: functional and cosmetic results. J Urol 2009;182:1736–43.
28. Hoag CC, Gotto GT, Morrison KB, et al. Long-term functional outcome and satisfaction of patients with hypospadias repaired in childhood. Can Urol Assoc J 2008;2:23–31.
29. Nelson CP, Bloom DA, Kinast R, et al. Long-term patient reported outcome and satisfaction after oral mucosa graft urethroplasty for hypospadias. J Urol 2005;174:1075–8.
30. Aho MO, Tammela OK, Somppi EM, et al. Sexual and social life of men operated in childhood for hypospadias and phimosis. A comparative study. Eur Urol 2000;37:95–100 [discussion: 101].
31. Berg R, Svensson J, Astrom G. Social and sexual adjustment of men operated for hypospadias during childhood: a controlled study. J Urol 1981;125:313–7.
32. Moriya K, Kakizaki H, Tanaka H, et al. Long-term cosmetic and sexual outcome of hypospadias surgery: norm related study in adolescence. J Urol 2006;176:1889–92 [discussion: 1892–3].
33. Mureau MA, Slijper FM, Nijman RJ, et al. Psychosexual adjustment of children and adolescents after different types of hypospadias surgery: a norm-related study. J Urol 1995;154:1902–7.
34. Avellan L. The development of puberty, the sexual debut and sexual function in hypospadiacs. Scand J Plast Reconstr Surg 1976;10:29–44.
35. Svensson J, Berg R, Berg G. Operated hypospadiacs: late follow-up. Social, sexual, and psychological adaptation. J Pediatr Surg 1981;16:134–5.

36. Dinneen MD, Duffy PG. Posterior urethral valves. Br J Urol 1996;78:275–81.
37. Smith GH, Canning DA, Schulman SL, et al. The long-term outcome of posterior urethral valves treated with primary valve ablation and observation. J Urol 1996; 155:1730–4.
38. Lopez Pereira P, Martinez Urrutia MJ, Jaureguizar E. Initial and long-term management of posterior urethral valves. World J Urol 2004;22:418–24.
39. Ansari M, Gulia A, Srivastava A, et al. Risk factors for progression to end-stage renal disease in children with posterior urethral valves. J Pediatr Urol 2010; 6(3):261–4.
40. Nguyen HT, Peters CA. The long-term complications of posterior urethral valves. BJU Int 1999;83(Suppl 3):23–8.
41. Lopez Pereira P, Espinosa L, Martinez Urrutina MJ, et al. Posterior urethral valves: prognostic factors. BJU Int 2003;91:687–90.
42. Peters CA, Bolkier M, Bauer SB, et al. The urodynamic consequences of posterior urethral valves. J Urol 1990;144:122–6.
43. Heikkila J, Rintala R, Taskinen S. Vesicoureteral reflux in conjunction with posterior urethral valves. J Urol 2009;182:1555–60.
44. McDougal WS. Metabolic complications of urinary intestinal diversion. J Urol 1992;147:1199–208.
45. Nguyen DH, Bain MA, Salmonson KL, et al. The syndrome of dysuria and hematuria in pediatric urinary reconstruction with stomach. J Urol 1993;150:707–9.
46. DeFoor WR, Heshmat S, Minevich E, et al. Long-term outcomes of the neobladder in pediatric continent urinary reconstruction. J Urol 2009;181:2689–93 [discussion: 2693–4].
47. Kristjansson A, Davidsson T, Mansson W. Metabolic alterations at different levels of renal function following continent urinary diversion through colonic segments. J Urol 1997;157:2099–103.
48. Gerharz EW, Turner WH, Kalble T, et al. Metabolic and functional consequences of urinary reconstruction with bowel. BJU Int 2003;91:143–9.
49. Fontaine E, Leaver R, Woodhouse CR. The effect of intestinal urinary reservoirs on renal function: a 10-year follow-up. BJU Int 2000;86:195–8.
50. Akerlund S, Campanello M, Kaijser B, et al. Bacteriuria in patients with a continent ileal reservoir for urinary diversion does not regularly require antibiotic treatment. Br J Urol 1994;74:177–81.
51. Nethercliffe J, Trewick A, Samuell C, et al. False-positive pregnancy tests in patients with enterocystoplasties. BJU Int 2001;87:780–2.
52. Hamid R, Greenwell TJ, Nethercliffe JM, et al. Routine surveillance cystoscopy for patients with augmentation and substitution cystoplasty for benign urological conditions: is it necessary? BJU Int 2009;104:392–5.

Urinary Tract Infections in Women

Elodi J. Dielubanza, MD*, Anthony J. Schaeffer, MD

KEYWORDS

• Urinary tract infection • Cystitis • Women • Recurrent

Urinary tract infection (UTI) is a pathogenic invasion of the urothelium with resultant inflammation, encompassing a spectrum of upper and lower urinary tract disease. Infections are classified as complicated or uncomplicated, based on host anatomy and comorbidities, and range clinically from benign self-limited cystitis to urosepsis. UTI is the most common extraintestinal infectious disease entity in women worldwide, and perhaps one of the most formidable challenges in clinical practice given its high prevalence, frequent recurrence, myriad associated morbidities, and rapidly evolving antimicrobial resistance. Achieving timely symptom relief and infection control while preventing morbidity, growth of resistant organisms, and recurrent infection are often difficult. The management of community-acquired UTI is plagued by a dearth of dependable culture data, accessible and updated local antimicrobial resistance patterns, and clear guidelines for treatment and prevention of recurrent UTI, as well as identification patterns of infection that warrant additional evaluation. This article

- Reviews epidemiology and pathogenesis of urinary tract infection in women,
- Characterizes common patterns of infection and clinical red flags and appropriate laboratory testing and imaging,
- Explores emerging patterns of antimicrobial resistance
- Reviews the updated guidelines for the treatment of uncomplicated UTI in women.

EPIDEMIOLOGY

The evaluation and treatment of community-acquired UTI commands a significant portion of health care resources. UTI is the chief complaint in eight million clinic and emergency department visits, leading to approximately 100,000 hospital admissions each year. Antimicrobial agents used for the treatment of UTI account for 15% of all outpatient prescriptions. The annual health care cost is an estimated $1.6 billion dollars and rising.[1] Women shoulder the greatest burden of disease, with a greater predilection for infection after the first year of life. According to the National Health

Department of Urology, Northwestern University, Feinberg School of Medicine, 303 East Chicago Avenue, Tarry 16-703, Chicago, IL 60611-3008, USA
* Corresponding author.
E-mail address: e-dielubanza@md.northwestern.edu

Med Clin N Am 95 (2011) 27–41
doi:10.1016/j.mcna.2010.08.023
0025-7125/11/$ – see front matter © 2011 Published by Elsevier Inc.

medical.theclinics.com

and Nutrition Examination Survey III (NHANES-III) data, the lifetime prevalence of UTI is 53,067 cases per 100,000 women, compared with 13,689 cases per 100,000 men. The widest gender gap occurs in young adulthood between ages 16 and 35 years, when women are about 35 times more likely to be affected. The gap narrows considerably after age 65, when the female-to-male ratio of infection declines to 2:1 due to sharp late-life increases in the incidence of benign prostatic hyperplasia, urinary retention, incontinence, and institutionalization in the male population (NHANES III). While male infection exhibits a bimodal distribution at the extremes of age, female infection displays a durable disease burden over a lifetime. The incidence of bacteriuria is about 1% in primary and middle school-aged girls, quadrupling to 4% by young adulthood, and increasing 1% to 2% per decade thereafter.[2,3] As such, one-third of women will have at least one symptomatic UTI by age 24, and more than one-half of women will be affected by the end of life.[4] While 90% of UTIs treated with appropriate antimicrobial therapy resolve, there is a strong tendency toward recurrence. In the literature, the recurrence rate of UTI in women ranges from 27% to 46% within 1 year.[5,6]

SUSCEPTIBILITY FACTORS

Increased female susceptibility to urinary tract infection is a function of basic anatomic factors as well as behavioral and physiologic factors that evolve over a woman's lifetime. The short female urethra provides an ideal bridge for invading pathogens and rapid ingress to the bladder. The longer male urethra facilitates urinary washout of ascending bacteria before entry to the bladder is permitted and is perhaps the most significant protective factor against infection in men. The proximity of the female urethra to hearty bacterial reservoirs in the rectum and vagina also plays a crucial anatomic role. Colonization of the periurethral mucosa with bacterial species from the bowel flora is inevitable in females. When enteropathogens infiltrate the bacterial milieu, the risk of symptomatic infection increases. A recent study of the microbiological events that precede *Escherichia coli* UTI found that the incidence of periurethral colonization with the causative bacterial strain increases from a baseline of 46% to 90% during the 14 days before the onset of symptoms.[7] Moreover, women with recurrent UTI are more likely to exhibit persistent colonization of the vaginal mucosa with enteropathogenic flora.[8] Variations in perineal anatomy among women also may affect susceptibility. Hooton and colleagues[9] demonstrated greater likelihood of anal to urethral distance of greater than 4.5 cm in women with recurrent UTI compared with controls, with an average difference of 0.2 cm between the two study populations, which persisted even when they controlled for body habitus. The authors contend that in the absence of other strong exogenous risk factors for recurrent UTI, this modest difference may play a significant in the pathogenesis of recurrent infection.

BEHAVIORAL FACTORS

Behavioral factors help microbes capitalize on female anatomic vulnerability. Several studies have found a dose-dependent relationship between sexual intercourse and the risk of UTI, findings which are corroborated by the spike in first infections among young adult women around the time of first sexual activity.[10] A prospective study of 796 sexually active young women found that the relative risk of UTI for sexual intercourse on 1, 3, and 5 of the previous 7 days was 1.42, 2.83, and 5.68, respectively.[11] The use of a spermicide, either alone or in conjunction with a barrier contraceptive (ie, diaphragm, cervical cap, male condom) also has been associated with increased risk of UTI.[11,12] Spermicides, especially those containing nonoxonol-9, alter vaginal flora, thereby facilitating periurethral colonization with uropathogens. Antimicrobial use in the previous month increases the risk of infection by the same mechanism. A study of two cohorts of premenopausal women, 326 women at a university health center and 425 women in a health maintenance organization (HMO), found that antimicrobial use in the prior 15 to 28 days was associated with odds ratios (ORs) of 2.57 and 5.83 for UTI in the two groups, respectively.[13] Furthermore, prior antimicrobial use increases the likelihood of subsequent infection with resistant organisms.[13–15] Extended treatment duration and inadvertent subtherapeutic dosing play a role in this phenomenon by increasing the probability of eradication of normal vaginal and rectal flora and selection for resistant organisms.[15,16] Considerable attention has been paid to the role hygiene practices in counseling women on risk reduction strategies. However, there has been no demonstrated benefit of employing the most commonly advised behavioral modifications: postcoital voiding, front-to-back wiping, increased fluid intake, avoidance of urine holding and douching, and proper tampon or sanitary napkin use.[17,18]

GENETIC FACTORS

Genetic predisposition to recurrent UTI is a well-supported concept, and women who suffer from recurrent infections often note maternal or other family history of infection. Schaeffer and colleagues[19] observed that women with recurrent UTI exhibit increased E coli binding receptivity that is not limited to the vaginal and urethral mucosa but also includes buccal mucosa, suggesting genetic differences in mucosal properties rather than differences in local milieu. Lewis blood group antigen nonsecretor and recessive phenotypes (ie, Le[a-b-] or Le[a+b-]) are associated with increased risk of recurrent infection. The Lewis antigen's protective effect against infection is related to its role in the fucosylation of uroepithelial surface proteins, which provides steric hindrance to microbial binding. Recessive and nonsecretor phenotypes are believed to be associated with increased density of available uroepithelial receptors for binding with bacterial adhesins. Shenfield and colleagues[20] found an OR of 3.4 for recurrent UTI among those with these phenotypes. Additionally, there is an observed association between human leukocyte antigen A3 (HLA-A3) expression and risk of recurrent UTI. Schaeffer and colleagues[21] found HLA A3 was present in 34% of patients with recurrent UTI compared with 8% of healthy controls in their study population.

AGE-SPECIFIC FACTORS

Estrogen status is perhaps the most important age-specific risk determinant for UTI. Estrogen promotes acidic vaginal pH and lactobacillus proliferation, which are the greatest host defenses against pathogenic colonization. Withdrawal of estrogen at the time of menopause leads to conversion of the predominant vaginal flora from lactobacillus to E coli and other Enterobacteriaceae, thus increasing the incidence of infection. A randomized, double-blind placebo-controlled trial of intravaginal estrogen replacement in postmenopausal women with recurrent UTI helped to illustrate the hormone's protective effect. Stamm and colleagues[22] found that 61% of the women treated with intravaginal estriol experienced restoration of lactobacilli colonization, a change that was not observed in any of the women in the placebo group. This translated into significant reduction in incidence of symptomatic UTI in the treatment group; 0.5 versus 5.9 episodes per patient year in the treatment group and controls, respectively. However, only intravaginal estrogen replacement has demonstrated risk reduction in the literature; oral replacement therapy confers no significant benefit.[23,24]

Surgical procedures to improve incontinence are associated with increased incidence of UTI. One study found that of 1356 women over age 65 who underwent urethral sling placement, one-third reported UTI within 3 months, and nearly half within 1 year of the procedure.[25] This difference is likely secondary to increased postvoid residual urine volumes and urinary stasis.[26]

Residence in a long-term nursing care facility bears a strong association with UTI in the elderly female population. Although the incidence of bacteriuria in independent elderly women is 2.8 to 8.6%, among institutionalized women it soars to 25% to 50%, as does the risk of symptomatic infection.[27] Much of the difference is attributable to greater prevalence of chronic comorbid conditions contributing to urodynamic abnormalities, elevated postvoid residual urine volume, poor functional status, and catheterization for incontinence. Distinguishing between symptomatic and asymptomatic infection in these patients also presents a clinical challenge given the frequent alterations in mental status and lack of localizing symptoms in this population. Thus, institutionalized women are more likely to be treated inappropriately with antimicrobial therapy for asymptomatic bacteriuria. Approximately 25% of antimicrobials given for UTI in the nursing home setting are given for asymptomatic infection.[28,29] As such, nursing homes are significant reservoirs for resistant organisms, and nursing home residents are at greater risk for symptomatic UTI with resistant organisms.

URINARY CATHETERIZATION

Indwelling urinary catheters and clean intermittent catheterization (CIC) are associated with high rates of bacteriuria. The incidence of bacteriuria is 3% to 6% per day with indwelling catheters and 1% to 3% per catheterization with CIC; thus virtually all patients using these modalities will have bacteriuria after 1 month.[30,31] Tambyah and colleagues[32] found that among patients with short-term indwelling catheters (ie, 2 to 4 days) placed during acute care admissions, the incidence of fever or other symptoms attributable to UTI is 7.7%. The incidence of fever related to urinary source in patients using long-term indwelling or intermittent cauterization is 1.1 episodes per 100 catheterized patient days.[33] Antimicrobial therapy in these patients should be undertaken only in the setting of symptoms. Antimicrobial prophylaxis schemes do not confer risk reduction for symptomatic UTI in patients with chronic indwelling catheters and function to increase the growth of resistant bacteria. The only risk-reduction strategy that has demonstrated significant benefit for patients with chronic indwelling catheters is maintaining a closed drainage system. Risk reduction in CIC is achieved best by compliance with proper cleaning technique, appropriately cleaning hands, catheter, and meatus before catheterization.

PREGNANCY

Pregnancy is an independent risk factor of upper UTI. While the incidence of asymptomatic bacteriuria is virtually identical in pregnant and nonpregnant women of childbearing age (2% to 7%), pregnancy-induced physiologic changes in the urinary tract increase the likelihood of upper UTI. Progesterone induces tonic relaxation of the ureteric smooth muscle, while blood volume and glomerular filtration rate (GFR) increase markedly to support the growing fetus, creating a permissive environment for renal pelviceal and ureteral dilation, vesicoureteral reflux, and urinary stasis. As such, 25% to 40% of pregnant women with untreated bacteriuria will develop pyelonephritis.[34] Previous history of UTI, low socioeconomic status, indigence, intercurrent diabetes, and sickle cell trait further increase this risk. The morbidity associated with upper tract UTI in pregnancy is significant and includes prematurity, low birth weight, preeclampsia, and cesarean delivery; therefore, screening and treatment for asymptomatic bacteriuria are the standard of care in pregnant patients.[35]

PATHOGENESIS

Most upper and lower UTIs result from bacterial ascent from the bowel or vaginal mucosa. The most common infecting pathogens are resident facultative anaerobes and gram-negative bacteria from the bowel and vaginal flora. *E coli* is the causative organism in nearly 85% of UTIs, *Staphylococcus saphrophyticus* represents 10% to 15% of cases, and *Enterobacteriaceae* species, *Proteus*, and *Klebsiella* comprise the remaining minority.[4]

E coli causes the greatest proportion of disease because of its acquisition of virulence factors that not only aid in mucosal adherence and ascent, but also evasion of host immune response. Central to the ability of pathogenic and nonpathogenic *E coli* subtypes to colonize the genitourinary tract is the expression of adhesins. Adhesins can be fimbrial or nonfimbrial, and mediate attachment to epithelial receptors. Mannose-sensitive, type-1 pili are expressed widely across *E coli* subtypes and appear to be among the most important adhesins for establishing colonization and infection. In animal models, bladder inoculation with type-1 piliated organisms resulted in greater colonization than inoculation with nonpiliated ones. Inoculation with antitype-1 pili antibodies and mannose-based competitive inhibitors conferred a protective effect against development of UTI in mice.[36,37]

Type-1 pili also facilitate intracellular translocation of the bacteria, enabling the establishment of intracellular bacterial communities (IBCs). These IBCs are shielded from antimicrobials and host immune response, yet undergo periodic shedding of bacteria into the bladder lumen, to renew surface colonization after immune eradication.[38] Mannose-resistant P-pili are fimbriated adhesins that confer tropism to the kidney and are expressed by most pyleonephritogenic strains of uropathogenic *E coli* (UPEC). The P-pili endow UPEC with a highly adhesive character and proficiency in the retrograde ureteral ascent implicated in the development of pyelonephritis. In one study, this adhesin was present in 91% of UPEC strains causing pyelonephritis, compared with only 19% of cystitis- associated strains and 14% of strains related to asymptomatic bacteriuria.[39]

Expression of type-1 and P-pili is not static. It undergoes phase variation, providing yet another means by which UPECs elude eradication by the host immune system. Piliated organisms, while invaluable to the establishment of both intracellular and extracellular colonies, promote phagocytosis, apoptosis, and neutrophil invasion. Nonpiliated organisms remain in solution in the urine without inciting a host immune response, acting as a local reservoir when adherent bacteria succumb to immune attack.[38,40]

The development of pyelonephritis usually depends on bacterial capacity for ascent as well as compromise in host anatomic defenses to facilitate colonization and ability to traverse the lengthy ureter without washout. Clustering of disease in pregnant women supports this assertion. During pregnancy, progesterone-mediated smooth muscle relaxation is believed to contribute to renal pelvis and ureteral dilation as well as impaired ureteral peristalsis, increased urinary retention, and increased bladder capacity, creating a permissive environment for bacterial ascent.[41] In healthy, nonpregnant women who are affected by pyelonephritis, cystitis-associated inflammatory changes in the bladder may induce a transient alteration in the competence of the ureterovesical junction, thereby facilitating distal ureteral colonization and enhancing the potential for upper tract infection.[4]

EVALUATION
Urinalysis and Urine Culture

Urinalysis is an array of biochemical assays and microscopic evaluations designed to aid in the presumptive diagnosis of UTI by facilitating the rapid identification of bacteriuria and pyuria. It is the most commonly used diagnostic modality in the outpatient evaluation of suspected UTI. Leukocyte esterase and nitrite are the most commonly referenced, and perhaps the most useful indices from the urine dipstick screening assay. The presence of leukocyte esterase suggests pyuria, indicative of host inflammatory response. Nitrite is the product of bacterial reduction of urine nitrate, and suggests the presence of gram-negative bacteria. When compared with urine cultures growing 10^3 CFU/mL or greater, the sensitivity and specificity for the finding of a positive result for both tests were 71% and 83%, respectively.[42]

False-negative results for leukocyte esterase can occur in the setting of early infection, when bacteriuria is present without hearty host inflammatory response. False-negative results for nitrite can occur in the setting of infection with gram-positive or other nonnitrate-reducing organisms. False-positive results in both tests can result from sample contamination. On microscopic evaluation, the presence or absence of bacteria is very important in determining the likelihood of infection however, the high incidence of contamination with clean-catch urine specimens and possibility for false-negative findings if bacterial colony count is lower than 10^5 CFU/mL are significant confounding factors. As such, the presence of white blood cells and the absence of vaginal epithelial cells in the urine sample can be vital to the presumptive diagnosis of UTI.

Urine culture is the gold standard diagnostic modality for UTI. However, obtaining reliable culture data and interpreting them appropriately can be challenging. The reliability of urine culture is directly related to the collection method employed. The collection method most commonly used in the outpatient setting, the midstream, clean catch voiding method, is also the least reliable. While it allows for collection without the aid of a skilled practitioner or the need for office appointment, creating convenience for patient and practitioner alike, it is mired by frequent contamination. Even when perineal cleansing is performed correctly, nearly one-third of these specimens can be contaminated.[43] Contamination is suggested by the presence of squamous epithelial cells on accompanying urinalysis or polymicrobial growth. For clean-catch voided specimens, convention dictates that the colony count should be at least 10^5 CFU/mL for a single organism. However, it is important to note that 20% to 40% of women presenting with cystitis will have low bacterial colony counts of 10^2 to 10^4 CFU/mL.[44,45] If voided urine specimens obtained for evaluation of recurrent or persistent symptoms suggest contamination, it may be prudent for the practitioner to consider catheterization for subsequent samplings in the interest of accurate bacterial identification. Catheterized urine specimens are far more sensitive than voided ones. When obtained in a sterile fashion, infection can be identified with as few as 100 CFU/mL. Suprapubic aspiration is the most sensitive modality, as it bypasses the colonizing organisms of perineum entirely. The presence of any bacteria is indicative of infection. This method is unlikely to be used in the management of uncomplicated UTI, but may be useful for patients with a particularly challenging body habitus that precludes sterile catheterization and the clinical need for pathogen isolation.

Radiographic Evaluation

Radiographic evaluation is not indicated for most women with recurrent infection. However, it can be an important component of the evaluation of women with concerning patterns of infection (ie, reinfection with same bacterial species as short time intervals, persistence of infection despite appropriate culture directed therapy). Kidney/ureter/ bladder plain film series (KUB), in conjunction with renal ultrasound, offer a basic examination of the urinary tract and remain an excellent first choice for evaluation for recurrent UTI. The size and contour of the kidneys and bladder, the presence of renal mass or abscess, certain renal and ureteral calculi, hydronephrosis suggestive of obstructive uropathy, and elevated postvoid residual urine can all be visualized using ultrasound. KUB can identify the presence of radio-opaque calculi along the genitourinary tract, especially proximal and distal ureteral stones that can be missed on ultrasound.

Any finding suggesting mass or complex fluid collection should prompt follow-up imaging with computed tomography (CT) or magnetic resonance imaging (MRI). CT offers very fine anatomic detail and is thus the superior study for evaluation of focal nephritis, renal or perirenal abscess and masses, and both radio-opaque and radiolucent stones. However, it also carries the greatest risk profile, exposing the patient to both intravenous contrast and ionizing radiation. This modality may be best reserved for a work-up for patients with hematuria or for patients who are acutely ill and in need of surgical or percutaneous interventions.[4]

APPROACH TO SPECIFIC PATTERNS OF INFECTION
Initial and Isolated Cystitis

The most common presenting symptoms for uncomplicated cystitis are urinary frequency, urgency, and dysuria. In a healthy patient presenting with initial or isolated clinical UTI (ie, no previous UTI in $\geq$1 year) it can be treated empirically on the basis of symptoms and positive urinalysis, provided that complicating factors have been thoroughly explored and excluded by history, physical examination, or imaging or ancillary tests as indicated. The clinical history is the physician's best first tool in the treatment of UTI, and should elucidate complicating factors, exclude other causes of genitourinary symptoms, and identify women at high risk for recurrent infection. Pregnancy, structural abnormalities of the genitourinary tract, urolithiasis, renal insufficiency, immune deficiency, diabetes mellitus, recent antibiotic therapy, or recent genitourinary instrumentation are important complicating factors to explore. These findings warrant upfront urine culture.

It is also important to carefully differentiate the lower urinary tract symptoms of cystitis from those of urethritis and vaginitis. Like cystitis, urethritis is associated with dysuria, frequency, and urgency; however, the onset of symptoms is generally more indolent, and vaginal discharge is often present. The most common infecting pathogens are *Neisseria gonorrhoeae, Chlamydia trachomatis*, and herpes simplex virus. The predominant symptoms of vaginitis are unpleasant vaginal odor, discharge, pruritus, and dyspareunia. The most common infecting pathogens are *Candida albicans, Gardenerella vaginalis,* and *Trichomonas vaginalis*.[46] History consistent with vaginitis or urethritis warrants pelvic examination, appropriate testing for pathogen isolation (ie, *Chlamydia trachomatis/Neisseria gonorrhea* urine polymerase chain reaction [PCR] assay, saline wet mount), and empiric therapy for patient and sexual partners as indicated. Of the women presenting with initial or isolated UTI, about one-third will experience recurrence of symptoms within 1 year, many within 6 months.[47]

Pyelonephritis

Pyelonephritis is an infection of the renal parenchyma and the clinical constellation of cystitis, flank pain, leukocytosis, and pyuria, with or without constitutional symptoms.

The initial evaluation of a patient with suspected pyelonephritis should include history and physical examination, complete blood count, and urine culture. Genitourinary imaging is required to rule out complicating factors such as nephrolithiasis and obstructive uropathy in septic, diabetic and immunocompromised patients, or those who remain febrile despite 72 hours of appropriate antibiotics. Ultrasound is an excellent first choice, and classic findings include renal enlargement and hypoechoic parenchyma secondary to edema.[4] In a clinically stable woman with mild, uncomplicated infection, outpatient oral antimicrobial therapy with close follow-up and repeat culture after the completion of therapy is an appropriate clinical approach. For patients with moderate-to-severe infections, admission for a short course of parenteral antimicrobial therapy with rapid transition to oral therapy guided by urine culture data is recommended.[48]

Unresolved UTI

Unresolved UTI is an infection in which symptoms and/or bacteriuria have failed to respond to antimicrobial therapy. This scenario should raise concern regarding antimicrobial agent and dosing, and warrants pathogen isolation via urine culture and physical examination to rule out obvious anatomic causes for persistent symptoms. Treatment failure is often a function of infection with a resistant organism or medication underdosing secondary to poor compliance.[4] Subsequent therapy should be culture-directed, and a follow-up urine culture should be obtained during the treatment course to confirm pathogen eradication. If culture-directed therapy fails to abolish infection, one should consider the possibility of poor antimicrobial tissue penetration, as in renal insufficiency or the presence of genitourinary abnormality, which permits continuous inoculation of the urine, as with fistula. Serum creatinine measurement and genitourinary tract imaging will aid in this determination. If symptoms persist in the setting of negative urine culture, urologic evaluation with cystoscopy may help to exclude noninfections causes of cystitis symptoms, such as malignancy and interstitial cystitis.

Recurrent UTI

Recurrent UTI is defined as reinfection of the urinary tract following eradication of infecting pathogens (ie, documented negative urine culture). By convention, the term recurrent UTI is reserved for a pattern of two or more infections within 1 year. There are two modes by which these recurrent infections occur: ascending reinfection from a source outside of the genitourinary tract (eg, vaginal reservoir, fistula) and reinoculation by persistent bacterial reservoir within the genitourinary tract (such as kidney stones, foreign bodies, and poorly draining regions of the urinary system). Variation in the causative pathogen in successive infections suggests ascending reinfection, while recurrent infections with the same microbial species suggest bacterial persistence.[4,5]

Initial evaluation of patients presenting with recurrent UTI should include a thorough history and physical examination to assess for associated risk factors. Important historical elements include timing of previous UTI, including temporal relationship with intercourse, barrier contraceptive use, menopausal status, recent antimicrobial use, and history of genitourinary instrumentation. On physical examination, key findings are vaginal atrophy, vaginal fullness characteristic of cystocele or uterine prolapse, and periurethral fullness consistent with urethral diverticula. Ancillary testing may include serum creatinine and postvoid residual measurements. Individuals presenting with recurrent infection with the same bacterial species at short time intervals should be referred for urologic evaluation, which will include imaging of the urinary tract and cystoscopy. These investigations are aimed at excluding the presence of urinary tract stones, urethral, bladder, or renal calyceal diverticula, and fistulas.

Although delay in the initiation of antimicrobial therapy for pathogen isolation would be an ideal therapeutic approach for recurrent infections, it is impractical in clinical practice where prompt symptom relief remains an important goal of care. The initiation of therapy will be empiric in most cases; however, it is important to obtain a urine specimen for culture at the time of presentation. These culture data will serve to confirm the appropriateness of empiric therapy, direct necessary alterations to empiric therapy, and characterize infection trends.

RED FLAGS

It is important to remain cognizant of several clinical scenarios in which classic signs and symptoms of cystitis belie a more complex underlying process:

Gross hematuria or persistent microscopic hematuria between documented infections should heighten the index of suspicion for underlying malignancy. Formal urologic evaluation should be pursued, including cystoscopy, urine cytology, and triphasic CT scan or renal ultrasound and retrograde pyelogram.

Recurrent symptoms of cystitis in the setting of negative urine culture may suggest mycobacterial infection, interstitial cystitis, or underlying malignancy. Pathogen isolation with mycobacterial culture should be undertaken if there is sufficient clinical suspicion. Otherwise, urologic evaluation with CT imaging cystoscopy is warranted.

Pyuria in the absence of bacteriuria is suggestive of mycobacterial infection or malignancy. If clinical suspicion warrants it, mycobacterial culture is an excellent preliminary evaluation. Otherwise urologic evaluation including upper and lower urinary tract imaging with cystoscopy and renal ultrasound may be warranted.

TREATMENT

Optimal antimicrobial agents for uncomplicated UTI are frequently in flux because of rapidly evolving antibiotic resistance patterns. The core principals of therapy for UTI, however, do not change. Timely administration of an agent that exhibits the appropriate spectrum of activity against the known or most likely infecting pathogen, with dose and therapy duration that are sufficient to affect bacterial eradication while minimizing the risk of adverse effects and the growth of resistant bacterial strains remain the paramount clinical priorities. Adherence to this core can be difficult in clinical practice, where culture data can be scarce, local resistance data out of reach, and selection of antimicrobial agent and treatment duration is often based on individual convention or gestalt rather than clear guidelines. These common therapeutic pitfalls are rendering many first-line therapies ineffective at rates that outstrip the development of new, effective antimicrobials. As the major prescribers of antibiotics for the treatment of UTI, the primary care provider will lead in the efforts to slow antimicrobial resistance.

DURATION OF THERAPY

Optimal antimicrobial therapy duration has been a well studied topic in the literature. The 3-day treatment regimen is widely advocated for the treatment of uncomplicated cystitis because of its excellent balance of effective symptom and pathogen eradication with minimal alterations in vaginal and bowel flora or adverse drug effects. A 2005 Cochrane review of randomized controlled trials comparing 3 days of oral antibiotic therapy with multiday therapy (5 days and longer) for uncomplicated cystitis in nonpregnant women found that long and short-term symptom cure rates were equivalent between groups, while rate of adverse effects were lower in the 3-day regimen groups. The incidence of recurrent bacteriuria at 4 to 10 weeks after therapy was more common in the 3-day therapy groups. However, prevention of asymptomatic bacteriuria in healthy, nonpregnant women is not indicated.[49]

Seven- to 10-day therapy regimens should be used for complicated infection depending on the clinical scenario. For the treatment of catheter-associated infections, the Infectious Disease Society of America guideline recommends 7 days of therapy for patients who exhibit prompt resolution of symptoms and 10 to 14 days of therapy for those with delayed clinical improvement.[48]

ANTIMICROBIAL AGENTS
Nitrofurantoin

With the incidence of uropathogen resistance rapidly exceeding 20% for trimethoprim-sulfamethoxazole (TMP-SMX, Bactrim, Septra) in many regions of the United States, nitrofurantoin (Macrobid, Macrodantin, Furodantin) has re-emerged on the clinical radar as viable first-line therapy for uncomplicated cystitis. The national rate of resistance is 0% to 7% throughout the literature, despite nitrofurantoin having been developed more than 50 years ago and being one of the first effective oral therapies for UTI.[50,51] Its spectrum covers non-methicillin-resistant *Staphylococcus aureus* (MRSA) staphylococcus, enterococci, and most *Enterobacteriaceae*, but most notably excludes *Acinetobacter, Serratia, Proteus,* and *Pseudomonas*. It is rapidly excreted in the urine, but exhibits poor tissue penetration throughout the body. Thus it has minimal effect on gastrointestinal (GI) and vaginal flora, but is not useful for upper tract infection or complicated infection. A regimen of nitrofurantoin monohydrate 100 mg by mouth, twice daily for 7 days is excellent first-line empiric therapy of uncomplicated cystitis.[50–52]

TMP-SMX

TMP-SMX has been a first-line therapy for UTI since the early 1990s, when the usefulness of beta-lactams like amoxicillin for empiric therapy was severely limited by widespread resistance. Over the intervening 20 years, the rate of resistance has more than tripled from approximately 7% in the 1990s to over 30% in some regions of the United States.[50,52] TMP-SMX is effective against many staphylococcus and streptococcus subspecies and most *Enterobacteriaceae*. It has excellent tissue penetration and can be used to treat upper UTIs with susceptible organisms. TMP-SMX 160/800 mg (double strength formulation) twice daily for 3 days is acceptable first-line empiric therapy for uncomplicated cystitis in geographic regions where resistance is below 20%. In regions where the rate of antibiotic resistance exceeds this threshold, the use of this agent should be culture-directed. A regimen of TMP-SMX 160/800 mg twice daily for 14 days can be used for outpatient therapy of acute pyelonephritis in the setting of urine culture-proven susceptibility.[52]

Fosfomycin Trometamol

Fosfomycin trometamol (Monurol) is a naturally occurring bacterial cell wall synthesis inhibitor that inhibits MurA enzyme and thus peptidoglycan biosynthesis. It exhibits a broad-spectrum of activity against *E coli, Enterobacteriaceae, Proteus mirabilis*, citrobacter subspecies, and extended beta-lactamase (ESBL)-producing organisms and vancomycin-resistant *Enterococcus* (VRE) and is delivered in a single 3 g oral dose. Fosfomycin is well-tolerated, and the rate of resistance among infecting pathogens is modest, making it an excellent agent for empiric therapy for UTI. The Antimicrobial Resistance Epidemiology in Females with Cystitis (ARESC) study, which surveyed resistance patterns among uropathogens from nine European nations and Brazil, found that 98.1% of the 2315 urine cultures that were positive for *E coli* exhibited sensitivity to fosfomycin.[53] A single 3 g dose of fosfomycin was compared with a 5-day regimen of nitrofurantoin 100 mg twice daily in one study and with a 5-day regimen of trimethoprim 200 mg twice daily in another.[54,55] Nitrofurantoin exhibited a superior early microbiological cure rate at 5 to 11 days following initiation of therapy, 86% versus 78%. However, early clinical cure at the same time point and late microbiological cure at 4 to 6 weeks were similar between the two agents. Ninety one percent of patients taking fosfomycin reported symptom improvement at 5 to 11 days compared with 95% of those on nitrofurantoin; follow-up urine culture at 4 to 6 weeks showed pathogen eradication in 96% of the fosfomycin group versus 91% of the nitrofurantoin group.[54] Minassian and colleagues[55] found an equivalent microbiological cure rate between fosfomycin and trimethoprim, 83% and 83.3% respectively. A single 3 g dose of fosfomycin can be used as a first-line agent for empiric therapy of cystitis. However, it exhibits poor tissue penetration and should not be used for treatment of pyelonephritis.

Fluoroquinolones

Over the past decade fluoroquinolones (ciprofloxacin, levofloxacin) have gone from being reserved for multidrug-resistant or otherwise complicated UTI, to one of the most commonly prescribed agents for empiric outpatient therapy of UTI. This practice shift is due in large part to explosive increase in bacterial resistance to TMP-SMX, and has led to the increase in the growth of resistant bacteria from 1% to 5% at the beginning of the last decade, to levels nearing 20% in some regions.[50] Furthermore, pathogens exhibiting fluoroquinolone resistance are often multidrug-resistant. In a study of 1858 *E coli* isolates from outpatient voided urine cultures, 54% exhibited resistance to two additional antimicrobial agents.[56] The bacterial spectrum is broad, and urinary excretion and tissue concentration are excellent among several members of this class of medications. It offers coverage of staphylococcus subspecies including *S aureus* and *S saprophyticus* and Enterobacteriaceae including *Pseudomonas aeruginosa*.

Given the broad spectrum, rapid rise in resistance, and relatively high incidence of adverse effects compared with other commonly used agents, the fluoroquinolones should be regarded as alternative agents for acute cystitis, reserved for therapy of resistant organisms or for use in patients with allergies to other first-line agents. Fluoroquinolones remain a good empiric therapy the acute pyelonephritis. Ciprofloxacin 500 mg twice daily for 7 days with or without an initial 400 mg intravenous dose may be used for the outpatient management of pyelonephritis in regions where resistance is less than 10%. If resistance exceeds 10%, an initial one-time dose of a long-acting antimicrobial, like ceftriaxone, should be given.[52]

MONITORING ANTIMICROBIAL RESISTANCE

Given the rapid rate at which antimicrobial resistance patterns are evolving, staying abreast of local patterns requires engagement with the literature and vigilance in one's own practice. It is a good practice to review one's outpatient urine culture results on a monthly or quarterly basis for trends in resistance in the immediate community.

ANTIMICROBIAL PROPHYLAXIS

For recurrent urinary tract infections, three antimicrobial regimens can effectively reduce the number and frequency of symptomatic infections. Continuous, symptom-dependent, and behavior-dependent prophylaxis schemes exist and confer similar risk reduction. Selection of an appropriate regimen is based largely upon patient lifestyle and compliance and patterns of infection.

Low-Dose Continuous Antimicrobial Prophylaxis

Low-dose continuous antimicrobial prophylaxis is appropriate for women with frequently symptomatic reinfections. It should be initiated in the setting of negative urine culture, and it consists of either a single daily or every other day dose of nitrofurantoin, TMP-SMX, or cephalexin. Breakthrough infections will occur in 5% of women using this regimen, and culture data should be obtained for any instance of breakthrough symptoms. These infections should be treated with a treatment-strength course of antibiotics. After culture-confirmed resolution of these infections, prophylaxis regimens can be resumed. It is important to note that infections with resistant organisms do not necessitate changing the prophylactic antimicrobial agent, provided the organism is eradicated with appropriate therapy. Prophylaxis is usually discontinued after 6 months duration and only restarted if reinfection occurs.

Postcoital Prophylaxis

Postcoital prophylaxis is excellent for women whose symptomatic infections cluster around periods of highest frequency of intercourse. It requires a single dose of the commonly used urinary antimicrobials following sexual activity. It is important to note that postcoital doses should not exceed a standard treatment dose if patients engage in intercourse more than once per day.

Self-Start Therapy

Self-start therapy is an excellent choice for highly motivated individuals. With this regimen, the patient collects a clean catch specimen for dip slide or conventional urine culture and begins a 3-day course of antibiotics at the onset of cystitis symptoms. It is an excellent choice for women who have discontinued continuous prophylaxis regimens. Schaeffer and colleagues[57] found that among a small cohort of 34 women employing this prophylactic strategy, symptom relief was achieved in 92% of episodes, and 86% were culture-conformed UTI.

SUMMARY

Nearly half of the world's women will experience a symptomatic UTI in their lifetime, and up to one-third of those affected will be plagued by recurrent infections. The management of UTI can be a formidable task given the prevalence of disease and high rate of recurrence, wide range of associated morbidity, rapidly evolving antimicrobial resistance and limited complement of antimicrobial agents, and necessity for timely symptom relief and infection control. Being organized and informed in one's approach to the care of women with UTI will give the treating physician the best chance at achieving the goals of care. A thorough and careful history will help characterize the pattern of infection and identify patients at risk for recurrence. Empiric therapy based on symptoms is an appropriate therapeutic approach for an isolated or initial uncomplicated UTI. Recurrent or persistent infection necessitates urine culture, physical examination, and possible radiologic evaluation. Recognizing red flags in the clinical history, physical examination, and laboratory evaluation will help to facilitate timely urologic evaluation and intervention for patients in whom symptoms belie a more serious process. Fluoroquinolone use as empiric therapy of uncomplicated cystitis should be minimized in favor of nitrofurantoin and fosfomycin and TMP-SMX in regions where resistance remains low. For patients with recurrent UTI, continuous antibiotic prophylaxis, self-start therapy, or postcoital therapy may be used to minimize the burden of frequent symptoms.

REFERENCES

1. Foxman B. Epidemiology of urinary tract infection infections: incidence, morbidity, and economic cost. Am J Med 2002;113(Suppl 1A):5S–13S.
2. Kunin CM, Zacha E, Paquin AJ. Urinary tract infections in schoolchildren: I. Prevalence of bacteriuria and associated urologic findings. N Engl J Med 1962;266: 1287–96.
3. Raz R. Asymptomatic bacteriuria: clinical significance and management. Int J Antimicrob Agents 2003;22(2):45–7.
4. Schaeffer AJ, Schaeffer EM. Infections of the urinary tract. In: Wein AJ, Kavoussi LR, editors. Campbell-Walsh urology. 9th edition. Philadelphia: Saunders Elsevier; 2007. p. 223–302.
5. Nicolle LE, Ronald AR. Recurrent urinary tract infection in women: diagnosis and treatment. Infect Dis Clin North Am 1987;1(4):793–806.
6. Harrison WO, Holmes KK, Belding ME, et al. A prospective evaluation of recurrent urinary tract infection in women. Clin Res 1974;125A.
7. Czaja CS, Stamm WE. Hooton TM. Prospective cohort study of microbial and inflammatory events immediately precede *Escherichia coli* recurrent urinary tract infection. J Infect Dis 2009;200:528–36.
8. Stamey TA, Timothy MM. Studies of introital colonization in women with recurrent urinary infections: I. The role of vaginal pH. J Urol 1975;114:261–3.
9. Hooton TM, Stapleton AE, Stamm WE. Perineal anatomy and urine-voiding characteristics of young women with and without recurrent urinary tract infections. Clin Infect Dis 1999;29:1600–1.
10. Foxman B, Geiger AM, Palin K, et al. First-time urinary tract infection and sexual behavior. Epidemiology 1995;6:162–8.
11. Hooton TM, Scholes D, Stamm WE. A prospective study of risk factors for symptomatic urinary tract infection in young women. N Engl J Med 1996;335:468–74.
12. Handley MA, Reingold AL, Shiboski S, et al. Incidence of acute urinary tract infection in young women and use of male condoms with and without Nonoxynol-9 spermicides. Epidemiology 2002;13:431–6.
13. Smith HS, Hughes JP, Hooton TM, et al. Antecedent antimicrobial use increases the risk of uncomplicated UTI in young women. Clin Infect Dis 1997;25:63–8.
14. Mazzulli T. Resistance trends in urinary tract pathogens and impact on management. J Urol 2002;168:1720–2.
15. Hillier S, Roberts Z, Dunstan F, et al. Prior antibiotics and risk of antibiotic-resistant community-acquired urinary tract infection: a case–control study. J Antimicrob Chemother 2007;60:92–9.
16. Colodner R, Kometiani, Chazan B, et al. Risk factors for community-acquired urinary tract infection due to quinolone-resistant *E coli*. Infection 2008;36:41.
17. Scholes D, Hooton TM, Roberts PL, et al. Risk factors for recurrent urinary tract infection in young women. J Infect Dis 2000;182:1777.
18. Beisel B, Hale W, Graves RS, et al. Clinical inquiries: does postcoital voiding prevent urinary tract infections in young women. J Fam Pract 2002;51(11):977.

19. Schaeffer AJ, Jones JM, Falkowski WS, et al. Adhesion of uropathogenic *E coli* to epithelial cells from women with recurrent urinary tract infection. Infection 1982; 10(3):186–91.

20. Shenfield J, Schaeffer AJ, Cordon-Cardo C, et al. Association of Lewis blood group phenotype with recurrent urinary tract infections in women. N Engl J Med 1989;320:773–7.

21. Schaeffer AJ, Radway RM, Chmiel JD. Human leukocyte antigens in women with recurrent urinary tract infections. J Infect Dis 1982;148(3):604.

22. Stamm WE, Raz R. Factors contributing to susceptibility of post-menopausal women to recurrent urinary tract infections. Clin Infect Dis 1999;28:723–5.

23. Raz R, Stamm WE. A controlled trial of intravaginal estriol in postmenopausal women with recurrent urinary tract infections. N Engl J Med 1993;329:753–6.

24. Orlander JD, Jick SS, Dean AD, et al. Urinary tract infections and estrogen use in older women. J Am Geriatr Soc 1992;40:817–20.

25. Anger JT, Litwin MS, Wang Q, et al. Complications of sling surgery among female medicare beneficiaries. Obstet Gynecol 2007;109:707–14.

26. Wullt B, Connell H, Rollano P, et al. Urodynamic factors influence the duration of Eschericia coli bacteria in deliberately colonized cases. J Urol 1998;159: 2057–62.

27. Nicole LE, Bradley S, Colgan R, et al. Infectious disease society of America guidelines for the diagnosis and treatment of asymptomatic bacteriuria in adults. Clin infect Dis 2005;40:643–54.

28. Nicolle LE, Bentley D, Garibaldi R, et al. Antimicrobial use in long-term care facilities. Infect Control Hosp Epidemiol 1996;17(2):119–28.

29. Nicolle LE. Urinary tract infections in long-term care facilities. Infect Control Hosp Epidemiol 2001;22:167–75.

30. King RB, Carlson CE, Mervine J, et al. Clean and sterile intermittent catheterization methods in hospitalized patients with spinal cord injury. Arch Phys Med Rehabil 1992;3(9):798–802.

31. Stamm WE. Urinary tract infections. Hospital infections. 4th edition. Philadelphia: Lippincott-Raven; 1998. p.477–85.

32. Tambyah PA, Maki DG. Catheter-associated urinary tract infection is rarely symptomatic: a prospective study of 1497 catheterized patients. Arch Intern Med 2000;160:678–82.

33. Warren JW, Damron D, Tenney JH, et al. Fever, bacteremia, and death as complications of bacteriuria in women with long-term indwelling urethral catheters. J Infect Dis 1987;155:1151–8.

34. Stamey TA. Pathogenesis and treatment of urinary tract infections. Baltimore (MD): Williams & Wilkins; 1980.

35. Mazor-Dray E, Levy A, Schlaeffer F, et al. Maternal urinary tract infection: is it independently associated with adverse pregnancy outcome. J Matern Fetal Neonatal Med 2009;22(2):124.

36. Aronson M, Medalia O, Schori L, et al. Prevention of colonization of the urinary tract of mice with *Escherichia coli* by blocking of bacterial adherence with methyl alpha-D-mannopyranoside. J Infect Dis 1979;139(3):329–32.

37. Hultgren SJ, Porter TN, Schaeffer AJ, et al. Role of type 1 pili and effects of phase variation on lower urinary tract infections produced by *Escherichia coli*. Infect Immun 1985;50(2):370–7.

38. Anderson GG, Martin SM, Hultgren SJ. Host subversion by formation of intracelluar bacterial communities in the urinary tract. Microbes Infect 2004;6: 1094–101.

39. Vaisanen V, Elo J, Tallgren LG, et al. Mannose-resistant haemagglutination and p antigen recognition are characteristic of *Escherichia coli* causing primary pyelonephritis. Lancet 1981;2:1366–9.
40. Silverblatt FJ, Dryer JS, Schauer S. Effect of pili on susceptibility to phagocytosis. Infect Immun 1979;24(1):218–23.
41. Ovalle A, Levancini A. Urinary tract infections in pregnancy. Curr Opin Urol 2001; 11(1):55–9.
42. Pfaller M, Rigenberg B, Rames L, et al. The usefulness of screening tests for pyuria in combination with urine culture in the diagnosis of urinary tract infection. Diagn Microbiol Infect Dis 1987;6(3):207–15.
43. Bent S, Saint S. Optimal use of diagnostic testing in women with acute uncomplicated cystitis. Am J Med 2002;113:21–8.
44. Kraft JK, Stamey TA. The natural history of symptomatic recurrent bacteriuria in women. Medicine (Baltimore) 1977;56:55–60.
45. Mabeck CE. Studies in urinary tract infections: I. The diagnosis of bacteriuria in women. Acta Med Scand 1969;186:35–8.
46. Stamm WE, Hooton TM. Management of urinary tract infections in adults. N Engl J Med 1993;329:1328–34.
47. Foxman B. Recurring urinary tract infection: incidence and risk factors. Am J Public Health 1990;80:331–3.
48. Warren JW, Abrutyn E, Hebel JR, et al. Infectious diseases society for the antimicrobial treatment of uncomplicated acute bacterial cystitis and acute pyelonephritis in women. Clin Infect Dis 1999;29:745–58.
49. Milo G, Katchman E, Paul M, et al. Duration of antibacterial treatment for uncomplicated urinary tract infections in women. Cochrane Database Syst Rev 2005;2:CD004682.
50. Zhanel GG, Hisanaga TL, Laing NM, et al. Antibiotic resistance in outpatient urinary isolates: final results from the North American urinary tract infection collaborative alliance (NAUTICA). Int J Antimicrob Agents 2006;27(6):468–75.
51. Kashanian J, Hakimian P, Shabsigh R. Nitrofurantoin: the return of an old friend in the wake of growing resistance. BJU Int 2008;102:1634–7.
52. Wagenlehner FM, Weidner W, Naber KG. An update on uncomplicated urinary tract infections in women. Curr Opin Urol 2009;19:268–74.
53. Schito GC, Naber KG, Botto H. The ARESC study: an international survey on the antimicrobial resistance of pathogens involved in uncomplicated urinary tract infections. Int J Antimicrob Agents 2009;34:407–13.
54. Stein GE. Comparison of single dose fosfomycin and a 7-day course of nitrofurantoin in female patients with uncomplicated urinary tract infection. Clin Ther 1999;2(11):1864–72.
55. Minassian MA, Lewis DA, Chattopadhyay D, et al. A comparison between single-dose fosfomycin trometamol (monuril) and a 5-day course of trimethoprim in the treatment of uncomplicated lower urinary tract infection in women. Int J Antimicrob Agents 1998;10(1):39–47.
56. Kalowsky JA, Hoban DJ, DeColby MR, et al. Fluroquinolone-resistant urinary isolates of Escherichia coli from outpatients are frequently multidrug resistant: results from the North American urinary tract infection collaborative alliance- quinolone resistance study. Antimicrob Agents Chemother 2006;50(6):2251–4.
57. Schaeffer AJ, Stuppy BA. Efficacy and safety of self-start therapy in women with recurrent urinary tract infection. J Urol 1999;161:207–11.

Urinary Infections in Men

Mathew C. Raynor, MD[a], Culley C. Carson III, MD[b],*

KEYWORDS

- Urinary infection • Sexually transmitted disease
- Pyelonephritis • Epididymitis • Abscess

Urinary tract infections (UTI) are one of the most common bacterial infections and account for significant morbidity and mortality. Additionally, evaluation and treatment of UTIs account for a significant amount of health care expenditures, estimated at more than $3 billion annually.[1,2] Most of these expenditures result from management of community-acquired infections, representing a common complaint among patients in an outpatient setting. Overall, the incidence of UTIs is higher in women, but men account for a large percentage of infections, especially complicated UTIs.

This review of urinary infections in men provides an overview of the general presentation, diagnosis, and management of common genitourinary infections in men. The focus of the article is on clinical presentation, basic diagnostic evaluation strategies, treatment options, and when referral to a specialist is warranted.

KIDNEY INFECTIONS
Pyelonephritis

Pyelonephritis refers to inflammation of the kidney and is considered an upper urinary tract infection. Acute pyelonephritis is a clinical diagnosis based on the classic presentation of fever (>100°F); chills; and flank or costovertebral angle pain. These signs and symptoms may be associated with urinary urgency, frequency, and dysuria. However, patients do not always present with classic symptoms. Gastrointestinal symptoms, such as nausea and emesis, may be present. Patients often have a history of previous UTI.

Diagnosis of acute pyelonephritis is based mainly on clinical symptoms. Laboratory diagnosis consists of urinalysis, urine culture, complete blood count, and serum chemistries. Urinalysis usually demonstrates evidence of inflammation and infection

The authors have nothing to disclose and report no conflicts of interest.
[a] Division of Urology, University of North Carolina School of Medicine, 2110 Physicians Office Building, CB 7235, Chapel Hill, NC 27599–7235, USA
[b] Division of Urology, University of North Carolina School of Medicine, 2113 Physicians Office Building, CB 7235, Chapel Hill, NC 27599–7235, USA
* Corresponding author.
E-mail address: culley_carson@med.unc.edu

Med Clin N Am 95 (2011) 43–54
doi:10.1016/j.mcna.2010.08.015
0025-7125/11/$ – see front matter © 2011 Elsevier Inc. All rights reserved.

with hematuria, pyuria, and bacteriuria. Leukocytosis is usually present with a predominance of neutrophils. Serum creatinine is usually normal. However, an elevated creatinine could indicate the presence of obstruction (bilateral obstruction or obstruction of a solitary kidney), dehydration, or severe infection. Blood cultures are not routinely drawn, unless the patient exhibits signs of significant illness (sepsis) or has risk factors for a complicated UTI. Blood cultures have been shown to be positive in about one quarter of patients with uncomplicated pyelonephritis in women.[3] However, this finding does not alter management decisions regarding therapy. Therefore, blood cultures can be omitted in cases of uncomplicated pyelonephritis.

The use of imaging studies in the diagnosis of acute pyelonephritis is a difficult clinical decision. The presence of urinary tract obstruction or stone in the setting of acute infection alters treatment strategies. However, most cases of uncomplicated pyelonephritis do not result from a stone or obstruction. Imaging options include plain radiograph, intravenous pyelogram, renal ultrasound, or CT. The use of plain radiograph has a very limited role in the management of the urinary tract. It may be useful to investigate other causes of abdominal pain. Likewise, intravenous pyelogram has fallen out of favor, given the routine availability and better anatomic detail with other modalities. Renal ultrasound is a useful screening tool to rule out the presence of hydronephrosis. CT can be performed with or without intravenous contrast agents to assess for hydronephrosis or calculus disease. There are no specific radiologic findings on CT to diagnose pyelonephritis. Some subtle findings to suggest the diagnosis include renal enlargement and perinephric fat stranding.

For practical purposes, if a patient presents with acute fever and flank or abdominal pain, most patients undergo cross-sectional abdominal imaging to evaluate for other causes, such as appendicitis, diverticulitis, or urolithiasis. Imaging should be strongly considered in a patient with clinical signs and symptoms of pyelonephritis and risk factors for complicated UTI. These include known functional or anatomic abnormalities in the urinary tract, the possibility of obstruction, recent instrumentation, recent antibiotic use, immunosuppression, or history of diabetes.

Management of acute pyelonephritis depends on properly classifying patients into uncomplicated and complicated groups. Any patient with presumed acute pyelonephritis without complicating factors and minimal symptoms without significant nausea or emesis can be treated as an outpatient. Empiric oral antimicrobial therapy should be initiated until results of urine cultures are finalized. In most cases, *Escherichia coli* are the causative bacteria. A much smaller percentage demonstrates gram-positive bacteria as the cause of pyelonephritis (*Staphylococcus epidermidis*, *Staphylococcus aureus*, and *Enterococcus faecalis*). Therefore, antimicrobial therapy can be chosen based on the presumed causative bacteria. Typically, a fluoroquinolone for 10 to 14 days is sufficient in an otherwise healthy man with a normal urinary tract. Alternatively, trimethoprim-sulfamethoxazole can be used for 10 to 14 days. If a gram-positive organism is suspected, amoxicillin or amoxicillin-clavulanic acid can be used.[4]

Patients who are severely ill or are suspected of having complicating factors require hospital admission. These patients should undergo abdominal imaging to evaluate for obstruction or other causes of illness. Urine and blood cultures should be obtained. Broad-spectrum parenteral antibiotics should be instituted, including a fluoroquinolone, aminoglycoside with or without ampicillin, or extended-spectrum cephalosporin with or without an aminoglycoside.[4] If there is any evidence of urinary tract abnormality or obstruction, urgent urologic consultation is needed because drainage of the urinary tract may be required with either ureteral stent or percutaneous nephrostomy. Parenteral antibiotic therapy should be continued until susceptibilities are returned or until the patient demonstrates clinical improvement. Patients may remain febrile after beginning antibiotics, but there tends to be a pattern of decreasing temperature spikes. Once improved and afebrile for more than 24 hours, oral antibiotics can be started and continued for a total of 14 days. If a patient remains febrile with or without persistent leukocytosis after 72 hours of therapy, repeat abdominal imaging is warranted to evaluate for possible renal or perinephric abscess. Additionally, repeat cultures from urine and blood should be obtained.

Follow-up urine culture should be obtained before completion of therapy and several weeks after completion of therapy to ensure urinary tract sterility. Relapse of infection can occur and usually requires a repeat 14-day course of culture-specific therapy.

Renal Abscess and Perinephric Abscess

Renal abscess refers to an abscess confined to the renal parenchyma. A perinephric abscess refers to an abscess cavity extending into or involving the perinephric space. Perinephric abscesses can result from extension of a renal abscess into the perinephric space or extension from another source, such as a psoas abscess, perforated appendicitis, or diverticulitis. Renal abscesses usually arise from ascending UTI and can often be associated with obstruction or calculus disease. Gram-negative bacteria account for most of renal abscesses. Gram-positive organisms can spread hematogenously and should be suspected in patients with symptoms of pyelonephritis and coexisting skin infections, endocarditis, or intravenous drug use. However, perinephric abscesses can often be polymicrobial.

Diagnosis of a renal or perinephric abscess is suspected in patients with fever and abdominal or flank pain. Additionally, renal or perinephric abscess should be suspected in patients with clinical pyelonephritis who have remained febrile for longer than 72 hours despite appropriate antimicrobial therapy. A marked and persistent leukocytosis is usually present. Urinalysis and urine culture can be misleading. These tests can be negative in a patient where the abscess cavity does not communicate with the collecting system. This situation most commonly occurs when there has been hematogenous spread of an infection. Blood cultures are usually positive in these cases.

Unlike cases of uncomplicated pyelonephritis, imaging is diagnostic for renal or perinephric abscess. Ultrasound is a very reliable and inexpensive method of diagnosis. However, CT is the imaging procedure of choice, given its excellent anatomic delineation (**Fig. 1**). Imaging features may demonstrate a rounded, slightly hypoattenuating lesion confined to the renal parenchyma. The rim of the abscess cavity may enhance with intravenous contrast. Perinephric abscesses demonstrate extension of the cavity through the renal capsule into the perinephric space and even into the psoas muscle. In severe cases, there may be significant parenchymal destruction and complete loss of the normal renal contour.

Management involves broad-spectrum antibiotics. Small (<3 cm) renal abscesses can often be managed in a manner similar to that of complicated pyelonephritis, with parenteral antibiotics and conversion to oral antibiotics with good clinical response. Follow-up imaging is needed to document improvement or resolution of the abscess. In cases of larger renal abscesses (>3–5 cm), smaller abscesses that do not respond to antimicrobial therapy, patients with diabetes, or in immunosuppressed patients, percutaneous aspiration and drainage of the abscess is indicated. Antibiotic regimens can be tailored to culture results. Urologic consultation is recommended in these cases because there may be a need for surgical drainage. Follow-up imaging is necessary. With today's improvements in imaging and image-guided therapy, surgical drainage is less frequently necessary.[5]

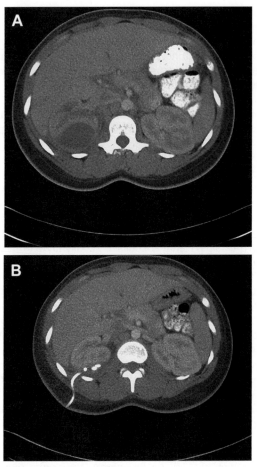

Fig. 1. Renal abscess. (*A*) Hypoattenuating fluid collection is seen with an enhancing rim confined to the renal parenchyma. (*B*) Imaging after percutaneous drainage and antibiotics demonstrates resolution.

Management of perinephric abscesses always requires drainage. These abscesses do not respond to antimicrobial therapy alone. Most of these cases can be aspirated and drained percutaneously. Surgical drainage is usually not required. However, in cases of large abscess cavities or a poorly functioning kidney, open drainage or nephrectomy may be necessary. Additionally, the presence of a perinephric abscess usually indicates an underlying problem. This could include an obstructed and infected kidney or a possible enteric communication. Further treatment directed at the underlying cause is needed once the abscess has been appropriately managed.

Emphysematous Pyelonephritis and Pyelitis

Emphysematous pyelonephritis is a rare and very serious infection involving gas-forming bacteria that results in renal parenchymal necrosis. This condition usually occurs in patients with diabetes and has a high mortality rate, ranging from 13% to 50%.[6] In addition to diabetes, many patients may have underlying poor renal function, urolithiasis, or urinary tract obstruction.

Diagnosis is made on the basis of clinical findings and, primarily, on imaging studies. Most patients are diabetic and present with high fever, flank pain, and vomiting. Laboratory studies show a significant leukocytosis and may demonstrate elevated serum creatinine, resulting from parenchymal necrosis and destruction. Urinalysis and urine culture usually demonstrate bacteriuria. The most common causative organism is *E coli*, followed by *Proteus* and *Klebsiella*. These patients are generally severely ill, with sepsis and hypotension common.

Imaging is diagnostic of emphysematous pyelonephritis. Plain radiograph or intravenous pyelogram is rarely used, but can demonstrate a collection of gas around the location of the kidney. This can be confused with bowel gas. CT is the imaging modality of choice. This demonstrates significant loculated gas throughout the renal parenchyma and even extending into the perinephric space. In severe cases, there can be complete destruction of the renal parenchyma. Emphysematous pyelonephritis must be differentiated from emphysematous pyelitis. This entity refers to the finding of gas within the collecting system of the kidney and not in the renal parenchyma. This condition is usually caused by a gas-forming bacterial UTI and does not require any special intervention. In cases of emphysematous pyelonephritis, a renal scan is recommended to assess split renal function.

Emphysematous pyelonephritis should be treated as an emergency situation. Patients are generally severely ill and require aggressive hydration, broad-spectrum antimicrobial therapy, and management of sepsis. Urologic consultation should be promptly obtained. Historically, emphysematous pyelonephritis was considered a surgical emergency and usually resulted in emergent nephrectomy. However, recent evidence suggests that medical management may actually improve outcomes and provide renal salvage. In general, management usually involves emergent drainage of the affected kidney with a percutaneous nephrostomy.[7] If conservative management fails, surgical therapy may be considered, but mortality rates after failure of conservative therapy are extremely high. Surgical therapy after successful conservative management may still be required if significant renal parenchymal destruction has occurred.

Management of Urinary Infection with Obstruction

In patients with evidence of UTI and imaging demonstrating obstruction of the urinary tract, urologic consultation is warranted. Obstruction causing hydronephrosis in the setting of an infection can lead to serious complications, including sepsis and death. The causes of obstruction include urolithiasis, ureteral stricture or scar, extrinsic compression, or significant bladder outlet obstruction resulting in urinary retention (**Fig. 2**). In the setting of obstruction and infection, pyonephrosis can occur. This term refers to a collection of purulent material in the collecting system proximal to the site of obstruction. This is essentially equivalent to an abscess in the urinary tract. Prompt intervention and drainage of the urinary tract is needed, usually including Foley catheter placement, ureteral stent placement, or nephrostomy drainage. Culture-specific antibiotics should be continued for at least 14 days and management of the underlying cause is needed.

Xanthogranulomatous pyelonephritis (XGP) represents a rare and severe form of renal deterioration secondary to obstruction and infection. Most patients present with flank pain, fever, and recurrent UTI with persistent bacteriuria. CT is the imaging modality of choice and usually demonstrates an enlarged, poorly functioning kidney with dilated calyces and thinning of the renal parenchyma. In most cases, the condition affects the entire kidney. The classic radiologic finding is a severely enlarged, hydronephrotic kidney with a thin rim of parenchyma and a centrally obstructing stone in the renal pelvis. Multiple renal or perinephric abscesses can occur (**Fig. 3**). Proteus

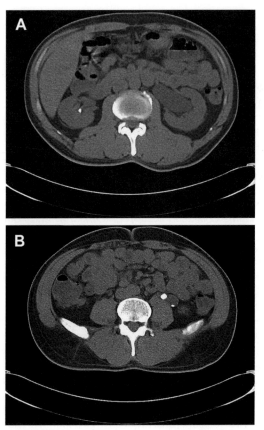

Fig. 2. Ureteral obstruction and infection. (*A*) Cross-sectional imaging shows hydronephrosis and perinephric fat-stranding. (*B*) A mid-ureteral obstructing stone was identified with proximal hydroureter.

and *E coli* are the most common causative bacteria.[8] Nuclear medicine renal function studies usually demonstrate severely diminished or no function in the affected kidney.

Management of XGP depends on the initial presentation and renal function of the affected kidney. Patients presenting as being acutely ill need medical stabilization and imaging to investigate for abscess or obstruction. Acute management of these patients usually involves broad-spectrum antibiotics and percutaneous drainage of the kidney. Once stabilized and treated with appropriate antibiotics, treatment then depends on renal function. If the kidney still maintains decent function, management of the obstructing stone and UTI can be pursued. Segmental involvement of XGP may be amenable to partial nephrectomy. If the kidney has little or no function, delayed nephrectomy is usually recommended.

BLADDER INFECTIONS
Uncomplicated Cystitis

Uncomplicated cystitis is uncommon in men. It is far more common in women. By definition, any bladder infection in a man is considered a complicated UTI. However, young men can experience acute uncomplicated cystitis without any underlying

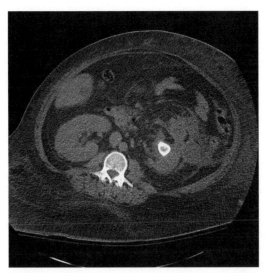

Fig. 3. Xanthogranulomatous pyelonephritis. Imaging shows a large centrally obstructing stone with complete obliteration of renal parenchyma and perinephric abscesses.

structural or functional abnormality. *E coli* are the most common causative organism, as it is in women.

Clinical presentation varies significantly and can include suprapubic or perineal pain, dysuria, frequency, urgency, and hematuria. In young sexually active men, sexually transmitted diseases (STD) should be considered. Urethritis can cause similar symptoms to those of acute cystitis.

Laboratory diagnosis includes urinalysis and urine culture. Microscopic examination of the urine may also show pyuria, hematuria, and bacteria. Routine dipstick urinalysis tests may show nitrite and leukocyte esterase positivity. These screening tests indicate the presence of bacteria that reduce nitrate to nitrite and pyuria. False-positive and false-negative tests can occur with these screening methods. Not all bacteria are capable of reducing nitrate to nitrite. Additionally, pyuria may be present in the absence of an infection. Any inflammation in the urinary tract can result in pyuria, such as recent instrumentation; foreign body (ureteral stent or nephrostomy); or stone. Improper collection of the specimen can also lead to false-positive results. Initial stream urine and improper cleansing before collection can lead to contamination of skin (especially in uncircumcised men) or distal urethral flora. Greater than 10^5 colony forming units (cfu) are strongly suggestive of an active infection. However, men may have less than 10^5 cfu but still have significant symptoms of cystitis. These men should be treated as having an active infection. Imaging is not needed in cases of uncomplicated cystitis unless an underlying cause is suspected.

Treatment of acute cystitis in younger healthy men involves a 7-day course of antibiotics. Typically, a fluoroquinolone or trimethoprim-sulfamethoxazole is the initial antibiotic of choice. Urine culture should be obtained and antimicrobial therapy altered based on susceptibilities. Follow-up urine culture to document urinary tract sterility is recommended in men and referral to a specialist is warranted if symptoms recur.

Recurrent UTI

In men with recurrent symptoms of cystitis and persistent bacteriuria, accurate diagnosis involves differentiating bacterial persistence from reinfection (with the same or usually a different organism) or inadequate treatment of the initial infection. Differentiating these causes can be quite difficult, especially in certain patient populations (eg, patients with neurogenic bladder, indwelling catheter, or asymptomatic bacteriuria).

Inadequate treatment of cystitis usually presents shortly after completing a course of antibiotics and urine culture demonstrates identical bacteria. Typically, treatment with a longer course of antibiotics and imaging to evaluate for a nidus of infection in men are warranted.

Reinfection simply refers to another infection after an adequate treatment response and posttreatment negative urine culture. Typically, these infections are caused by different bacteria and there tends to be a longer time-interval between infections. These types of infections in men should warrant urologic evaluation to look for any functional or structural abnormality creating a reservoir or sanctuary site in the urinary tract. These infections can be managed medically with antibiotics as a complicated UTI.

Bacterial persistence usually refers to reinfection or persistent infection from the same strain of bacteria. These infections warrant further urologic evaluation. Typically, bacterial persistence indicates a source of bacteria within the urinary tract that has evaded eradication. These bacteria may arise from infection stones, an atrophic nonfunctional kidney, bacterial prostatitis, foreign body, or other structural abnormality in the urinary tract. Imaging is warranted in these patients. CT or other cross-sectional imaging technique is the modality of choice. Treatment should be culture-specific and, ultimately, referral to a specialist and management of the underlying cause. In rare cases, men may benefit from long-term antimicrobial use. This could include intermittent self-start therapy or antibiotic prophylaxis.

Catheter-associated UTI

Management of infections associated with urinary catheters can be somewhat confusing. It is well-known that bacterial colonization of urinary catheters is routine. In patients with long-term indwelling catheters (>30 days), 100% of patients had bacteria present.[9] This is also true in men who perform intermittent catheterization.

In general, there are two groups of men with an indwelling urinary catheter who warrant treatment: those men who are symptomatic and those men who are undergoing urologic intervention. If a patient has symptoms consistent with cystitis and has an indwelling catheter or is on intermittent catheterization, urine culture should be obtained and treatment begun for a complicated UTI.[9] If a patient with an indwelling catheter has no symptoms, then treatment of bacteriuria is not warranted. If a patient is scheduled to undergo a urologic procedure, then culture should be obtained and the infection treated appropriately before intervention to reduce the risk of hematogenous spread.

ORCHITIS AND EPIDIDYMITIS

Orchitis and epididymitis can be difficult clinical conditions to recognize, properly diagnose, and treat. By definition, orchitis and epididymitis refer to inflammation of the testis and epididymis, respectively. The source of inflammation could be bacterial, viral, fungal, traumatic, autoimmune, or idiopathic. The clinical presentation of men can range from acute and severe illness to chronic pain. Infectious orchitis may coexist with epididymitis. Bacterial epididymo-orchitis is most commonly caused by urinary pathogens, including *E coli*, and STDs, including *Neisseria gonorrhea* and *Chlamydia trachomatis*. Viral etiologies include mumps and mononucleosis. Mycobacterial infections, including tuberculosis, can also affect the testis and epididymis.

Men presenting with acute-onset testicular pain should undergo evaluation with scrotal ultrasound to evaluate for testicular torsion or malignancy. Patients may also present with signs and symptoms suggestive of an infectious etiology. Laboratory tests should include urinalysis and urine culture. A screen for STDs is needed, if suspected. Infectious bacterial etiologies usually respond to antibiotics. A fluoroquinolone is usually adequate. However, other antibiotics to cover possible STDs in at-risk patients also can be used. Chronic epididymo-orchitis is a much more difficult scenario. Usually, conservative measures are undertaken with scrotal support and analgesics. Surgery is rarely needed for recalcitrant pain.

SEXUALLY TRANSMITTED DISEASES
Chlamydia

Chlamydia is the most common bacterial STD in the United States and the most common cause of epididymitis in young men. It is also a common cause of nongonococcal urethritis. Symptoms typically include dysuria and mucopurulent urethral discharge. Some infections may be asymptomatic.

Diagnosis typically involves obtaining an intraurethral swab for analysis. Swab culture, nucleic acid amplification tests (NAAT), and nucleic acid hybridization tests (NAHT) are used to diagnose *C trachomatis*. NAAT is preferred because of its higher sensitivity. NAAT can also be performed on a urine sample, but culture and NAHT require intraurethral swab.

Treatment involves antibiotic therapy to cover both *Chlamydia* and gonorrhea, because these two infections commonly coexist. A single dose of ceftriaxone, 125 mg intramuscularly, or a single dose of cefixime, 400 mg orally, covers gonorrhea. Treatment for *Chlamydia* involves one single dose of azithromycin, 1 g orally, or a 7-day course of doxycycline, 100 mg twice daily. Follow-up cultures or evaluation is not needed, unless symptoms recur. Partner notification for evaluation and treatment is recommended.

Gonorrhea

Gonorrhea is the second most common bacterial STD, behind *Chlamydia*. Gonococcal urethritis in men typically produces symptoms of significant urethral discharge and dysuria, prompting evaluation.

Diagnosis can be made by Gram stain of urethral discharge, demonstrating gram-negative intracellular diplococci. Urethral swab can also be obtained for culture, NAHT, or NAAT.

Treatment involves one single dose of ceftriaxone, 125 mg intramuscularly, or a single dose of cefixime, 400 mg orally. Fluoroquinolone can also be used for treatment of *N gonorrhea*, but resistant strains have increased in incidence (especially in California and Hawaii). Cotreatment for *Chlamydia* is also recommended. Partner notification for evaluation and treatment is recommended.

Chancroid

Chancroid is one of several STDs that cause a genital ulcer and is the most common STD worldwide. Symptoms include a painful ulcer along with painful or tender inguinal adenopathy. Chancroid is caused by *Haemophilus ducreyi*, a gram-negative rod in short, parallel chains. Coinfection with syphilis and herpes simplex virus (HSV) are approximately 10%. Additionally, men diagnosed with chancroid have a higher rate of HIV infection.

Diagnosis of chancroid is mainly clinical. Examination of the exudates or serologic testing to evaluate for syphilis is required. Special culture media is needed to identify *H ducreyi*. Polymerase chain reaction testing can be used, but is not approved by the Food and Drug Administration.

Treatment for chancroid is usually curative. A single dose of azithromycin, 1 g orally, or ceftriaxone, 250 mg intramuscularly, is sufficient. Alternatively, ciprofloxacin, 500 mg twice daily for 3 days, or erythromycin base, 500 mg orally three times daily for 7 days, can be used. Patients should be tested for syphilis and HIV at the time of diagnosis and 3 months after treatment.

Lymphogranuloma Venereum

Lymphogranuloma venereum is caused by C trachomatis serotypes L1, L2, and L3. This STD is rare in the United States. Symptoms include a small painless genital ulcer or papule that is usually self-limited. Painful and suppurative inguinal or femoral adenopathy can then develop. This adenopathy is usually unilateral.

Diagnosis is difficult because cultures are routinely nondiagnostic. Immunofluorescence or nucleic acid detection can be used. Treatment is generally recommended if the clinical presentation is suggestive of lymphogranuloma venereum.

Treatment involves a 3-week course of doxycycline, 100 mg twice daily, as the preferred method. Alternatively, erythromycin base, 500 mg four times daily, can be used for 3 weeks.

Syphilis

Syphilis is caused by the spirochete *Treponema pallidum*. The incubation period can range from 10 days to 3 months. Typically, primary syphilis is characterized by a single painless and indurated ulcer usually located on the glans penis. Nontender inguinal adenopathy may be present. Primary syphilis may go unnoticed and untreated. These symptoms usually persist for 4 to 6 weeks. Latent syphilis refers to patients with serologic evidence of infection but no clinical evidence of disease. Secondary syphilis may present anywhere from 2 months to 2 years after the primary ulcer. Symptoms usually consist of a maculopapular rash on the trunk and arms associated with nontender adenopathy. The palms and soles may also be involved. Condyloma lata refers to enlarged and eroded papules in the intertriginous areas and are quite infectious. Tertiary syphilis can develop in untreated patients. This stage of disease is quite rare, except in patients with HIV. In this stage, syphilis can affect any organ system.

Diagnosis of early syphilis involves darkfield examination and direct fluorescent antibody testing of ulcer exudate tissue. These methods are considered definitive for the diagnosis of syphilis. Serologic testing methods are frequently used to provide a presumptive diagnosis of syphilis. Nontreponemal (VDRL and rapid plasma reagin) and treponemal tests (fluorescent treponemal antibody absorption test) are used. Nontreponemal tests can produce false-positive results in the presence of certain medical conditions (acute febrile illness, recent immunization, autoimmune disorders, intravenous drug use, and chronic liver disease). VDRL or rapid plasma reagin is measured as titers and can be used to follow response to therapy. Treponemal tests (fluorescent treponemal antibody absorption test) usually remain positive for life after diagnosis, regardless of treatment.

Treatment for syphilis in any stage is penicillin G, administered parenterally. The dose and length of treatment depend on the clinical stage and symptoms of the disease.

Herpes Simplex

Genital herpes is a common infection in the United States. There are two types of herpes virus: HSV-1 and HSV-2. Most cases of genital herpes are caused by HSV-2, but up to 50% of cases of primary genital herpes may be caused by HSV-1. Primary infection is characterized by painful ulcers on the genitalia associated with painful inguinal adenopathy and flulike symptoms. The ulcers are usually small and multiple vesicular lesions with an erythematous base. Asymptomatic viral shedding and recurrences are common and vary by viral type.

Definitive diagnosis involves viral culture from an active lesion. However, this test has low sensitivity. Polymerase chain reaction assays are more sensitive tests but have not been approved for genital lesions. Type-specific serologic tests have been developed based on specific viral proteins.

Treatment involves the use of antiviral agents. Acyclovir (400 mg three times a day for 7–10 days), famciclovir (250 mg three times a day for 7–10 days), or valacyclovir (1 g twice a day for 7–10 days) are recommended for use in primary outbreaks. Suppressive therapy can be used to minimize recurrences.

Human Papilloma Virus

Genital warts (condylomata acuminata) are caused by human papilloma virus. There are over 100 types of human papilloma virus. Types 6 and 11 cause most visible warts, but there are types that have a higher risk of malignant transformation (types 16, 18, 31, 33, and 35). The lesions can range in number and size.

Diagnosis is based mainly on clinical evaluation of the typical wartlike lesion. Biopsy is usually not necessary, unless there is significant burden of disease that may need surgical excision. Some lesions may spontaneously regress. Recurrence is common.

Treatment can take many forms, depending on burden of disease, location, and patient or physician preference. Topical treatment can be applied by the patient or physician. Patient-applied treatment includes topical 0.5% podofilox gel or 5% imiquimod cream. Physician-applied treatments include podophyllin resin, trichloroacetic acid, liquid nitrogen, or laser therapy. Surgical excision is also an option for larger lesions. Referral to a specialist is recommended for large lesions or lesions surrounding the urethral meatus.

Molluscum Contagiosum

Molluscum contagiosum virus is a member of the Pox family and is most commonly transmitted by sexual contact in adolescents and adults. There is an incubation period of 2 to 4 weeks. The diagnosis is based mainly on clinical evidence of small pearly papules with central umbilication usually present on the genitalia, inguinal region, and lower abdomen. The disease process is usually self-limited. Treatment is usually not needed. However, these lesions can be treated with cautery or cryotherapy, if desired.

Diagnostic and treatment guidelines for STDs are available at the Centers for Disease Control and Prevention Web site (www.cdc.gov/std).

SUMMARY

Infections in the genitourinary tract in men can range from acute, life-threatening illnesses to chronic conditions. Clinical presentation, previous history, physical examination findings, and laboratory studies can be used to generate possible diagnoses. Appropriate use of imaging can further aid in identifying potential causes. In the presence of complicating factors or evidence of obstruction of the urinary tract, urologic consultation is recommended for further evaluation and management.

REFERENCES

1. Griebling TL. Urologic Diseases in America Project: trends in resource use for urinary tract infections in men. J Urol 2005;173:1288–94.

2. Griebling TL. Urologic Diseases in America Project: trends in resource use for urinary tract infections in women. J Urol 2005;173:1281–7.

3. Velasco M, Martinez JA, Moreno-Martinez A, et al. Blood cultures for women with uncomplicated acute pyelonephritis: are they necessary? Clin Infect Dis 2003;37:1127–30.

4. Warren JW, Abrutyn E, Hebel JR, et al. Guidelines for antimicrobial treatment of uncomplicated acute bacterial cystitis and acute pyelonephritis in women. Infectious Diseases Society of America (IDSA). Clin Infect Dis 1999;29:745–58.

5. Shu T, Green JM, Orihuela E. Renal and perirenal abscesses in patients with otherwise anatomically normal urinary tracts. J Urol 2004;172:148–50.

6. Somani BK, Nabi G, Thorpe P, et al. Is percutaneous drainage the new gold standard in the management of emphysematous pyelonephritis? Evidence from a systematic review. J Urol 2008;179:1844–9.

7. Pontin AR, Barnes RD. Current management of emphysematous pyelonephritis. Nat Rev Urol 2009;6:272–9.

8. Korkes F, Favoretto RL, Broglio M, et al. Xanthogranulomatous pyelonephritis: clinical experience with 41 cases. Urology 2008;71:178–80.

9. Hooton TM, Bradley SF, Cardenas DD, et al. Diagnosis, prevention, and treatment of catheter-associated urinary tract infection in adults: 2009 international clinical practice guidelines from the Infectious Diseases Society of America. Clin Infect Dis 2009;50:625–63.

Bladder Pain Syndrome

Philip Hanno, MD, MPH[a],*, Jørgen Nordling, MD, DrMedSci, FEBU[b],
Magnus Fall, MD, PhD[c]

KEYWORDS

- Bladder pain syndrome • Interstitial cystitis
- Painful bladder syndrome • Chronic pelvic pain

> We have all met, at one time or another, patients who suffer chronically from their bladder; and we mean the ones who are distressed, not only periodically but constantly, having to urinate often, at all moments of the day and of the night, and suffering pains every time they void.
>
> –Bourque JP.

NOMENCLATURE

"If names be not correct, language is not in accordance with the truth of things. If language be not in accordance with the truth of things, affairs cannot be carried on to success." *The Analects of Confucius*, Book 13, Verse 3.[1]

In 1915, Guy L. Hunner[2,3] described red bleeding areas high on the bladder wall in female patients with severe urinary urgency, frequency, and pelvic pain. He named these lesions elusive ulcers because the cystoscopic equipment at that time was not of today's standard. However, these inflammatory infiltrates are not ulcers,[4] and this characterization has caused much confusion and underdiagnosing of the condition. The first to call the disease "interstitial cystitis" was Alexander J.C. Skene[5] in 1887: "When the disease has destroyed the mucous membrane partly or wholly and extended to the muscular parietes, we have what is known as interstitial cystitis." Many patients with urinary urgency, frequency, and pelvic pain do not present with such inflammatory lesions, and for lack of another designation, they were also given a diagnosis of interstitial cystitis. Unfortunately, this broadened concept of interstitial cystitis never had a proper diagnosis, so it was up to the physician to decide which patients they felt had the disease. It is easy to imagine that this has resulted in confusion

[a] Perelman Center for Advanced Medicine, Hospital of the University of Pennsylvania, West Pavilion 3rd Floor, 3400 Civic Center Boulevard, Philadelphia, PA 19104, USA
[b] Department of Urology, Koebenhavns AMT, Herlev, Hospital of the University of Copenhagen, 75 Herlev Ringvej, DK-2730, Herlev, Denmark
[c] Department of Urology, Institute of Clinical Sciences, Sahlgrenska Academy, University of Gothenburg, Sahlgrenska University Hospital, Gothenburg SE 41345, Sweden
* Corresponding author.
E-mail address: hannop@uphs.upenn.edu

Med Clin N Am 95 (2011) 55–73
doi:10.1016/j.mcna.2010.08.014
0025-7125/11/$ – see front matter © 2011 Elsevier Inc. All rights reserved.

medical.theclinics.com

and frustration for both doctors and patients because nobody knew how to make the diagnosis and therefore it was used with huge individual and geographic variances.

In 1978, Messing[6] introduced submucosal petecchial bleeding or glomerulations noted during bladder distention as a cardinal finding in patients with interstitial cystitis. This was incorporated in the revised National Institute of Diabetes and Digestive and Kidney Diseases (NIDDK) criteria from 1990[7] demanding 2 positive inclusion criteria for the diagnosis:

1. Bladder pain or urinary urgency
2. Glomerulations at bladder dilatation or Hunner ulcer and a long list of exclusion criteria.

The NIDDK criteria were too restrictive to be used clinically, and were designed only to be used for the selection of patients for research to obtain reasonably comparable patient groups. Sixty percent of patients with a clinical diagnosis of interstitial cystitis do not fulfill the NIDDK criteria.[8] Nevertheless, they have had widespread use as diagnostic criteria for interstitial cystitis even up to today.[9] Furthermore, it has been demonstrated that 45% of asymptomatic females and 20% of men with lower urinary tract symptoms (LUTS) demonstrate glomerulations at bladder distension[10,11] and 10% to 34% of patients with a diagnosis of interstitial cystitis do not demonstrate glomerulations at bladder distension.[12,13] Hunner ulcer is present in only about 10% of patients with a diagnosis of interstitial cystitis, leaving bladder pain or urinary urgency as the only valid inclusion criteria. Many patients have therefore received the diagnosis on the basis of urinary urgency, although this is the diagnostic symptom for overactive bladder syndrome (OAB).

Because the nomenclature has been so variable in the literature to date, in this article the terms BPS, PBS, and IC will be used interchangeably to refer to the same condition, which has yet to be crystallized as to name and definition worldwide. The reader will no doubt see all of these terms in recent and past references.

DEFINITION

In an attempt to solve these problems, the International Incontinence Society (ICS) in 2002 focused on bladder pain in this condition and introduced the term painful bladder syndrome (PBS) as suprapubic pain related to bladder filling accompanied by other symptoms such as increased daytime and nighttime frequency in the absence of proven urinary tract infection (UTI) or other obvious pathology.[14] Interstitial cystitis (IC) was defined as "painful bladder syndrome with typical cystoscopic and histologic features," which were left undefined. It was shown however, that this definition had a sensitivity of only 64% when tested on patients with a clinical diagnosis of interstitial cystitis.[15] It was primarily because of the criteria "suprapubic" and "related to bladder filling" that patients failed to meet the syndrome definition.

In 2008, the European Society for the Study of Interstitial Cystitis proposed a new definition, and for purposes of a more consistent taxonomy proposed the name bladder pain syndrome (BPS), which would be diagnosed on the basis of chronic pelvic pain, pressure, or discomfort perceived to be related to the urinary bladder accompanied by at least one other urinary symptom such as persistent urge to void or urinary frequency. Confusable diseases as the cause of the symptoms must be excluded.

Further documentation and classification of BPS might be performed according to findings at cystoscopy with hydrodistension and morphologic findings in bladder biopsies. The presence of other organ symptoms, as well as cognitive, behavioral, emotional, and sexual symptoms should be addressed.[16]

With the designation of pelvic pain perceived to be related to the bladder as the key feature of the syndrome, the cognitive, behavioral, emotional, and sexual consequences of a pain syndrome must therefore be taken care of by the care provider(s). These aspects are as important as in other pain syndromes such as irritable bowel syndrome, fibromyalgia, and chronic fatigue syndrome, all of which have been shown to be associated with BPS.[17]

Prevalence

It has been estimated that the prevalence of chronic pain owing to benign causes in the population is at least 10%.[18] Prevalence studies of BPS are hampered by many problems.[19] The lack of an accepted definition, the absence of a validated diagnostic marker, and questions regarding etiology and pathophysiology make much of the literature difficult to interpret.

Over time, estimates of prevalence of symptoms compatible with a diagnosis of BPS have suggested that the magnitude of the problem has been underestimated in the past. Two recent investigations sponsored by the National Institutes of Health illustrate the point. The Boston Area Community Health Survey suggested a prevalence of BPS symptoms of 1% to 2% of the population depending on the definition used.[20] The Rand Corporation's $5 million epidemiology study, which is ongoing, estimates a prevalence of 2.7% of the female population older than 18 years using a high specificity definition.[21] Neither study includes any random subset with clinical confirmation of the diagnosis. It is clear that the prevalence of BPS symptoms is much greater than the prevalence of a physician diagnosis of the syndrome.

Natural History

Although all symptoms fluctuate, there appears to be no evidence of significant change in overall disease severity over a 5-year period.[22] Longer longitudinal studies are lacking. Symptom onset is typically acute or subacute, with symptoms initially misinterpreted as being the result of a urinary tract infection. Symptoms usually stabilize with periods of flare and remission, often unrelated to specific therapies used. Long-term progression of symptom severity is thought to occur in only 10% of cases. No effects on pregnancy outcomes have been noted.[23] Bladder cancer has not been associated with the syndrome, although the irritative voiding symptoms associated with some forms of bladder cancer can be misdiagnosed for BPS. It is essential that anyone with microhematuria be evaluated by a urologist with appropriate imaging studies and cystoscopy to rule out the possibility of a urothelial malignancy.

There is an associated high incidence of comorbidity including depression, chronic pain, and anxiety and overall mental health.[24] All domains of female sexual function including sexually related distress, desire, and orgasm frequency can be affected.[25] Numerous associated disorders have been described,[26–28] and BPS should be considered as a concomitant diagnosis when patients with associated diseases are evaluated. Inflammatory bowel disease was found in more than 7% of the IC population that Alagiri[26] studied, a figure 100 times higher than in the general population. Although unexplained at this time, abnormal leukocyte activity has been implicated in both conditions.[29,30]

Etiology

The hypotheses of etiologies of BPS range from increased urothelial permeability, immunologic or neurogenic abnormalities, to pelvic floor dysfunction and even sexual abuse (**Fig. 1**). It is important to note observations of comorbidities; in many cases of chronic bladder pain, there are associations to conditions such as irritable bowel syndrome, fibromyalgia, Sjögren syndrome, anxiety disorders, and chronic pain in other locations than the bladder. Thus, a large number of patients seem to suffer from a more general nerve dysfunction rather than a distinct and defined disease confined to the urinary bladder. Central nervous system mechanisms are probably very important.

It is likely that BPS has a multifactorial etiology that may act predominantly through one or more pathways resulting in the typical symptom complex.[31–35] There are an abundance of theories regarding its pathogenesis, but confirmatory evidence gleaned from clinical practice has proven sparse. Among numerous proposals are "leaky epithelium," mast cell activation, and neurogenic inflammation, or some combination of these and other factors leading to a self-perpetuating process resulting in chronic bladder pain and voiding dysfunction.[36] Irritable bowel syndrome, fibromyalgia, chronic fatigue syndrome, and various other chronic pain disorders may precede or follow the development of BPS in some patients, but development of associated

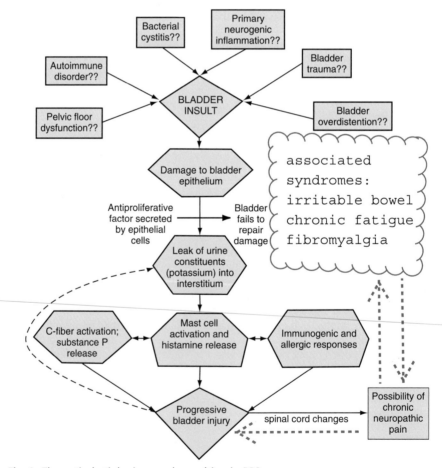

Fig. 1. Theoretical etiologic cascade resulting in BPS.

syndromes is not inevitable by any means, and their relationship to etiology is currently unknown.[37,38]

Both stress and pelvic floor dysfunction can contribute to BPS symptom severity and may be targets for treatment. Whether they can be contributing initiators of the syndrome complex is unclear at this time. The 5:1 female preponderance suggests hormonal involvement in etiology.

Focused history and physical examination, as well as urine tests and culture, common blood tests, urodynamics, and cystoscopy may be necessary in the evaluation of patients with bladder pain.[39] The completion of these steps may require collaboration among the primary care physician, the urologist, and the gynecologist (see **Table 1** for a list of confusable diseases).

History
A general thorough medical history should be taken with special emphasis given to the following:

Previous pelvic operations
Previous UTI
Bladder history/urologic diseases
Location of pelvic pain (referred pain) and relation to bladder filling/emptying; characteristics of pain onset, correlation with other events, and description of pain
Previous pelvic radiation treatment
Autoimmune diseases
Use of tiaprophenic acid.

Physical examination
A common physical examination should be performed, including palpation of the lower abdomen for bladder fullness and tenderness:

Standing: kyphosis, scars, hernia
Supine: abduction/adduction of the hips, hyperesthetic areas.

In females, physical examination should include a vaginal examination with pain mapping of the vulvar region and vaginal palpation for tenderness of the bladder, urethra, and levator and adductor muscles of the pelvic floor. Tenderness might be graded as mild, moderate, or severe.

Pain mapping inspection
Vulva
Exclusion of vulvar/vestibular diseases (vulvitis, dermatosis, and so forth)
Evaluation of introital area (endometriosis)
Tenderness of vestibular glands or vulvar skin (Touch Test: use wet cotton stick or finger tip)
Vagina
Tenderness during insertion and opening of speculum
Cervical pathology
Vaginal fornices (endometriosis)
Bimanual physical examination
Tenderness of urethra, trigone, and bladder
Superficial/deep vaginal tenderness
Tenderness of pelvic floor muscles (levator, adductor)
Tenderness in adnexal areas.

Table 1 Confusable diseases	
Confusable Disease	**Excluded or Diagnosed by**
Bladder carcinoma	Urine cytology, cystoscopy, and biopsy
Carcinoma in situ	Urine cytology, cystoscopy, and biopsy
Infection with:	
Common intestinal bacteria	Routine bacterial culture
Mycobacterium tuberculosis	Dipstick; if "sterile" pyuria culture for M tuberculosis
Chlamydia trachomatis	Special culture
Ureaplasma urealyticum	Special culture
Mycoplasma hominis	Special culture
Mycoplasma genitalis	Special culture
Corynebacterium urealyticum	Special culture
Candida species	Special culture
Herpes simplex	Physical examination
Human papilloma virus	Physical examination
Radiation	Medical history
Chemotherapy, including	
Immunotherapy with cyclophosphamide	Medical history
Anti-inflammatory therapy with tiaprophenic acid	Medical history
Bladder neck obstruction	Flowmetry and ultrasound post void residual
Neurogenic outlet obstruction	Medical history, flowmetry, and ultrasound post void residual
Bladder stone	Imaging or cystoscopy
Lower ureteric stone	History and/or hematuria; imaging
Urethral diverticulum	Medical history and physical examination
Urogenital prolaps	Medical history and physical examination
Endometriosis	Medical history and physical examination
Vaginal candidiasis	Medical history and physical examination
Cervical, uterine and ovarian cancer	Medical history and physical examination
Incomplete bladder emptying	Ultrasound post void residual
Overactive bladder	Medical history and urodynamics (urology)
Prostate cancer	Physical examination and prostate specific antigen
Benign prostatic obstruction	Flowmetry and pressure-flow studies (urology)
Chronic bacterial prostatitis	Medical history, physical examination, culture
Chronic nonbacterial prostatitis	Medical history, physical examination, culture
Pudendal nerve entrapment	History, physical examination, nerve block (pain management)
Pelvic floor muscle–related pain	Medical history, physical examination

Many conditions and diseases might cause pain perceived to be related to the bladder. Many of these have specific causes of which most can be treated, and it is therefore important to exclude these diseases as the cause of the patient's symptoms.[16] This does not mean that bladder pain syndrome cannot coexist with a confusable disease.

In males, digital rectal examination (DRE) should be performed with pain mapping of the scrotal–anal region and palpation of tenderness of the bladder, prostate, levator and adductor muscles of the pelvic floor, and the scrotal contents.

Laboratory tests

Urine dipstick (red blood cells, pH, leucocytes, nitrate)
Urine culture in all; if sterile pyuria, culture for tuberculosis
Urine cytology in risk groups
Investigations for vaginal Ureaplasma and *Chlamydia* in females and prostatitis in men are optional.

Symptom evaluation

Voiding diary with volume intake and output for 3 days at initial evaluation
At follow-up, only number of voids during day and nighttime is necessary
A Symptom Score and Quality-of-Life Score are useful
Pain should be recorded using a Visual Analog Scale (VAS) for pain during the preceding 24 hours (to fit with the voiding diary). Separate scores for the average, mildest, and worst pain might be obtained.

Urodynamics

Filling cystometry is helpful when overactive bladder (OAB) is suspected. In females, flow rate calcuation, post void residual urine volume, and pressure-flow study are optional. In males, a flow rate should be done in all, and if maximum flow is less than 20 mL/s a pressure-flow study and measure of residual urine volume should be done.

Cystoscopy and morphology

Cystoscopy under local anesthesia might be part of the general urologic workup to exclude diagnoses other than BPS.

Cystoscopy under anesthesia, either spinal or general, is controversial. The findings of glomerulations are of questionable value as mentioned previously, but bladder capacity under anesthesia does give information about potential functional capacity. Moreover, the finding of a Hunner lesion offers the possibility of a specific and often highly effective local treatment and a Hunner lesion is often best recognized using bladder distension.[40–42]

Bladder biopsies might give information about confusable diseases as in carcinoma in situ. More specific findings such as mast cell infiltration and bladder wall fibrosis might give some information about disease severity and prognosis.[12] Morphologic investigation should also use the technique described by the International Society for the Study of Bladder Pain Syndrome (ESSIC).[39] Staining for detrusor mastocytosis can be done in accordance with daily practice.[43]

Because cystoscopic and morphologic findings are controversial and not always obtained as a part of the routine evaluation, a classification system has been proposed to characterize patients and make comparisons between patient groups possible (**Table 2**).[16] The finding of glomerulations (type 2) may already be obsolete because findings of glomerulations have no specificity or sensitivity for the diagnosis of BPS, the choice of treatment, or prognosis.[12,44]

Taxonomy issues

A clinical term should have clear diagnostic features that translate to known patho-physiological processes to facilitate identification of rational treatment. Unfortunately, the latter has certainly not been the case for many pelvic pain states, and the literature

Table 2					
ESSIC Classification of bladder pain syndrome (BPS) types					
		Cystoscopy with Hydrodistension			
		Not Done	Normal	Glomerulations[a]	Hunner Lesion[b]
Biopsy	Not done	XX	1X	2X	3X
	Normal	XA	1A	2A	3A
	Inconclusive	XB	1B	2B	3B
	Positive[c]	XC	1C	2C	3C

Abbreviation: ESSIC, International Society for the Study of Bladder Pain Syndrome.
[a] Cystoscopy: glomerulations grades 2–3.
[b] With or without glomerulations.
[c] Histology showing inflammatory infiltrates and/or detrusor mastocytosis and/or granulation tissue and/or intrafascicular fibrosis.

has been flooded with a wide variety of diagnostic expressions with obscure meaning, such as interstitial cystitis, prostatodynia, dysaesthetic vulvodynia, and proctalgia fugax. For the most part these "diagnoses" describe syndromes that do not have recognized standard definitions, yet their names seem to infer knowledge of a pathophysiological cause for the patient's symptoms. It has been emphasized repeatedly during the past few years that these organ-based diagnoses are misleading and may promote erroneous thinking about diagnosis and treatment on the part of physicians, surgeons, and not the least, patients. Even Confucious knew that this is not just an intellectual problem because such terminology can lead to measures and therapies that are misguided or even harmful.[1,45]

As a consequence of this growing awareness, several organizations and working groups are involved in systematic efforts to create a correct and practically useful taxonomy that is descriptive in nature while taking pain location into account. The International Continence Society (ICS) has an ambitious terminology project ongoing since the 1970s. Within this framework, the first initiative was taken to use descriptive terms without implying organ-centered assumptions.[14] The ICS terminology report introduced 7 genito-urinary pain syndromes: painful bladder syndrome, urethral pain syndrome, vulvar pain syndrome, vaginal pain syndrome, scrotal pain syndrome, perineal pain syndrome, and pelvic pain syndrome, while also describing their substance. Shortly thereafter, guidelines on chronic pelvic pain were published by the European Association of Urology (EAU) (www.uroweb.org) in their comprehensive set of urology guidelines. These were followed by a short form in *European Urology* 1 year later,[46] and recently revised.[47] These guidelines recognized that pelvic and genito-urinary pain often overlap and that pain conditions cannot always be presented as distinct separate entities. The EAU guidelines included definitions for chronic pelvic pain states extending the definitions presented by the ICS. The taxonomy was based on the axial structure used by the International Association for the Study of Pain (IASP).[37] To conform to the structure of this taxonomy, BPS was introduced as a preferred term instead of PBS for better concordance with other pelvic pain conditions (**Table 3**).

What are the merits of the ongoing efforts? Let us look at 2 examples of transition from previous to current taxonomy.

Example 1, "prostatitis" and "prostatodynia" These terms imply different symptoms to different people but point to a prostate origin that may not be certain. To arrive at

Table 3

EAU classification of chronic urogenital pain syndromes[a]

Axis I Region		Axis II System	Axis III End Organ Pain Syndrome as Identified from Hx, Ex, and Ix			Axis IV Referral Characteristics	Axis V Temporal Characteristics	Axis VI Character	Axis VII Associated Symptoms	Axis VIII Psychological Symptoms
Chronic pelvic pain	Pelvic pain syndrome	Urologic	Bladder pain syndrome	(See Table 2 on ESSIC classification)		Suprapubic	ONSET	Aching	URINARY	ANXIETY
			Urethral pain syndrome			Inguinal	Acute	Burning	Frequency	About pain or putative cause of pain
			Prostate pain syndrome	Type A inflammatory		Urethral	Chronic	Stabbing	Nocturia	
				Type B noninflammatory		Penile/clitoral	ONGOING	Electric	Hesitance	Other
			Penile pain syndrome	Testicular pain syndrome		Perineal	Sporadic	Other	Poor flow	DEPRESSION
				Epididymal pain syndrome		Rectal	Cyclical		Pis en deux	Attributed to pain/ impact of pain
				Postvasectomy pain syndrome		Back	Continuous		Urge	Attributed to other causes or
		Gynecological	Endometriosis associated pain syndrome			Buttocks	TIME		Urgency	unattributed
			Vaginal pain syndrome				Filling		Incontinence	SHAME, GUILT related to disclosed pain
			Vulvar pain syndrome	Generalized Vulvar Pain Syndrome	Vestibular pain syndrome		Emptying		Other	syndrome or undisclosed sexual
				Localized vulvar pain syndrome	Clitoral pain syndrome		Immediate post		GYNECOLOGICAL eg, Menstrual	experience/s
							Late post		SEXUAL eg, Female	PTSD SYMPTOMS
							PROVOKED		dyspareunia impotence	Reexperiencing
									Gastrointestinal	Avoidance
		Anorectal							MUSCULAR	Hyperarousal
		Neurologic	eg, Pudendal pain syndrome						Hyperalgesia	
		Muscular							CUTANEOUS	
	Non pelvic pain syndrome	Neurologic	eg, Pudendal neuralgia						Allodynia	
		Urologic								

Abbreviations: ESSIC, International Society for the Study of Bladder Pain Syndrome; Ex, examination; Hx, history; Ix, investigation; PTSD, posttraumatic stress disorder.

[a] The table presented is not comprehensive; for the purpose of this document the main emphasis has been on the urologic pain syndromes.

This classification represents the efforts of many groups, as indicated in the main text. The work is in progress and further changes in this classification system are likely.

the diagnosis of *prostate pain syndrome,* the prostate would have to be tender and appropriate sexual and urinary symptoms would be present. A substantial number of patients could have idiopathic painful prostate syndrome where no cause could be identified. To arrive at even more specific terms, abnormal inflammatory parameters and/or infection would need to be identified from prostatic secretions or tissue to justify the term *prostatitis.* However, if the pain cannot objectively be associated with the individual organ, the syndrome would be described in terms of the symptoms. It is therefore proposed to change "prostatodynia" to *perineal pain.* The latter describes only where the patient feels the pain and leaves the possibility of different origins and pathologies as etiologic for the patient's symptoms.

Example 2, "interstitial cystitis" As mentioned, prevalence figures are conflicting and vary widely depending on which prevalence survey is considered; the wide range reasonably depends on difficulties in uniformly defining the disease. There is one well-defined, but in most clinics not so frequently reported, subset of this painful condition that should be separated out, characterized by a panmural inflammation with a characteristic pattern of inflammatory cell involvement, perineural cell infiltrates, defective urothelium, granulation tissue, and typical cystoscopic lesions seen in the bladder at distension,[48] the classic Hunner[2,3] type of disease. The word "interstitial cystitis" denotes inflammatory changes in the bladder wall interstitium, ie, an inflammation extending beyond the mucosa. The category in question fulfills the requirements. However, the term "interstitial cystitis" has become more widely used, as its definition has become symptom-based rather than based on identification of the specific form of inflammation by cystoscopic appearance and histologic features. In 1987, in an effort to bring order from the existing chaos, the US National Institutes of Health arranged a workshop and subsequently published an arbitrary definition designed to categorize patients suitable for clinical trials.[49] There were no compulsory histologic criteria for making the diagnosis of IC and subsequently the symptom criteria, after exclusion of a number of well-defined diseases, were found sufficient for the diagnosis. Since then, it has been repeatedly claimed that even without histologic abnormalities, the diagnosis of interstitial cystitis can be made.[50] Comparison of various studies as to composition of series and the subsequent treatment results has been hampered or even made impossible although no doubt we are dealing with a heterogeneous concept.[27,51] That is why the initiative of the International Society for the Study of Bladder Pain Syndrome is so important.[16]

Significance of cystoscopic findings

There seems to be at least one category of patients with a more generalized autonomous nerve dysfunction and rather uncharacteristic, maybe secondary effects to be seen when examining the bladder endoscopically. There is also a more well-defined entity in the form of specific inflammatory lesions of the bladder, although associated with general immunologic features as well.[48]

Bladder pain syndrome/interstitial cystitis is divided into the classic inflammatory type and nonulcer disease, respectively. The 2 presentations are different in terms of demographic, endoscopic, histologic, and neurobiological findings as well as in the response to various types of treatment. The classic type presents Hunner-type lesions. These lesions typically display reddened mucosal areas with small vessels radiating toward a central scar, fibrin deposit, or coagulum (**Fig. 2**), this site rupturing with increasing bladder distension with petechial oozing of blood from the ulcer and the mucosal margins (**Fig. 3**). A slightly bullous edema develops post distension, possibly as a result of mast cell degranulation.[48,51] On the other hand, cystoscopy in nonulcer IC

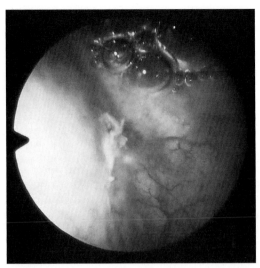

Fig. 2. Cystoscopic appearance of Hunner lesion before bladder distension: circumscript inflammatory reaction with radiating vessels and central scar with fibrin deposit. (*From* Johansson SL, Fall M. Clinical features and spectrum of light microscopic changes in interstitial cystitis. J Urol 1990;143(6):1118–24; with permission.)

can show a totally normal-appearing urothelium or multiple glomerulations after hydrodistension (**Fig. 4**) and, in some patients, the development of small, multiple, superficial mucosal cracks or a slight general edema. These findings are not specific for nor pathognomonic of BPS. A series of 130 patients with classic and 101 with nonulcer disease, diagnosed according to NIDDK criteria, were evaluated as to possible differences. Symptoms and bother were equally severe in the 2 groups. Patients with nonulcer disease were younger at diagnosis (P<.0001) and at symptom onset. Furthermore,

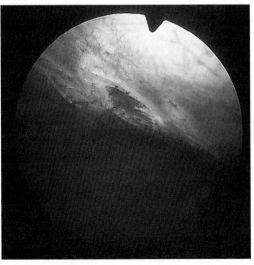

Fig. 3. Lesion during bladder distension in general anesthesia: mucosal rupture at the lesion site with waterfall-like bleeding.

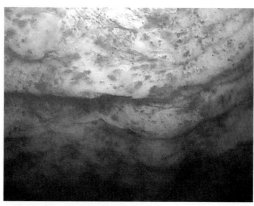

Fig. 4. Bladder pain syndrome of so-called nonulcer type. Multiple punctuate submucosal bleedings (glomerulations) following bladder distension during anesthesia and mild general edema. Normal bladder mucosa before distension.

there was a marked and significant difference in bladder capacity while patients were under general anesthesia ($P<.0001$). Patients with the classic type had smaller bladder capacity; some of them even a contracted bladder. This was not seen in patients with nonulcer disease. Bladder contracture is an expression of the destructive nature of the inflammatory involvement of the bladder wall seen in classic Hunner type.

The current observations together with previous findings clearly demonstrated that the 2 presentations represent separate entities. They should be evaluated separately in clinical studies.[52]

The issue of phenotyping

Obviously, there are at least 2 categories of BPS differing in a number of features: endoscopic findings, histopathology, clinical course, and response to various treatments. However, the picture may be even more complicated. At this stage, to be able to move forward, relevant phenotyping is essential, and this requires systematic collection and analysis of objective and subjective data and consensus on what the relevant data are. It is worth remembering the maxim "the better you describe a disease, the better you understand it."

ESSIC was the first to attack this vital question. They have made strenuous attempts to define, investigate, and name categories of patients within the spectrum of chronic bladder pain by means of standard investigations.[16,39] These ESSIC efforts are ongoing. The issue of phenotyping has been explored from another angle, looking into various domains of the complex according to the so-called UPOINT (Urinary, Psychosocial, Organ specific, Infection, Neurologic/systemic, and Tenderness) classification system.[17,38] Such a classification may in the future help to direct multimodal therapy and improve treatment outcomes. Genetic factors are relevant and have also been taken into account.[53]

Treatment

Once the diagnosis has been made, one must decide whether to institute therapy or use policy of conservative "watchful waiting" (**Fig. 5**). If the patient has not had an empiric course of antibiotics for his or her symptoms, such a trial is reasonable. Doxycycline has been reported efficacious in a Swiss study.[54] Further attempts to alleviate symptoms with antibiotics are unlikely to be worthwhile and are not recommended in the

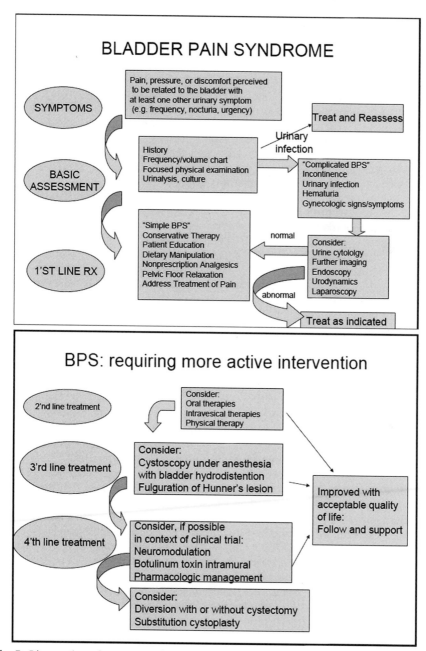

Fig. 5. Diagnostic and treatment algorithm for BPS suggested by the International Consultation on Incontinence. (*From* Hanno P, Lin AT, Nordling J, et al. Bladder pain syndrome. In: Abrams P, Cardozo L, Khoury S, et al, editors. Incontinence. Paris: Health Publication Ltd; 2009. p. 1459–518; with permission.)

absence of positive cultures. Stress reduction, exercise, warm tub baths, and efforts by the patient to maintain a normal lifestyle all contribute to improving overall quality of life.[55] Biofeedback, soft tissue massage, and other physical therapies may aid in muscle relaxation of the pelvic floor.[56–60] This is a reasonable intervention given the association of pelvic floor dysfunction and BPS.[61] A preliminary NIDDK trial has suggested the efficacy of such physical therapy when compared with global therapeutic massage.[62]

Elaborate dietary restrictions are unsupported by any studies, but many patients do find that their symptoms are adversely affected by specific foods and do well to avoid them.[28,63] These may include caffeine, alcohol, artificial sweeteners, hot pepper, and beverages like cranberry juice that might acidify the urine.[64] Anecdotal association of BPS with many foods has spawned the recommendation of various "interstitial cystitis diets" with little in the way of any objective, scientific basis.

Few of the oral therapies commonly used for the treatment of BPS have been supported by unequivocal evidence of efficacy in large, multicenter, randomized controlled clinical trials. There is little evidence that any change the natural history of the disease, although many are effective in relieving symptoms in individual patients. Amitriptyline, a tricyclic antidepressant, has become a staple of oral treatment and is used in dosages starting at 10 mg daily that are slowly increased over several weeks to up to 50 to 75 mg daily as tolerated. Amitryptiline has several pharmacologic properties that may diminish pain, increase bladder capacity, block the actions of histamine, act as a mild antimuscarinic, and aid sleep.[65,66] Hydroxyzine at dosages of 25 to 50 mg daily helps a small proportion of patients.[67] Sodium pentosanpolysulphate, the only oral therapy approved by the Food and Drug Administration (FDA), has efficacy in a subset of patients that may drop below 30% of those initially treated and can take up to 6 months to show any benefit.[68,69] The appropriate long-term use of analgesic medications forms an integral part of the treatment of a chronic pain condition like BPS.

The potential for high efficacy combined with safety and low side-effect profile that is gained by applying a treatment directly to the bladder lining has made intravesical therapy an important treatment option. Dimethylsulfoxide (DMSO) has the longest history of use for this problem and is often combined in intravesical cocktails that are administered weekly or biweekly. The solution may include lidocaine, heparin, and/or sodium bicarbonate. There is no study to definitively show that the cocktail solutions are any more effective than DMSO alone. DMSO is the only intravesical therapy approved by the FDA for BPS (still termed interstitial cystitis by FDA). It is an organic solvent, a by-product of the paper pulp industry, and has analgesic and anti-inflammatory properties.[70,71] A variety of intravesical cocktails usually combining a local analgesic and a mucopolysaccharide like heparin have been used.[72,73]

Off-label therapies have included neuromodulation (approved for frequency and urgency syndrome) and Intradetrusor botulinum toxin injections.[74,75] Surgical destruction of Hunner lesions has proven effective in relieving symptoms for up to 12 months or more in the patients who have the Hunner type of disease.[41,76]

Major surgery for BPS is an aggressive but reasonable option for patients with severe symptoms who have failed standard attempts at treatment and when the disease course suggests that spontaneous remission of symptoms is unlikely. Patients with a small bladder capacity under anesthesia are less likely to respond to conservative attempts at therapy. Patients with a Hunner lesion may have the best results with major surgery. If one conceptualizes BPS as 2 disorders, one of pain and the other of frequency, it becomes easier for the patient and physician to rationalize the decision. Conduit urinary diversion will resolve the frequency symptoms. Diversion, and even cystectomy with diversion, cannot guarantee a pain-free result,[77] and it is critical for the patient to factor this into the decision about this often irrevocable step.

The diversity of BPS/IC therapies underscores the lack of understanding about the treatment of this syndrome.[78] It has not only been a difficult condition to diagnose, but also a difficult condition for which to assess therapeutic impact. There is a 50% incidence of temporary remission unrelated to therapy, with a mean duration of 8 months.[21] A somewhat surprising finding from the Interstitial Cystitis Database was that there was no evidence of a long-term change in average symptom severity over the 4-year course of follow-up, although there was initial improvement in symptoms partially because of regression to the mean[79] and the intervention effect.[22] In a chronic, devastating condition with primarily subjective symptomatology, no known cause, and no cure, patients are desperate and often seem to respond to any new therapy. They are often victims of unorthodox health care providers with untested forms of therapy, some medical, some homeopathic, and some even surgical.

The treatment of this chronic condition is very complex, and is best undertaken by a physician with a special interest in the syndrome.[80] Primary care physicians need to be aware of its existence, and not "write-off" persistent pelvic pain and frequency as a variant of normal or as a persistent urinary tract infection to be treated with a never-ending litany of antibiotics.

The International Consultation on Incontinence has recommended the following[81]:

Initial Treatment

Patient education, dietary manipulation, nonprescription analgesics, and pelvic floor relaxation techniques comprise the initial treatment of BPS. The treatment of pain needs to be addressed directly, and in some instances referral to an anesthesia/pain center can be an appropriate early step in conjunction with ongoing treatment of the syndrome. When conservative therapy fails or symptoms are severe and conservative management is unlikely to succeed, oral medication, intravesical treatment, or physical therapy can be prescribed. It is recommended to initiate a single form of therapy and observe results, adding another modality or substituting another modality as indicated by degree of response or lack of response to treatment. Excellence can be the enemy of good.

Secondary Assessment

If initial oral or intravesical therapy fails, or before beginning such therapy, it is reasonable to consider further evaluation, which can include urodynamics, pelvic imaging, and cystoscopy with bladder distention and possible bladder biopsy under anesthesia. Findings of bladder overactivity suggest a trial of antimuscarinic therapy. Findings of a Hunner lesion suggest therapy with transurethral resection or fulguration of the lesion. Distention itself can have therapeutic benefit in 30% to 50% of patients, although benefits rarely persist for longer than a few months.

Refractory BPS

Those patients with persistent, unacceptable symptoms despite oral and/or intravesical therapy are candidates for more aggressive modalities. Many of these are best administered within the context of a clinical trial if possible. These may include neuromodulation, intradetrusor botulinum toxin, or newly described pharmacologic management techniques. At this point, most patients will benefit from the expertise of an anesthesia pain clinic. The last step in treatment is usually some type of surgical intervention aimed at increasing the functional capacity of the bladder or diverting the urinary stream. Urinary diversion with or without cystectomy has been used as a last resort with good results in selected patients. Augmentation or substitution cystoplasty seems less effective and more prone to recurrence of chronic pain.

REFERENCES

1. Ware J. The analects of Confucious. New York: New American Library; 1955. Mentor Religious Classic.
2. Hunner GL. A rare type of bladder ulcer. Further notes, with a report of eighteen cases. JAMA 1918;70(4):203–12.
3. Hunner GL. A rare type of bladder ulcer in women; report of cases. Boston Med Surg J 1915;172:660–4.
4. Peterson A, Hager B. Interstitial cystitis: report of cases. Cal West Med 1929; 31(4):262–7.
5. Skene AJC. Diseases of the bladder and urethra in women. New York: William Wood; 1887.
6. Messing EM. The diagnosis of interstitial cystitis. Urology 1987;29(Suppl 4):4–7.
7. Wein A, Hanno PM, Gillenwater JY. Interstitial cystitis: an introduction to the problem. In: Hanno PM, Staskin DR, Krane RJ, et al, editors. Interstitial cystitis. London: Springer-Verlag; 1990. p. 3–15.
8. Hanno PM, Landis JR, Matthews-Cook Y, et al. The diagnosis of interstitial cystitis revisited: lessons learned from the National Institutes of Health Interstitial Cystitis Database study. J Urol 1999;161(2):553–7.
9. Homma Y, Ueda T, Tomoe H, et al. Clinical guidelines for interstitial cystitis and hypersensitive bladder syndrome. Int J Urol 2009;16(7):597–615.
10. Furuya R, Masumori N, Furuya S, et al. Glomerulation observed during transure-thral resection of the prostate for patients with lower urinary tract symptoms suggestive of benign prostatic hyperplasia is a common finding but no predictor of clinical outcome. Urology 2007;70(5):922–6.
11. Waxman JA, Sulak PJ, Kuehl TJ. Cystoscopic findings consistent with interstitial cystitis in normal women undergoing tubal ligation. J Urol 1998;160(5):1663–7.
12. Richter B, Hesse U, Hansen AB, et al. Bladder pain syndrome/interstitial cystitis in a Danish population: a study using the 2008 criteria of the European Society for the Study of Interstitial Cystitis. BJU Int 2010;105(5):660–7.
13. Simon LJ, Landis JR, Erickson DR, et al. The Interstitial Cystitis Data Base Study: concepts and preliminary baseline descriptive statistics. Urology 1997;49(Suppl 5A):64–75.
14. Abrams PH, Cardozo L, Fall M, et al. The standardisation of terminology of lower urinary tract function: report from the standardisation sub-committee of the inter-national continence society. Neurourol Urodyn 2002;21:167–78.
15. Warren JW, Meyer WA, Greenberg P, et al. Using the International Continence Society's definition of painful bladder syndrome. Urology 2006;67(6):1138–42.
16. van de Merwe JP, Nordling J, Bouchelouche P, et al. Diagnostic criteria, classifi-cation, and nomenclature for painful bladder syndrome/interstitial cystitis: an ESSIC proposal. Eur Urol 2008;53(1):60–7.
17. Nickel JC, Tripp DA, Pontari M, et al. Psychosocial phenotyping in women with interstitial cystitis/painful bladder syndrome: a case control study. J Urol 2010; 183(1):167–72.

18. Verhaak PFM, Kerssens JJ, Dekker J, et al. Prevalence of chronic benign pain disorder among adults: a review of the literature. Pain 1998;77:231–9.
19. Bernardini P, Bondavalli C, Luciano M, et al. [Interstitial cystitis: epidemiology]. Arch Ital Urol Androl 1999;71(5):313–5 [in Italian].
20. Clemens JQ, Link CL, Eggers PW, et al. Prevalence of painful bladder symptoms and effect on quality of life in black, Hispanic and white men and women. J Urol 2007;177(4):1390–4.
21. Berry SH, Stoto M, Elliot M, et al. Prevalence of interstitial cystitis/painful bladder syndrome in the United States. J Urol 2009;181(4):20–1.
22. Propert KJ, Schaeffer AJ, Brensinger CM, et al. A prospective study of interstitial cystitis: results of longitudinal followup of the interstitial cystitis data base cohort. The Interstitial Cystitis Data Base Study Group. J Urol 2000;163(5):1434–9.
23. Onwude JL, Selo-Ojeme DO. Pregnancy outcomes following the diagnosis of interstitial cystitis. Gynecol Obstet Invest 2003;56(3):160–2.
24. Hanno P, Baranowski A, Fall M, et al. Painful bladder syndrome (including interstitial cystitis). In: Abrams PH, Wein AJ, Cardozo L, editors. Incontinence, vol. 2. 3rd edition. Paris: Health Publications Limited; 2005. p. 1456–520. Chapter 23.
25. Ottem DP, Carr LK, Perks AE, et al. Interstitial cystitis and female sexual dysfunction. Urology 2007;69(4):608–10.
26. Alagiri M, Chottiner S, Ratner V, et al. Interstitial cystitis: unexplained associations with other chronic disease and pain syndromes. Urology 1997;49(Suppl 5A): 52–7.
27. Hand JR. Interstitial cystitis: report of 223 cases (204 women and 19 men). J Urol 1949;61:291–310.
28. Koziol JA. Epidemiology of interstitial cystitis. Urol Clin North Am 1994;21(1): 7–20.
29. Bhone AW, Hodson JM, Rebuck JW, et al. An abnormal leukocyte response in interstitial cystitis. J Urol 1962;88:387–91.
30. Kontras SB, Bodenbender JG, McClave CR, et al. Interstitial cystitis in chronic granulomatous disease. J Urol 1971;105(4):575–8.
31. Erickson DR. Interstitial cystitis: update on etiologies and therapeutic options. J Womens Health Gend Based Med 1999;8(6):745–58.
32. Holm-Bentzen M, Nordling J, Hald T. Etiology: etiologic and pathogenetic theories in interstitial cystitis. In: Hanno PM, Staskin DR, Krane RJ, et al, editors. Interstitial cystitis. London: Springer-Verlag; 1990. p. 63–77.
33. Keay SK, Szekely Z, Conrads TP, et al. An antiproliferative factor from interstitial cystitis patients is a frizzled 8 protein-related sialoglycopeptide. Proc Natl Acad Sci U S A 2004;101(32):11803–8.
34. Mulholland SG, Byrne DS. Interstitial cystitis. J Urol 1994;152(3):879–80.
35. Levander H. [Sensory sensitization, part II: pathophysiology in dysfunctional disorders. Understanding the inner life of the nerve pathways may explain hitherto unexplainable symptoms]. Lakartidningen 2003;100(18):1618–9 [in Swedish].
36. Elbadawi A. Interstitial cystitis: a critique of current concepts with a new proposal for pathologic diagnosis and pathogenesis. Urology 1997;49(Suppl 5A):14–40.
37. Merskey H, Bogduk N. Classification of chronic pain. Seattle (WA): IASP Press; 1994.
38. Nickel JC, Shoskes D, Irvine-Bird K. Clinical phenotyping of women with interstitial cystitis/painful bladder syndrome: a key to classification and potentially improved management. J Urol 2009;182(1):155–60.
39. Nordling J, Anjum FH, Bade JJ, et al. Primary evaluation of patients suspected of having interstitial cystitis (IC). Eur Urol 2004;45(5):662–9.

40. Peeker R, Fall M. Treatment guidelines for classic and non-ulcer interstitial cystitis. Int Urogynecol J Pelvic Floor Dysfunct 2000;11(1):23–32.
41. Rofeim O, Hom D, Freid RM, et al. Use of the neodymium: YAG laser for interstitial cystitis: a prospective study. J Urol 2001;166(1):134–6.
42. Shanberg AM, Malloy TR. Use of lasers in interstitial cystitis. In: Sant GR, editor. Interstitial cystitis. Philadelphia: Lippincott-Raven; 1997. p. 215–8.
43. Larsen MS, Mortensen S, Nordling J, et al. Quantifying mast cells in bladder pain syndrome by immunohistochemical analysis. BJU Int 2008;102:204–7.
44. Erickson DR, Tomaszewski JE, Kunselman AR, et al. Do the National Institute of Diabetes and Digestive and Kidney Diseases cystoscopic criteria associate with other clinical and objective features of interstitial cystitis? J Urol 2005; 173(1):93–7.
45. Abrams P, Baranowski A, Berger R, et al. A new classification is needed for pelvic pain syndromes—are existing terminologies of spurious diagnostic authority bad for patients? J Urol 2006;175:1989–90.
46. Fall M, Baranowski A, Fowler CJ, et al. EAU guidelines on chronic pelvic pain. Eur Urol 2004;46:681–9.
47. Fall M, Baranowski A, Elneil S, et al. European Association of urology guidelines on chronic pelvic pain. Eur Urol 2010;57(1):35–48.
48. Johansson SL, Fall M. Clinical features and spectrum of light microscopic changes in interstitial cystitis. J Urol 1990;143(6):1118–24.
49. Gillenwater JY, Wein AJ. Summary of the National Institute of Arthritis, Diabetes, Digestive and Kidney Diseases Workshop on Interstitial Cystitis, National Institutes of Health, Bethesda, Maryland, August 28–29, 1987. J Urol 1988;140(1): 203–6.
50. Rosamilia A, Igawa Y, Higashi S. Pathology of interstitial cystitis. Int J Urol 2003; 10(Suppl):S11–5.
51. Fall M, Johansson SL, Aldenborg F. Chronic interstitial cystitis: a heterogeneous syndrome. J Urol 1987;137(1):35–8.
52. Peeker R, Fall M. Toward a precise definition of interstitial cystitis: further evidence of differences in classic and nonulcer disease. J Urol 2002;167(6): 2470–2.
53. Dimitrakov J, Guthrie D. Genetics and phenotyping of urological chronic pelvic pain syndrome. J Urol 2009;181(4):1550–7.
54. Burkhard FC, Blick N, Hochreiter WW, et al. Urinary urgency and frequency, and chronic urethral and/or pelvic pain in females. Can doxycycline help? J Urol 2004; 172(1):232–5.
55. Whitmore KE. Self-care regimens for patients with interstitial cystitis. Urol Clin North Am 1994;21(1):121–30.
56. Holzberg A, Kellog-Spadt S, Lukban J, et al. Evaluation of transvaginal theile massage as a therapeutic intervention for women with interstitial cystitis. Urology 2001;57(6 Suppl 1):120.
57. Lukban J, Whitmore K, Kellogg-Spadt S, et al. The effect of manual physical therapy in patients diagnosed with interstitial cystitis, high-tone pelvic floor dysfunction, and sacroiliac dysfunction. Urology 2001;57(6 Suppl 1):121–2.
58. Markwell SJ. Physical therapy managment of pelvi/perineal and perianal syndromes. World J Urol 2001;19:194–9.
59. Meadows E. Treatments for patients with pelvic pain. Urol Nurs 1999;19:33–5.
60. Mendelowitz F, Moldwin R. Complementary approaches in the management of interstitial cystitis. In: Sant GR, editor. Interstitial cystitis. Philadelphia: Lippincott-Raven; 1997. p. 235–40.

61. Peters KM, Carrico DJ, Kalinowski SE, et al. Prevalence of pelvic floor dysfunction in patients with interstitial cystitis. Urology 2007;70(1):16–8.
62. FitzGerald MP, Anderson RU, Potts J, et al. Randomized multicenter feasability trial of myofascial physical therapy for the treatment of urological chronic pelvic pain syndromes. J Urol 2009;182(2):570–80.
63. Koziol JA, Clark DC, Gittes RF, et al. The natural history of interstitial cystitis: a survey of 374 patients. J Urol 1993;149(3):465–9.
64. Shorter B, Lesser M, Moldwin RM, et al. Effect of comestibles on symptoms of interstitial cystitis. J Urol 2007;178(1):145–52.
65. Foster H, Kreder K, FitzGerald MP, et al. Effect of amitriptyline on symptoms in newly diagnosed patients with interstitial cystitis/painful bladder syndrome. J Urol 2010;183:1853–8.
66. Hanno PM. Amitriptyline in the treatment of interstitial cystitis. Urol Clin North Am 1994;21(1):89–91.
67. Theoharides TC, Sant GR. Hydroxyzine therapy for interstitial cystitis. Urology 1997;49(Suppl 5A):108–10.
68. Hanno PM. Analysis of long-term Elmiron therapy for interstitial cystitis. Urology 1997;49(Suppl 5A):93–9.
69. Jepsen JV, Sall M, Rhodes PR, et al. Long-term experience with pentosanpolysulfate in interstitial cystitis. Urology 1998;51:381.
70. Stewart BH, Branson AC, Hewitt CB, et al. The treatment of patients with interstitial cystitis, with special reference to intravesical DMSO. Trans Am Assoc Genitourin Surg 1971;63:69–74.
71. Stewart BH, Shirley SW. Further experience with intravesical dimethyl sulfoxide in the treatment of interstitial cystitis. J Urol 1976;116(1):36–8.
72. Weaver RG, Dougherty TF, Natoli CA. Recent concepts of interstitial cystitis. J Urol 1963;89:377–83.
73. Welk BK, Teichman JM. Dyspareunia response in patients with interstitial cystitis treated with intravesical lidocaine, bicarbonate, and heparin. Urology 2008;71(1):67–70.
74. Schmidt RA. Urodynamic features of the pelvic pain patient and the impact of neurostimulation on these parameters. World J Urol 2001;19:186–93.
75. Apostolidis A, Dasgupta P, Denys P, et al. Recommendations on the use of botulinum toxin in the treatment of lower urinary tract disorders and pelvic floor dysfunctions: a European consensus report. Eur Urol 2009;55(1):100–19.
76. Fall M. Conservative management of chronic interstitial cystitis: transcutaneous electrical nerve stimulation and transurethral resection. J Urol 1985;133(5):774–8.
77. Baskin LS, Tanagho EA. Pelvic pain without pelvic organs. J Urol 1992;147(3):683–6.
78. Rovner E, Propert KJ, Brensinger C, et al. Treatments used in women with interstitial cystitis: the interstitial cystitis data base (ICDB) study experience. The Interstitial Cystitis Data Base Study Group. Urology 2000;56(6):940–5.
79. Sech SM, Montoya JD, Bernier PA, et al. The so-called "placebo effect" in benign prostatic hyperplasia treatment trials represents partially a conditional regression to the mean induced by censoring. Urology 1998;51:242–50.
80. Fall M, Oberpenning F, Peeker R. Treatment of bladder pain syndrome/interstitial cystitis 2008: can we make evidence-based decisions? Eur Urol 2008;54(1):65–75.
81. Hanno P, Lin A, Nordling J, et al. Bladder Pain Syndrome Committee of the International Consultation on Incontinence. Neurourol Urodyn 2010;29(1):191–8.

Prostatitis and Chronic Pelvic Pain Syndrome in Men

Naji J. Touma, MD, FRCS(C)*, J. Curtis Nickel, MD, FRCS(C)

KEYWORDS
- Prostatitis • Chronic pelvic pain syndrome
- Urology • Primary care practice

EPIDEMIOLOGY

Prostatitis is the most common urologic diagnosis in men aged younger than 50 years and the third most common urologic diagnosis in men aged older than 50 years after benign prostate hyperplasia and prostate cancer. There were almost 2 million US physician visits annually from 1990 to 1994 with prostatitis listed as the diagnosis.[1] Of all prostatitis visits, 46% and 47% were to urologists and primary care physicians, respectively. Based on both a physician survey study in Dane County, Wisconsin and a survey of younger men from a Wisconsin National Guard unit, it was estimated that 5% of men (aged 20 to 50 years) have a history of prostatitis.[2] Symptoms of prostatitis wax and wane with approximately one-third to one-half of patients experiencing relief of symptoms over a 1-year period.[3]

Many men developing either an acute or chronic prostatitis condition present initially to their primary care physicians or to emergency. It is generally recognized that the most appropriate diagnosis and effective treatment strategy is associated with first presentation. Therefore, primary care physicians have an important role in the diagnosis and management of prostatitis.

CLASSIFICATION OF PROSTATITIS SYNDROMES

The National Institutes of Health (NIH) developed a classification system for prostatitis syndromes according to presumed etiology and clinical findings, including culture and microscopic findings from expressed prostatic secretions, preprostatic and postprostatic massage urine sediment, or semen analysis (**Box 1**).[4] This classification system was developed to standardize clinical research and has been adopted by the urologic

Department of Urology, Queen's University, Kingston General Hospital, 76 Stuart Street, Kingston, ON K7L 2V7, Canada
* Corresponding author.
E-mail address: njtouma@gmail.com

Med Clin N Am 95 (2011) 75–86
doi:10.1016/j.mcna.2010.08.019
0025-7125/11/$ – see front matter © 2011 Elsevier Inc. All rights reserved.

Box 1
NIH Classification of the prostatitis syndromes

This system, developed for clinical research purposes, can be simplified for use in primary care practice (see text)

Category I, or acute bacterial prostatitis (ABP), is an acute infection of the prostate and is manifested by systemic signs of infection and a positive urine culture.

Category II, or chronic bacterial prostatitis (CBP), is a chronic bacterial infection where bacteria are recovered in significant numbers from a purulent prostatic fluid. This bacteria is thought to be the most common cause of recurrent urinary tract infection in men.

Category III, or chronic pelvic pain syndrome (CPPS), is diagnosed when no pathogenic bacteria can be localized to the prostate (culture of expressed prostatic fluid or postprostatic massage urine specimen) and is further divided into IIIa and IIIb. Category IIIa refers to inflammatory CPPS where a significant number of white blood cells (WBCs) are localized to the prostate; whereas, Category IIIb is noninflammatory.

Category IV refers to asymptomatic inflammatory prostatitis where bacteria or WBCs are localized to the prostate, but patients are asymptomatic.

---

community in describing patients in clinical practice. With modifications it can prove useful in clinical primary care practice.

Acute and chronic bacterial prostatitis (Category I and II), or ABP and CBP, respectively, are based on chronicity and cultures. Category I is characterized by sick patients with clinical evidence of an acute infection of the lower urinary tract invariably associated with a positive urine culture. Category II chronic prostatitis is typically diagnosed in a man with a history of recurrent urinary tract infections (UTI), usually lower tract and not associated with systemic signs and symptoms, such as seen in Category I. Many times patients are asymptomatic between these episodes and often only culture of prostate-specific specimens (see postprostate massage urine specimen collection later) is positive.

Category III chronic prostatitis/chronic pelvic pain syndrome (CP/CPPS) is a chronic lower urinary tract and pelvic pain syndrome that is not associated with UTI or infection. The primary care physician should not concern himself whether patients have Category IIIA or IIIB because that differentiation has little impact on treatment decisions.

Category IV, defined as inflammatory asymptomatic prostatitis, is not generally considered an important category for primary care physicians.

ETIOLOGY OF PROSTATITIS SYNDROMES

ABP and CBP (Categories I and II) are mostly caused by gram-negative Enterobacteriaceae and enterococci species that originate in the gastrointestinal flora. The most common organism is *Escherichia coli*, which is identified in the majority of infections.[5] Pseudomonas aeruginosa, Serratia species, Klebsiella species, and Enterobacter aerogenes make up most of the rest of the gram-negative cultured organisms.[6] Nonbacterial prostatitis (CP/CPPS) syndromes are caused by an inter-related cascade of inflammatory, immunologic, neuroendocrine, and neuropathic mechanisms that begin with an initiator (perhaps an initial infection) in a genetically or anatomically susceptible man.[7] In many or most cases the pathology extends beyond the prostate gland itself.

EVALUATION OF THE MAN PRESENTING WITH PROSTATITIS
Evaluation of Acute Prostatitis

Patients suspected of having ABP (Category I) present with symptoms of a severe lower urinary tract infection with variable obstructive voiding symptoms and commonly systemic symptoms largely of fever, and occasionally, of nausea and vomiting. Evaluation consists of a complete physical examination, including digital rectal examination (very tender, possibly hot, prostate), urinalysis (evidence of infection), and a urine culture to confirm the diagnosis. A vigorous digital rectal examination in this setting is to be avoided because of the risk of systemic bacterial dissemination.

Evaluation of Chronic Prostatitis and Chronic Pelvic Pain Syndrome

History
The physician should obtain a history that may include previous UTI, sexually transmitted diseases, past lower urinary tract problems, and previous urologic instrumentation and surgery. The most important history is comprised of a discussion of the pain (location, severity, and frequency), voiding symptoms (obstructive and irritative), and the impact this condition is having on the patients' activities and quality of life (**Fig. 1**).

Pain or Discomfort

1. In the last week, have you experienced any pain or discomfort in the following areas?

	Yes	No
a. Area between rectum and testicles (perineum)	❑ 1	❑ 0
b. Testicles	❑ 1	❑ 0
c. Tip of the penis (not related to urination)	❑ 1	❑ 0
d. Below your waist, in your pubic or bladder area	❑ 1	❑ 0

2. In the last week, have you experienced:

	Yes	No
a. Pain or burning during urination?	❑ 1	❑ 0
b. Pain or discomfort during or after sexual climax (ejaculation)?	❑ 1	❑ 0

3. How often have you had pain or discomfort in any of these areas over the last week?

❑ 0 Never
❑ 1 Rarely
❑ 2 Sometimes
❑ 3 Often
❑ 4 Usually
❑ 5 Always

4. Which number best describes your AVERAGE pain or discomfort on the days that you had it, over the last week?

❑ ❑ ❑ ❑ ❑ ❑ ❑ ❑ ❑ ❑ ❑
0 1 2 3 4 5 6 7 8 9 10
NO   PAIN AS
PAIN   BAD AS
                              YOU CAN
                              IMAGINE

Urination

5. How often have you had a sensation of not emptying your bladder completely after you finished urinating, over the last week?

❑ 0 Not at all
❑ 1 Less than 1 time in 5
❑ 2 Less than half the time
❑ 3 About half the time
❑ 4 More than half the time
❑ 5 Almost always

6. How often have you had to urinate again less than two hours after you finished urinating, over the last week?

❑ 0 Not at all
❑ 1 Less than 1 time in 5
❑ 2 Less than half the time
❑ 3 About half the time
❑ 4 More than half the time
❑ 5 Almost always

Impact of Symptoms

7. How much have your symptoms kept you from doing the kinds of things you would usually do, over the last week?

❑ 0 None
❑ 1 Only a little
❑ 2 Some
❑ 3 A lot

8. How much did you think about your symptoms, over the last week?

❑ 0 None
❑ 1 Only a little
❑ 2 Some
❑ 3 A lot

Quality of Life

9. If you were to spend the rest of your life with your symptoms just the way they have been during the last week, how would you feel about that?

❑ 0 Delighted
❑ 1 Pleased
❑ 2 Mostly satisfied
❑ 3 Mixed (about equally satisfied and dissatisfied)
❑ 4 Mostly dissatisfied
❑ 5 Unhappy
❑ 6 Terrible

Scoring the NIH-Chronic Prostatitis Symptom Index Domains

Pain: Total of items 1a, 1b, 1c, 1d, 2a, 2b, 3, and 4 = _____

Urinary Symptoms: Total of items 5 and 6   = _____

Quality of Life Impact: Total of items 7, 8, and 9   = _____

Fig. 1. NIH Chronic Prostatitis Symptom Index: NIH-CPSI.

CBP (Category II) is suggested by a history of recurrent urinary tract infection (many times the patients are asymptomatic between these episodes but as they become more frequent, symptoms tend to persist). Patients with CP/CPPS (Category III) present with waxing and waning genitourinary and pelvic pain, typically characterized by perineal discomfort or pain as well as pain/discomfort associated with ejaculation. Patients also complain of pain or discomfort in the penis (including dysuria), testes, suprapubic area, and many times in the groin/thighs and back. Patients do need to be asked how the symptoms impact on their daily activities and general quality of life.

The Chronic Prostatitis Symptom Index (CPSI) (see **Fig. 1**) is a useful clinical questionnaire because objective parameters in this condition are often lacking.[8] The CPSI consists of 9 questions evaluating 3 domains that should be evaluated: pain, urinary function, and quality of life. Pain, which is usually the most important feature of CP/CPPS, is captured in 4 questions assessing location, severity, and frequency. Urinary function is evaluated with 2 questions assessing obstructive and irritative symptoms. Quality of life is evaluated with 3 questions looking at the impact of symptoms on activities of daily living. The CPSI allows the physician to document the most important variables associated with a diagnosis of chronic prostatitis. The total score is extremely useful in determining potential response to treatment in a condition characterized largely by symptoms and not associated with cure in many cases, but only long-term amelioration of symptoms that wax and wane.

Physical examination

The physical examination is an important part of the evaluation of CP/CPPS, although it is usually unhelpful in diagnosing or further classifying it. The physical examination consists of an abdominal examination (including suprapubic area), followed by careful examination and palpation of the groin, spermatic cord, epididymis, and testes. The clinician is looking for areas of pain/discomfort, for unexpected masses, and for the possibility of urinary retention. The focused examination is completed with a modified digital rectal examination (DRE) that not only evaluates the prostate for tenderness, consistency, pain/discomfort, nodules, and any irregularities but also includes palpation of the perineum, pelvic floor, and pelvic sidewalls noting any muscle spasm or myofascial tenderness.

Laboratory evaluation

In patients suspected of acute bacterial prostatitis, a urine culture is mandatory before initiating antibiotic therapy. To further classify chronic prostatitis, cultures of urine before and after a prostatic massage are necessary. A simple 2-glass technique has been shown to be a highly effective and practical collection method to rule out infection (Category II CBP).[9] It consists of a midstream urine followed by collection of the first 10 mL of urine after a vigorous prostate massage. A prostate massage consists of index finger palpation starting at the lateral edge of each lobe and rolling it toward the midline. It should be performed bilaterally and at the level of the base and the apex of the prostate. Significant bacteriuria in the postprostatic massage urine specimen or an increased bacterial count compared with that in the preprostatic massage specimen indicates localization of infection in the prostate (Category II). Most patients will have negative or nonlocalizing cultures (Category III CP/CPPS). Microscopy on the spun sediment of these specimens is not especially useful as there are no criteria on how to use this information.

The diagnosis of prostatitis of all categories often overlaps with that of benign prostatic hyperplasia and even prostate cancer. Prostate-specific antigen (PSA) testing is not recommended as part of a workup for prostatitis/CPPS. In fact, during both acute and chronic bacterial prostatitis episodes, PSA levels can be falsely elevated.[10] The disruption in the normal prostate tissue architecture caused by inflammation most likely accounts for this spurious rise. This PSA elevation can persist anywhere from 1 to 6 months after the initial infection episode. It seems prudent, therefore, to wait for 6 months before PSA testing for the purposes of prostate cancer screening or case detection is pursued.[11] On the other hand, PSA levels do not seem to be significantly affected in chronic pelvic pain syndrome (Category III).[12] As per the American Urological Association guidelines on PSA testing, a baseline PSA can be discussed with patients at 40 years of age, taking into account the results of the DRE examination, family history of prostate cancer, and ethnicity.[13] There is no role for imaging in the diagnosis of prostatitis. However, a CT scan of the pelvis or an ultrasound can be performed for patients with ABP who are unresponsive to antibiotics to look for a potential prostatic abscess.

TREATMENT
General Concepts of Treatment in Primary Care

Once the physician has established a diagnosis of prostatitis, decided whether it is acute or chronic, made an attempt to culture the appropriate urine specimens, and classified the individual patient, treatment can be initiated. Patients with acute prostatitis require antibiotics, supportive therapy (fluids, analgesics, antipyretics), and possibly short-term urethral catheterization. Catheterization should only be performed in the setting of urinary retention, as a theoretical risk of bacteremia does exist, especially with traumatic catheterization. Chronic prostatitis warrants 1 trial of antibiotic therapy and if that fails, no further antibiotics should be prescribed. Those who fail antibiotic therapy should be educated about this chronic condition and counseled in regard to conservative measures they can take to help. These measures include diet modification (avoidance of food or drink that exacerbate the pain and voiding symptoms, such as coffee, spicy foods, and so forth), an exercise program (avoid high-impact exercise or activities that result in perineal pressure, such as bicycle riding), the use of perineal support (ring cushion), and local heat therapy (hot water bottle or heating pad applied to perineum). Definitive therapies, including their rationale and evidence for efficacy, are subsequently listed.

Antimicrobial Agents

Antimicrobials are the most commonly prescribed agents for all categories of prostatitis. Although their use for acute and chronic bacterial prostatitis can be understandable based on objective culture results, they have remained the first-line treatment for other categories of prostatitis based on a belief that most CP syndromes may be at least initially caused by bacteria. For the most part, antibiotics (after a possible empiric treatment trial) are not recommended unless specific cultures as described previously are positive for a uropathogenic organism.

Trimethoprim-sulfamethoxazole (TMP-SMX) or trimethoprim alone were widely used in previous decades for prostatitis, both acute and chronic. Bacterial eradication was reported to be in the range of 30% to 50% in most studies with a longer duration of treatment providing better results (90 days).[14,15] The fluoroquinolones have demonstrated improved therapeutic results. One review examining the effect of quinolones, including norfloxacin, ciprofloxacin, ofloxacin, and lomefloxacin, on chronic bacterial prostatitis found a bacterial eradication rate of 57% to 77%.[16] Typically, the duration of treatment is about 1 month and the effects are superior to the effects of TMP-SMX in category II CBP.

Although strong evidence exists that ciprofloxacin and levofloxacin are ineffective in patients with Category III CPPS who have been symptomatic for many years and who have been heavily treated previously, there is moderate but still weak evidence that empiric use of antibiotics during initial presentation in patients who are antibiotic naïve may result in significant amelioration of symptoms in some patients.[17] However, the nonbacterial chronic prostatitis syndromes (CPPS) do not respond to further antibiotic treatment if initial empiric therapy is unsuccessful.

Alpha Blockers

Anatomic or neurophysiologic obstruction at the level of the bladder outlet results in high-pressure dysfunctional flow patterns. This high-pressure voiding could result in intraprostatic ductal reflux, which is hypothesized to be a major factor in the pathogenesis of both bacterial and nonbacterial prostatitis.[18] The bladder neck and prostate are rich in alpha receptors. It is thought that alpha blockade may reduce outflow obstruction, improve urinary flow, and even diminish intraprostatic ductal reflux. The clinical evidence examining the effects of alpha blockers on Category III CPPS, however, has been conflicting. Four small, randomized trials examining the effects of alfuzosin, terazosin, tamsulosin, and doxazosin have confirmed a beneficial effect of alpha blockade in patients with recent onset of the disease who have not been heavily pretreated and with voiding cosymptoms.[19–22] Treatment must be continued for at least 6 weeks.

Conversely, 2 recent, large, NIH-sponsored, randomized trials did not confirm these findings. Alexander and colleagues[23] examined the effects of tamsulosin, ciprofloxacin, and combination therapy on heavily pretreated subjects with chronic symptoms. Tamsulosin studied in heavily pretreated subjects, with or without ciprofloxacin, was not shown to be effective versus placebo; whereas, alfuzosin evaluated in an alpha-blocker naïve subject population diagnosed within 2 years failed to show any improvement in symptom reduction over placebo.[24]

These seemingly conflicting results highlight the difficulty of conducting studies on subjects with heterogeneous symptoms. Within each group, the number of subjects whose main bothersome symptoms were urinary in nature, and who were likely to respond to alpha blockers, was likely different. The suggestion then, is to consider alpha-blocker therapy in men with obstructive or irritative voiding symptoms.

Antiinflammatory Agents and Immune Modulators

Given the inflammatory nature of class IIIA prostatitis, various nonsteroidal antiinflammatories, corticosteroids, and immunosuppressants have been looked at as potential therapies for this condition. Short-term cyclooxygenase type 2 therapy has shown a modest dose-dependent response for reducing pain symptoms and improving quality of life.[25,26] However, long-term cyclooxygenase type 2 therapy is not recommended. Short-term nonsteroidal antiinflammatories are worth considering in the early stage of the condition.

Other Medical Therapies

Skeletal muscle relaxants have been advocated as adjuncts for CPPS as pelvic floor neuromuscular dysregulation has been hypothesized as a possible cause for some of the symptoms. Baclofen, for instance, has shown some benefit in 1 small trial in subjects with chronic abacterial prostatitis.[27] Other suggested skeletal muscle relaxants include diazepam and cyclobenzaprine. The 5-alpha reductase inhibitors, finasteride and dutasteride, may be helpful in older patients with concurrent benign prostatic hyperplasia, although they cannot be recommended as monotherapy.[28]

Several phytotherapeutic agents, such as Cernilton, a pollen extract; Quercetin, a natural bioflavonoid; and Serenoa repens, an extract of the Saw Palmetto berry, provide modest benefit in some patients.[29–31] Neuromodulatory intervention (for example tricyclic antidepressants and gabapentinoids) show some promise for refractory patients who develop a chronic pelvic neuropathic type of pain.[32]

Physical Therapy

Prostatic massage is the oldest traditional form of therapy for prostatitis. Evidence supporting repetitive prostate massage therapy is conflicting, and a consensus panel concluded that prostatic massage could be used as an adjunct form of therapy only in selected patients. Frequent ejaculation may achieve the same.[33] Heat therapy; physiotherapy massage; ischemic compression; stretching; anesthetic injections; acupuncture; electroneural modulation; and mind-body interactions, such as progressive relaxation exercises, yoga, and hypnosis, have all been tried, although more scientific scrutiny is necessary to understand the role of these interventions in the treatment of CP/CPPS.[34]

Psychological Support

Chronic pain of CP/CPPS has been associated with poor quality of life and depression. A cognitive-behavioral program has been developed, which specifically targets empirically supported biopsychosocial variables (such as pain catastrophizing, depressive thinking, social support) and encourages patients to critically evaluate their patterns of thinking and to entertain novel thinking and behavioral responses to their troublesome symptoms. The end objective is to improve overall quality of life.[35]

Surgical Intervention

Surgery for the chronic bacterial prostatitis syndromes should be reserved only for those with definite indications (such as urethral stricture, bladder neck obstruction, and so forth). Transurethral resection of the prostate gland is not recommended. Although radical prostatectomy may prevent the recurrent urinary tract infections associated with Category II CBP, it is considered a drastic step. Microwave thermotherapy of the prostate has shown some promise in CPPS, but the evidence for this is not strong.

EMERGING CONCEPT OF HETEROGENEOUS CLINICAL PHENOTYPES IN CHRONIC PROSTATITIS SYNDROMES

Patients with acute bacterial prostatitis are similar in presentation and response to therapy. On the other hand, a single treatment that fits all patients with chronic prostatitis does not work in clinical practice. It is becoming increasingly clear that patients with CBP and CPPS are not a homogenous group with identical etiologic mechanisms, genitourinary pain, voiding symptoms, or psychosexual problems, but rather a heterogeneous group of individual patients with widely differing clinical phenotypes. Therefore, a panacea that cures this challenging clinical entity will likely never be found. Rather, the challenge is to identify which subgroup of patients will respond to a particular therapy. A clinically practical phenotyping classification system for patients diagnosed with urologic chronic pelvic pain syndromes has recently been proposed (UCPPS).[36] UPOINT is a 6-point clinical classification system that categorizes the phenotype of patients with UCPPS (which includes the chronic prostatitis syndromes) into 1 or more of 6 clinically identifiable domains: urinary, psychosocial, organ specific, infection, neurologic/systemic, and tenderness (muscle). A physician

Table 1
The UPOINT clinical phenotyping strategy for patients presenting with urologic chronic pelvic pain syndromes, including men with CPPS

UPOINT Domain	Clinical Findings	Therapies
Urinary	Urinary frequency, urgency, obstructive voiding	Anticholinergics, alpha blockers
Psychosocial	Depression, anxiety, poor coping mechanisms, catastrophizing	Amitriptyline, counseling, referral to psychologist
Organ specific	Gently palpating prostate exacerbates typical symptoms	Consider initial antibiotic, quercetin, pollen extract, finasteride/dutasteride
Infection	Recurrent UTI, bacterial localization	Antibiotics
Neurologic/ systemic	Pelvic neuropathic pain, other associated conditions (irritable bowel syndrome, fibromyalgia)	Tricyclic antidepressants, gabapentinoids
Tenderness	Tenderness or spasm of perineum or pelvic floor	Skeletal muscle relaxants, physiotherapy, local heat therapy, donut cushion, massage therapy

Box 2
Practical advice for the primary care physician

1. Categorize patients:

   Decide if it is acute or chronic prostatitis.

   Conduct a focused physical examination (including DRE).

   Rule out infection (premassage and postmassage urine culture).

   Consider CPSI to document symptoms at presentation and during therapy.

   Determine UPOINT phenotypes (or at least nonprostate centric associated conditions).

2. Provide education and conservative therapy for all patients (see text).

3. Use empiric trial of antibiotics for only an initial presentation.

4. Consider alpha-blocker therapy for those with voiding symptoms.

5. Consider short-term nonsteroidal antiinflammatory drugs for pain.

6. Consider muscle relaxants, amitriptyline (or gabapentinoid), or physiotherapy for patients with pelvic floor tenderness or neuropathic pain.

7. Be aware of associated psychosocial associations and refer appropriately if identified (particularly depression).

8. Refer to urologist if previous plan fails.

9. When condition settles down, consider a prostate-specific antigen test in patients older than 40 years of age to reassure patients and yourself that cancer is not an issue (this suggestion is in constant flux and the PSA screening debate continues).

10. Consider initial presentation as an acute, self-limited problem; consider patients with long-term problems as having a chronic pain condition that may not be curable.

11. Remember that for chronic, treatment refractory patients, amelioration of symptoms and improvement in quality of life is the goal of management.

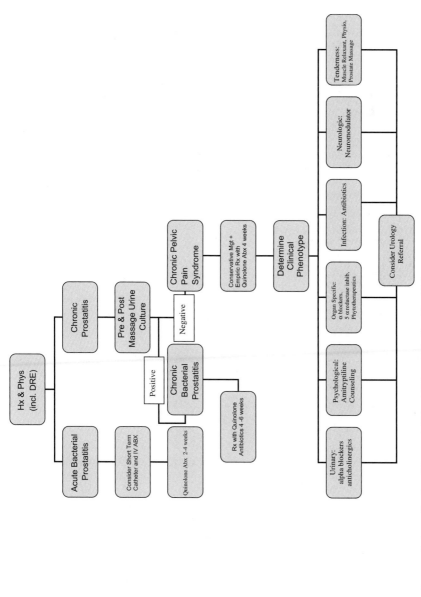

Fig. 2. Approach to patients with prostatitis. ABX, antibiotics; Hx, history.

can easily and quickly categorize patients into 1 or more of these UPOINT domains and then develop an individually designed therapeutic plan specifically addressing the clinical phenotypes identified. Most patients will be categorized with more than 1 UPOINT domain and will require multimodal therapy. **Table 1** outlines this concept.

SUMMARY

Primary care physicians can and should diagnose, classify, and treat patients presenting with acute and chronic prostatitis syndromes. Although the chronic syndromes are a challenge to manage, this review article provides the necessary background to allow primary care physicians to take on this task. **Box 2** and **Fig. 2** provide practical advice to the primary care physician based on this article. Patients who are unfortunate to be diagnosed with a prostatitis syndrome have the best chance for successful therapy at initial presentation. Those patients will ultimately benefit from an informed and educated physician.

REFERENCES

1. McNaughton-Collins M, Stafford RS, O'Leary MP, et al. How common is prostatitis? A national survey of physician visits. J Urol 1998;159:1224–8.
2. Moon TD. Questionnaire survey of urologists and primary care physicians' diagnostic and treatment practices for prostatitis. Urology 1997;50:543–7.
3. Propert KJ, McNaughton-Collins M, Leiby E, et al. A prospective study of symptoms and quality of life in men with chronic prostatitis/chronic pelvic pain syndrome: the national institutes of health chronic prostatitis cohort study. J Urol 2006;175:619–23.
4. Krieger JN, Nyberg LJ, Nickel JC. NIH consensus definition and classification of prostatitis. JAMA 1999;282:236–7.
5. Stamey TA. Urinary tract infection in males. In: Stamey TA, editor. Pathogenesis and treatment of urinary tract infections. Baltimore (MD): Williams and Wilkins; 1980. p. 343–429.
6. Meares EM Jr. Acute and chronic prostatitis: diagnosis and treatment. Infect Dis Clin North Am 1987;1:855–73.
7. Pontari MA, Ruggieri MR. Mechanisms in prostatitis/chronic pelvic pain syndrome. J Urol 2004;172(3):839–45.
8. Litwin MS, McNaughton-Collins M, Fowler FJ, et al. The national institutes of health chronic prostatitis symptom index: development and validation of a new outcome measure. J Urol 1999;162(2):369–75.
9. Nickel JC. The pre and post massage test (PPMT): a simple screen for prostatitis. Tech Urol 1997;3:38–43.
10. Tchetgen MB, Oesterling JE. The effect of prostatitis, urinary retention, ejaculation, and ambulation on the serum prostate-specific antigen concentration. Urol Clin North Am 1997;2:283–91.
11. Kawakami J, Siemens DR, Nickel JC. Prostatitis and prostate cancer: implications for prostate cancer screening. Urology 2004;64(6):1075–80.
12. Nadler RB, Schaeffer AJ, Knauss JS, et al. Total prostate specific antigen is elevated and statistically, but not clinically significant, in patients with chronic pelvic pain syndrome/prostatitis (abstract). J Urol 2003;169(Suppl 4):27.
13. Greene KL, Albertsen PC, Babaian RJ, et al. Prostate specific antigen best practice statement: 2009 update. J Urol 2009;182(5):2232–41.
14. Meares EM Jr. Long-term therapy of chronic bacterial prostatitis with trimethoprim-sulfamethoxazole. Can Med Assoc J 1975;112(Suppl):22–5.

15. McGuire EJ, Lytton B. Bacterial prostatitis: treatment with trimethoprim-sulfame-thoxazole. Urology 1976;7(5):499–500.
16. Naber KJ. Antibiotic treatment of chronic bacterial prostatitis. In: Nickel JC, editor. Textbook of prostatitis. Oxford (UK): ISIS Medical Media Ltd; 1999. p. 283–92.
17. Nickel JC, Downey J, Clark J, et al. Levofloxacin treatment for chronic prostatitis/chronic pelvic pain syndrome (CP/CPPS) in men: a randomized placebo controlled multi-center trial. J Urol 2003;62:614–7.
18. Kirby RS, Lowe D, Bultitude MI, et al. Intraprostatic urinary reflux: an aetiological factor in abacterial prostatitis. Br J Urol 1982;54:729–31.
19. Cheah PY, Liong ML, Yuen KH, et al. Terazosin therapy for chronic prostatitis/chronic pelvic pain syndrome: a randomized, placebo controlled trial. J Urol 2003;169(2):592–6.
20. Mehik A, Alas P, Nickel JC, et al. Alfuzosin treatment for chronic prostatitis/chronic pelvic pain syndrome: a prospective, randomized, double-blind placebo controlled pilot study. J Urol 2003;62(3):425–9.
21. Nickel JC, Narayan P, MacKay J, et al. Treatment of chronic prostatitis/chronic pelvic pain syndrome with tamsulosin: a randomized double blind trial. J Urol 2004;171:1594–7.
22. Evliyaoğlu Y, Burgut R. Lower urinary tract symptoms, pain and quality of life assessment in chronic non-bacterial prostatitis patients treated with alpha-blocking agent doxazosin; versus placebo. Int Urol Nephrol 2002;34(3):351–6.
23. Alexander RB, Propert KJ, Schaeffer AJ, et al. Chronic prostatitis collaborative research network. ciprofloxacin or tamsulosin in men with chronic prostatitis/chronic pelvic pain syndrome: a randomized, double-blind trial. Ann Intern Med 2004;141(8):581–9.
24. Nickel JC, Krieger JN, McNaughton-Collins M, et al. Alfuzosin and symptoms of chronic prostatitis-chronic pelvic pain syndrome. N Engl J Med 2008;359(25): 2663–73.
25. Nickel JC, Pontari M, Moon T, et al. A randomized, placebo controlled multi-center study to evaluate the safety and efficacy of rofecoxib in the treatment of chronic non-bacterial prostatitis. J Urol 2003;169:1401–5.
26. Zeng X, Ye Z, Yang W, et al. [Clinical evaluation of celecoxib in treating type IIIA chronic prostatitis]. Zhonghua Nan Ke Xue 2004;10(4):278–81 [in Chinese].
27. Osborn DE, George NJ, Rao PN. Prostatodynia–physiological characteristics and rational management with muscle relaxants. Br J Urol 1981;53(6):621–3.
28. Nickel JC, Downey J, Pontari MA, et al. A randomized placebo-controlled multi-centre study to evaluate the safety and efficacy of finasteride for male chronic pelvic pain syndrome (category IIIa chronic nonbacterial prostatitis). BJU Int 2004;93(7):991–5.
29. Rugendorff EW, Weidner W, Ebeling L. Results of treatment with pollen extract (Cernilton N) in chronic prostatitis and prostatodynia. Br J Urol 1993;71:433–8.
30. Shoskes DA, Zeitlin SI, Shahed A, et al. Quercetin in men with category III chronic prostatitis: a preliminary prospective, double-blind, placebo control trial. Urology 1999;54(6):960–3.
31. Reissigl A, Djavan B, Pointner J. Prospective placebo-controlled multicenter trial on safety and efficacy of phytotherapy in the treatment of chronic prostatitis/chronic pelvic pain syndrome [abstract 233]. J Urol 2004;171(4):61.
32. Pontari MA, Krieger JN, Litwin MS, et al. A randomized placebo-controlled multi-centre trial of Pregabalin for the treatment of men with chronic prostatitis/chronic pelvic pain syndrome [abstract 340]. J Urol 2009;181(4):123.

33. Mishra VC, Browne J, Emberton M. Role of repeated prostatic massage in chronic prostatitis: a systematic review of the literature. Urology 2008;72:731–5.
34. Potts JM. Chronic pelvic pain syndrome: a non-prostatocentric perspective. World J Urol 2003;21(2):54–6.
35. Nickel JC, Mullins C, Tripp DA. Development of an evidence-based cognitive behavioural treatment program for men with chronic prostatitis/chronic pelvic pain syndrome. World J Urol 2008;26:167–72.
36. Shoskes DA, Nickel JC, Dolinga R, et al. Clinical phenotyping of patients with chronic prostatitis/chronic pelvic pain syndrome and correlation with symptom severity. Urology 2009;73(3):538–42.

Male Lower Urinary Tract Symptoms (LUTS) and Benign Prostatic Hyperplasia (BPH)

Claus G. Roehrborn, MD

KEYWORDS

- Lower urinary tract symptoms (LUTS)
- Benign prostatic hyperplasia (BPH) • Medical therapy
- α blocker • 5-α-Reductase inhibitors • Antimuscarinics

DEFINITIONS AND NOMENCLATURE OF MALE LOWER URINARY TRACT SYMPTOMS/BENIGN PROSTATIC HYPERPLASIA

In addressing male lower urinary tract symptoms (LUTS) and benign prostatic hyperplasia (BPH), the first objective must be to establish a common set of definitions and nomenclature. In the past terms such as prostatism were used to describe men with LUTS from any cause, unduly drawing conclusions regarding a possible causal relationship between the symptoms and the prostate. In the more recent literature and clinical jargon, men were labeled as having BPH even though BPH is merely a histologic condition without inherent pathognomonic significance. Attempts to focus on the symptoms and deemphasize the perceived role and/or causality of any specific organ in the etiology of such symptoms have only been made recently. Nonetheless, the International Code of Diseases (ICD) still maintains organ-specific codes in addition to symptom-driven codes that were added in later years. In addition, most medications approved for the treatment of men with male LUTS by the US Food and Drug Administration specifically state the approval for "signs and symptoms of BPH" in their label, although in clinical practice they are used to treat male LUTS independent of whether or not BPH is actually present.[1]

There are 3 broad categories of male LUTS: storage (irritative) symptoms, voiding (obstructive) symptoms, and postmicturition symptoms (**Table 1**). Some of these symptoms have specific representation in the categories of ill-defined symptoms

Conflicts of interest: The author is or has been investigator or consultant to companies and organizations studying, manufacturing and/or marketing products for the treatment of male LUTS and BPH: Eli Lilly, GSK, Pfizer, Sanofi Aventis, Merck, Watson Pharmaceuticals, NIH/NIDDK.
Department of Urology, UT Southwestern Medical Center, 5323 Harry Hines Boulevard, J8 142, Dallas, TX 75390-9110, USA
E-mail address: claus.roehrborn@utsouthwestern.edu

Med Clin N Am 95 (2011) 87–100
doi:10.1016/j.mcna.2010.08.013
0025-7125/11/$ – see front matter © 2011 Elsevier Inc. All rights reserved.

Table 1 Male LUTS		
Storage	**Voiding**	**Postmicturition**
Urgency	Hesitancy	Postvoid dribble
Frequency	Poor flow	Sense of incomplete emptying
Nocturia	Intermittency	
Urgency incontinence	Straining	
Other incontinence	Terminal dribble	

Data from Abrams P, Cardozo L, Fall M, et al. The standardisation of terminology of lower urinary tract function: report from the Standardisation Sub-committee of the International Continence Society. Am J Obstet Gynecol 2002;187(1):116–26.

within ICD-9 codes from 780 to 799. It is estimated that nearly two-thirds of men presenting with male LUTS have a mixture of storage and voiding symptoms.[2] A specific term, overactive bladder (OAB), which is used in both men and women, is defined as urgency, with or without urgency incontinence, usually with frequency and nocturia (International Continence Society [ICS] 2002 definition).[3]

EPIDEMIOLOGY AND NATURAL HISTORY

From the foregoing discussion it is clear that BPH itself is actually only a histologic diagnosis that does not have much clinical significance. However, it becomes a clinical entity when associated with bothersome LUTS, significant prostatic enlargement, and/or bladder outlet obstruction. **Fig. 1** illustrates this complex relationship. Of all men older than 40 years, about 50% will develop histologic hyperplasia or BPH in an age-dependent manner[4]; of these 30% to 50% will have bothersome LUTS, which may also be caused by other conditions[5–9]; some will develop a significant enlargement of the prostate (EP), which can only exist in men with histologic BPH; some will develop bladder outlet obstruction (BOO), which may also arise from causes other than BPH and EP.

BOO can be measured by invasive pressure flow urodynamic studies, or by performing a noninvasive urinary flow rate recording. A rule of thumb is that a maximum flow rate of 15 mL/s or greater is normal, one between 10 and 15 mL/s is a diagnostic gray zone, and a maximum flow rate of less than 10 mL/s indicates obstruction with more than two-thirds of men falling into this category found to have obstruction when undergoing pressure flow studies. However, the maximum urinary flow rate declines with advancing age as a result not only of BPH and EP but also as a result of a weakening of the detrusor muscle. Treatment choices should take into consideration whether the patient has LUTS with or without EP and with or without BOO as different therapies provide different aspects of relief for these different conditions.

As more and more men have histologic BPH with increasing age, the incidence of bothersome symptoms measured as more than 7 points on the standardized International Prostate Symptoms Score[10] (IPSS) increases with advancing age to a similar degree among men of different cultural and ethnic origins.[5] It is convenient to consider that whereas 50% of all men have some element of BPH, 50% of those have bothersome symptoms, which amounts to approximately 25% of the total male population. Of course, this represents some simplification and the incidence rates for all proportions increase with age.

Although there is no strong correlation between prostate size, symptoms, and urinary flow rates in large studies on male LUTS and BPH, there are several important relationships. First, in men with BPH and no evidence of cancer, serum prostate-specific

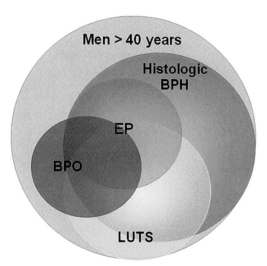

Fig. 1. Of all men older than 40 years, in an age-dependent manner, about 50% will develop histologic hyperplasia or BPH; of those 50% will have bothersome LUTS, which may also be caused by other conditions; some will develop a significant enlargement of the prostate (EP), which can only exist in men with histologic BPH; some will develop bladder outlet obstruction (BOO), which may also arise from causes other than BPH and EP. Treatment should take into consideration whether the patient has LUTS with or without EP and with or without BOO.

antigen (PSA) level correlates with total prostate volume, with the strength of the correlation being approximately $r = 0.5$ to 0.7, implying that nearly 50% of the volume variability may be explainable by serum PSA level.[11–14] The importance of this correlation lies in the observation that prostate volume and serum PSA level both to a similar degree predict some of the natural history of male LUTS, BPH, EP, and BOO. In other words, men with larger glands and higher serum PSA values are more likely to experience further volume increases in their prostate, increasing severity of symptoms, maximum urinary flow rate decreases, and ultimately progression to acute urinary retention (AUR; the total inability to void requiring a catheterization of the bladder) and subsequent prostate surgery.[11,15]

Because most primary care providers do not have access to ultrasound-based measurement of the prostate volume, a convenient rule of thumb is to consider a serum PSA level of 1.5 ng/dL as a threshold above which most men with male LUTS will have a prostate volume of greater than 30 mL or grams.[16] A serum PSA level of 1.5 or greater and a volume greater than 30 mL have been strongly associated with accelerated progression of BPH, male LUTS, EP, BOO, and ultimately AUR with possible need for surgery. Although similar relationships exist for the free PSA value, the ratio of free to total PSA expressed in percent, often used to assess the risk for prostate cancer, is not affected by prostate volume.

BASIC ASSESSMENT OF MALE LUTS FOR PRIMARY CARE PROVIDERS

A basic evaluation should be done on every patient presenting to a health care provider with male LUTS (**Fig. 2**).[1]

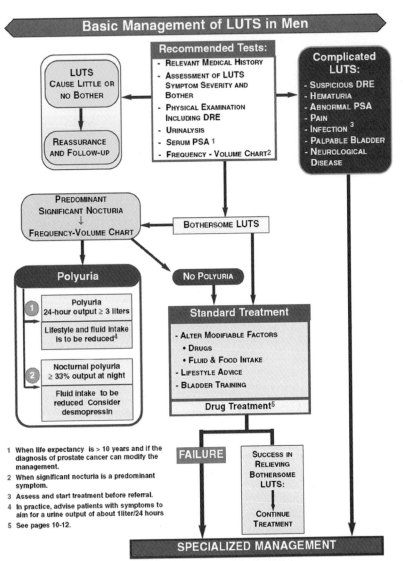

Fig. 2. Basic management of male LUTS. (*From* Abrams P, Chapple C, Khoury S, et al. Evaluation and treatment of lower urinary tract symptoms in older men. J Urol 2009;181(4):1779–87; with permission.)

History

A relevant medical history should be obtained focusing on the nature and duration of reported genitourinary tract symptoms, previous surgical procedures (in particular as they affect the genitourinary tract), general health issues, sexual function history, medications currently taken, and patient fitness for possible surgical procedures or other treatments.

Assessment of Symptoms and Bother

At least a semi-quantitative assessment of symptoms and bother is strongly recommended to grade the severity of LUTS and to understand the degree of bother caused by those symptoms. Excellent quantitative assessment tools such as the IPSS with bother score have been developed and validated (**Table 2**). The IPSS score and a single disease-specific quality of life question are the most widely used diagnostic tools in urology, and they are widely available, validated, and translated in many languages. The questionnaires may be filled in by the patient at home before the appointment, or in the waiting area or consult room, but as little as possible interference from health care provider and personnel is recommended. A score of 7 or less points is considered mildly symptomatic, 8 to 19 points as moderate, and a score of 20 to 35 points as severely symptomatic. However, not all patients are equally bothered by similar symptom scores. The quality of life question addresses this issue by asking "how would you feel if you would have to live with your symptoms the way they are right now for the rest of your life," with the answers ranging from "delighted, pleased, mostly satisfied, mixed (about equally satisfied and dissatisfied), mostly dissatisfied, unhappy to terrible" or from 0 to 6 points. The answer to this single question often guides the provider's discussion with the patient as it indicates the degree of bother the patient experiences.

Physical Examination and Digital Rectal Examination

A focused physical examination should be performed to assess the suprapubic area to rule out bladder distention, and overall motor and sensory function focused on the perineum and lower limbs. Digital rectal examination (DRE) should be performed to evaluate anal sphincter tone and the prostate gland with regard to approximate size, consistency, shape, and abnormalities suggestive of prostate cancer. It is difficult even for an experienced examiner to correctly estimate prostate size.[17–19] For prediction of natural history and treatment choices, the serum PSA level is a convenient proxy parameter with reasonable clinical correlation to prostate volume (see section on Epidemiology and Natural History).

Urinalysis

Urine should be analyzed using any of the widely available dipstick tests. These tests are done to determine if the patient has hematuria, proteinuria, pyuria, or other pathologic findings (eg, glucosuria, ketonuria, positive nitrite test, and so forth). Examination of the urinary sediment and culture is indicated if the result of the dipstick is abnormal. The results of urinalysis may guide further testing independent of the evaluation for LUTS.

Serum PSA Level

The benefits and risks of PSA testing should be discussed with the patient including the possibility of false-positive and false-negative results regarding cancer, the possible complications of subsequent transrectal ultrasound-guided biopsy, and the possibility of a false-negative biopsy. PSA testing in patients with male LUTS may also be beneficial in terms of providing an estimate for prostate volume, and thus for the prediction of the natural history and for treatment selection.

Frequency Volume Charts

Frequency volume charts (FVC; voiding diary or time and amount voiding charts) are particularly useful when nocturia is the dominant symptom. The time and voided volume are recorded for each micturition during several 24-hour periods (usually 3), and help to identify patients with nocturnal polyuria or excessive fluid intake, which are common in the aging male.

Table 2
International Prostate Symptom Score (IPSS)

Urinary Symptoms	Not at All	Less Than 1 Time in 5	Less Than Half the Time	About Half the Time	More Than Half the Time	Almost Always
1. In the past month, how often have you had a sensation of not emptying your bladder completely after you finished urinating?	0	1	2	3	4	5
2. In the past month, how often have you had to urinate again less than 2 hours after you finished urinating?	0	1	2	3	4	5
3. In the past month, how often have you found you stopped and started again several times while urinating?	0	1	2	3	4	5
4. In the past month, how often have you found it difficult to postpone urination?	0	1	2	3	4	5
5. In the past month, how often have you had a weak urinary stream?	0	1	2	3	4	5
6. In the past month, how often have you had to push or strain to begin urination?	0	1	2	3	4	5
7. In the past month, how many times did you typically get up to urinate from the time you went to bed until the time you got up in the morning?	Never 0	1 time 1	2 times 2	3 times 3	4 times 4	5 or more times 5
Total for urinary symptoms						

From Barry MJ, Fowler FJ Jr, O'Leary MP, et al. The American Urological Association symptom index for benign prostatic hyperplasia. The Measurement Committee of the American Urological Association. J Urol 1992;148(5):1549–57 [discussion: 1564]; with permission.

MANAGEMENT

If the assessment demonstrates the presence of male LUTS associated with findings of DRE suspicious of prostate cancer, hematuria, abnormal PSA level, pain, recurrent infection (infection should be assessed and treatment started by the practitioner before referral), palpable bladder, or neurologic disease, the patient should be referred to a specialist (urologist) for appropriate evaluation before advising treatment (see **Fig. 2**).

WATCHFUL WAITING

Patients who score 7 or less points on the IPSS questionnaire are considered mildly symptomatic. Patient with mild symptoms or those with moderate symptoms (8–19 points) who are not particularly bothered by these symptoms, as assessed by the quality of life question, are in most cases best advised to pursue a watchful waiting strategy consisting of annual reassessment, as well as lifestyle and fluid management recommendations.

ACTIVE THERAPY OPTIONS

Any health care provider can discuss treatment options with the patient based on the results of the initial assessment (see **Fig. 2**). In primary care there should be a discussion of the benefits and risks involved with each of the recommended treatment alternatives (watchful waiting, medical treatment, interventional therapy, surgical, or nonsurgical treatment). The choice of treatment is reached in a shared decision-making process between physician and patient.

If the patient has predominantly significant nocturia and gets out of bed to void 2 or more times per night then he should be asked to complete an FVC for 3 days. The FVC will show 24-hour polyuria or nocturnal polyuria when present. Pokyuria has been defined as output greater than 3 L. In practice, patients with symptoms are advised to aim for a urine output of 1 L per 24 hours. Nocturnal polyuria is diagnosed when more than 33% of the 24-hour urine output occurs at night. The patient should be treated according to the nocturia algorithm. If symptoms do not improve sufficiently, the patient should be treated along the same lines as men without predominant nocturia.

If the patient has no polyuria and medical treatment is considered, the physician can proceed with therapy based mainly on first altering modifiable factors such as concomitant drugs, regulation of fluid intake especially in the evening, lifestyle changes (avoiding a sedentary lifestyle), and dietary advice (avoiding dietary indiscretions such as excessive intake of alcohol and highly seasoned or irritative foods).

Phytotherapy

Most men with male LUTS are already taking over-the-counter supplements in an effort to improve their symptoms when presenting to a health care provider.[20] Despite their widespread use, however, there is no good evidence in the peer-reviewed literature to indicate their efficacy and safety particularly compared with placebo. The best planned and executed placebo-controlled study using Saw Palmetto extract, the most common phytotherapeutic agent, failed to show any efficacy in any parameter measured after a 12-month treatment period.[21] The American Urological Association (AUA), the European Association of Urology (EAU), and the International Consultation for Urological Diseases (ICUD) guidelines for the management of male LUTS do not recommend the use of any of these supplements.[1,22,23]

α Adrenergic Receptor Blocker (α Blocker)

The lower urinary tract, and specifically the bladder neck and prostate, are richly innervated with α adrenergic receptor endings, most of which are α 1a receptors.[24] Acknowledging the risk of oversimplification, by blocking these receptors with α blocking drugs, the smooth muscle tissue relaxes allowing for improved urine flow and improved LUTS.

The drugs that are currently available in the United States are terazosin (1, 2, 5, and 10 mg, requiring dose titration, generic); doxazosin (1, 2, 4, and 8 mg, requiring dose titration, generic); tamsulosin (0.4 mg, titration optional to twice a day dosing, generic in 2010); alfuzosin (10 mg slow-release formulation, brand Uroxatral); silodosin (4 and 8 mg, brand Rapaflo). There are countless meta-analyses and guideline documents available to testify that overall the efficacy of the available α blocker drugs is comparable.[22,24–26] Improvements from baseline in the IPSS score of 4 to 6 points can be expected, and the difference from placebo in controlled trials may be as high as 3 points.

The α blocker drugs differ in their side-effect profile. The titratable terazosin and doxazosin have a higher incidence of orthostatis, hypotension, dizziness and so forth; the more α 1a–specific drugs tamsulosin and silodosin have a higher incidence of absence of emission, also often incorrectly labeled as retrograde ejaculation.

Cost, convenience of single dose versus dose titration, and desire to avoid cardiovascular adverse events in the elderly population may be the deciding factors when choosing one α blocker over another. Floppy iris syndrome, first described to occur with tamsulosin, may occur with any of the α blockers. Patients must discontinue taking α blockers before undergoing cataract surgery and resume them thereafter.[27,28]

Long-term medical therapy studies such as Medical Therapy of Prostatic Symptoms (MTOPS) and Alfuzosin Long Term Efficacy and Safety Study (ALTESS) have demonstrated that α blocker drugs have long-term efficacy in terms of symptom improvement, but they allow ongoing prostate growth, and thus do not reduce the risk of progression to AUR and need for surgery.[15]

5-α-Reductase Inhibitors

In contrast to the α blocker drugs, 5-α-reductase inhibitors (ARIs) work on the hormonal control of prostate growth and BPH development. There are 2 available drugs in this class: finasteride (5 mg, generic, brand Proscar) and dutasteride (0.5 mg, brand Avodart). Both have the same mechanism of action and block the 5-α-reductase isoenzymes from converting testosterone to the more potent dihydrotestosterone (DHT) hormone. This in turn leads to a reduction in the androgenic drive in the prostate, and over a period of 3 to 6 months an approximately 25% reduction in prostate volume, a 50% reduction in total serum PSA level, and an improvement in symptoms and urinary flow rate. The 2 drugs differ in several points: finasteride inhibits the type II 5-α-reductase enzyme, whereas dutasteride inhibits both types I and II. This leads to a greater reduction in serum DHT (>90% for dutasteride vs ~70% for finasteride) and in intraprostatic DHT (~95 % vs ~85%).[29] Furthermore, finasteride has a serum half-life of less than 1 day, whereas the half-life of dutasteride is about 5 weeks. The side-effect spectrum of both drugs is similar. In many large and long-term trials, erectile dysfunction, reduced libido and decreased ejaculate volume occur in about 5% to 10% of patients, and breast enlargement and nipple tenderness may occur in 1% to 2% of patients.[22]

The improvement in IPSS and in maximum urinary flow rate with ARIs has always been viewed as inferior to that achieved with α blocker drugs, an observation based on studies in which a direct comparison was made (such as the VA COOP study,[30] the European PREDICT study,[31] or the MTOPS study over 5 years[32]).

In understanding the mechanism of action of the ARIs, it becomes clear that they may work better in patients with larger glands, and (by proxy) higher serum PSA values. The recently concluded CombAT study (Combination of Avodart and Tamsulosin) verified this theory.[33] Because of the enrollment requirements of a prostate volume greater than 30 g and a serum PSA level greater than 1.5 ng/dL the baseline prostate volumes and serum PSA values were higher than in most other studies on male LUTS and BPH. In turn, after about 1 to 2 years on study drug, the patients treated with dutasteride had greater improvements in IPSS and maximum flow rate compared with those treated with tamsulosin.

Antimuscarinics

The detrusor muscle of the bladder is partially under parasympathetic and cholinergic control. In the past, it was considered risky to administer anticholinergic (antimuscarinic) drugs to men with male LUTS and BPH for fear of decreasing detrusor efficiency, and thus increasing postvoid residual urine (PVR) and ultimately causing AUR. Recognizing the prevalence of storage symptoms and that the OAB syndrome is as common in men as it is in women,[2] appropriate studies (including men obstructed by urodynamic criteria) showed that at least in the short to intermediate term these drugs did not carry an excessive risk of increasing PVR or AUR.[34–36] A large population-based study from the United Kingdom suggests that if such risk exists, it would manifest itself in the first 3 months of treatment. Thus, baseline and follow-up PVR checks are recommended when starting patients with male LUTS on such drugs.[37]

There are many drugs available in the United States that are in this category, but not all have been tested in male patients. The largest numerical experience exists for tolterodine (various dosages and long-acting preparation, brand Detrol), but studies have also been conducted with fesoterodine (4 and 8 mg, brand Toviaz) and oxybutinin (various dosages from 5 to 15 mg and extended release preparation, generic). Other drugs in this class are darifenacin (7.5 and 15 mg sustained release, brand Enablex), trospium (20 mg and 60 mg sustained release, brand Sanctura), and solifenacin (5 and 10 mg, brand Vesicare). Based on the effect of these drugs in women, one might assume a class effect and similar efficacy (and safety) of all drugs in the class in patients with male LUTS.[38]

The most common use of antimuscarinics in patients with male LUTS is in a scenario in which treatment with α blocker drugs partially succeeded in improving the voiding symptoms, but failed to relieve the storage symptoms sufficiently well. Several admittedly uncontrolled studies have found that this add-on therapy provides measurable improvement in this difficult to treat group of patients.[39–41]

The adverse event spectrum is similar to that observed in women with OAB, and by and large, the changes in PVR, maximum flow rate, and other urodynamic changes are minimal.[42]

Combination(s) of Different Drugs

Although it might seem natural and logical to combine 2 of the 3 drug classes for enhanced efficacy, early trials failed to show superiority of a combination of an α blocker with an ARI drug. Specifically, the 12-month VA COOP and PREDICT studies found the efficacy of the α blocker alone was similar to that in the combination therapy arm, but associated with more adverse events.[30,31] The failure of these studies was attributed to a lack of synergy between the 2 drug classes, patient selection, and the duration of the trials. Only the 5-year MTOPS trial demonstrated that, even in a population of men with male LUTS and average prostate size, combination therapy was superior to either monotherapy in terms of preventing overall progression of disease.[32] Detailed analyses showed that in men with larger glands and higher serum PSA levels, the superiority of the combination therapy became significant even earlier, and thus, in the end it was found to be a matter of both patient selection and duration of treatment.[15,43]

The CombAT trial took advantage of these insights and enrolled only men with a prostate volume greater than 30 g and PSA level greater than 1.5 ng/dL.[33,44,45] As a result, the combination therapy arm proved to be superior to the α blocker arm in terms of improvement in symptoms and flow rate and prevention of symptom progression and AUR/surgery both earlier in the trial and to a larger degree than in MTOPS. Combination therapy with both an α blocker and an ARI is therefore a reasonable strategy for men with larger glands and higher serum PSA values (**Fig. 3**).

The other combination that has been studied is that of α blocker plus antimuscarinic, specifically in men with predominantly storage or OAB type symptoms. Although several smaller studies had already documented the potential of adding the antimuscarinic drug to α blocker therapy for men with residual storage symptoms, the TIMES study and its subset analyses showed that this combination may be the best therapeutic choice from the start in men with significant bother and storage symptoms.[46–48]

SUMMARY

- Male LUTS, BPH, EP, and BOO are common among aging men and will increase in socioeconomic and medical importance at a time of increased life expectancy and aging of the baby boomer generation.
- Although still not perfectly understood, it is clear that the male androgenic steroid hormones testosterone and dihydrotestosterone (DHT) play a major permissive role in the development of BPH together with a host of growth factors and other causative factors.
- In many men the condition is progressive as measured by symptoms and deterioration in urinary flow rate, increase in prostate size, and ultimately AUR and need for surgery.
- Baseline assessment parameters (including age, symptom severity, urinary flow rate, prostate size, and/or serum PSA) may help in identifying men at greater risk

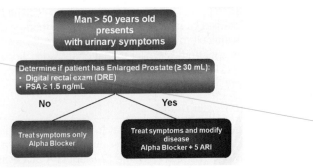

Fig. 3. A practical algorithm to determine the choice of medical therapy in men with male LUTS and BPH. (*From* Kaplan S. A practical algorithm for the diagnosis and management of EP. Weill Medical College of Cornell University Reports on Men's Urologic Health 2006;1:1–8; with permission.)

of progression who may benefit from more aggressive medical management using combination therapy.

- Excellent and widely accepted guidelines are available for the primary care provider to help in the assessment of men with male LUTS and BPH, and in choosing from a variety of treatment options.
- Watchful waiting remains a reasonable strategy for many patients with mild or moderate symptoms.
- In patients with moderate to severe symptoms and bother caused by these symptoms, providers can make educated and differential choices between several classes of drugs, alone or in combination, to effectively treat and improve the symptoms in most men.
- Despite the efficacy of medical therapy, there will be patients who require referral to a urologist either early to rule out prostate cancer and other conditions, or later, after initial medical therapy and lifestyle management has failed. Perhaps as many as 30% of patients fail to achieve sufficient symptom improvement with medication, lifestyle adjustment, and fluid management.

REFERENCES

1. Abrams P, Chapple C, Khoury S, et al. Evaluation and treatment of lower urinary tract symptoms in older men. J Urol 2009;181(4):1779–87.
2. Irwin DE, Milsom I, Hunskaar S, et al. Population-based survey of urinary incontinence, overactive bladder, and other lower urinary tract symptoms in five countries: results of the EPIC study. Eur Urol 2006;50(6):1306–14 [discussion: 1314–5].
3. Abrams P, Cardozo L, Fall M, et al. The standardisation of terminology in lower urinary tract function: report from the Standardisation Sub-committee of the International Continence Society. Urology 2003;61(1):37–49.
4. Roehrborn C, McConnell J. Etiology, pathophysiology, epidemiology and natural history of benign prostatic hyperplasia. In: Wein A, Kavoussi LR, Novick A, et al, editors. Campbell-Walsh urology, vol. 2. 9th edition. Philadelphia: Saunders; 2007. p. 2727–65.
5. Oishi K, Boyle P, Barry M, et al. Epidemiology and natural history of benign prostatic hyperplasia. 4th International Consultation on Benign Prostatic Hyperplasia. Plymouth (UK): Plymbridge Distributors Ltd; 1998. p. 23–59.
6. Girman CJ. Natural history and epidemiology of benign prostatic hyperplasia: relationship among urologic measures. Urology 1998;51(Suppl 4A):8–12.
7. Girman CJ, Epstein RS, Jacobsen SJ, et al. Natural history of prostatism: impact of urinary symptoms on quality of life in 2115 randomly selected community men. Urology 1994;44(6):825–31.
8. Girman CJ, Jacobsen SJ, Guess HA, et al. Natural history of prostatism: relationship among symptoms, prostate volume and peak urinary flow rate. J Urol 1995; 153(5):1510–5.
9. Girman CJ, Jacobsen SJ, Rhodes T, et al. Association of health-related quality of life and benign prostatic enlargement. Eur Urol 1999;35(4):277–84.
10. Barry MJ, Fowler FJ Jr, O'Leary MP, et al. The American Urological Association symptom index for benign prostatic hyperplasia. The Measurement Committee of the American Urological Association. J Urol 1992;148(5):1549–57 [discussion: 1564].
11. Roehrborn CG. The utility of serum prostatic-specific antigen in the management of men with benign prostatic hyperplasia. Int J Impot Res 2008;20(Suppl 3): S19–26.

12. Bohnen AM, Groeneveld FP, Bosch JL. Serum prostate-specific antigen as a predictor of prostate volume in the community: the Krimpen study. Eur Urol 2007;51(6):1645–52 [discussion: 1652–3].

13. Lieber MM, Jacobsen SJ, Roberts RO, et al. Prostate volume and prostate-specific antigen in the absence of prostate cancer: a review of the relationship and prediction of long-term outcomes. Prostate 2001;49(3):208–12.

14. Roehrborn CG, Boyle P, Gould AL, et al. Serum prostate-specific antigen as a predictor of prostate volume in men with benign prostatic hyperplasia. Urology 1999;53(3):581–9.

15. Roehrborn CG. BPH progression: concept and key learning from MTOPS, ALTESS, COMBAT, and ALF-ONE. BJU Int 2008;101(Suppl 3):17–21.

16. Gould AL, Roehrborn CG, Boyle P. Relationship between prostate volume and serum prostate specific antigen (PSA) in men with clinical BPH. J Urol 1998; 159:109A.

17. Roehrborn CG, Sech S, Montoya J, et al. Interexaminer reliability and validity of a three-dimensional model to assess prostate volume by digital rectal examination. Urology 2001;57(6):1087–92.

18. Yanoshak SJ, Roehrborn CG, Girman CJ, et al. Use of a prostate model to assist in training for digital rectal examination. Urology 2000;55(5):690–3.

19. Roehrborn CG. Accurate determination of prostate size via digital rectal examination and transrectal ultrasound. Urology 1998;51(Suppl 4A):19–22.

20. Meyer JP, Gillatt DA. Alternative medications for benign prostatic hyperplasia available on the Internet: a review of the evidence for their use. BJU Int 2002; 90(1):41–4.

21. Bent S, Kane C, Shinohara K, et al. Saw palmetto for benign prostatic hyperplasia. N Engl J Med 2006;354(6):557–66.

22. AUA Practice Guidelines Committee. AUA guideline on management of benign prostatic hyperplasia (2003). Chapter 1: diagnosis and treatment recommendations. J Urol 2003;170(2 Pt 1):530–47.

23. Madersbacher S, Alivizatos G, Nordling J, et al. EAU 2004 guidelines on assessment, therapy and follow-up of men with lower urinary tract symptoms suggestive of benign prostatic obstruction (BPH guidelines). Eur Urol 2004;46(5):547–54.

24. Roehrborn CG, Schwinn DA. Alpha1-adrenergic receptors and their inhibitors in lower urinary tract symptoms and benign prostatic hyperplasia. J Urol 2004; 171(3):1029–35.

25. Clifford G, Farmer R. Medical therapy for benign prostatic hyperplasia: a review of the literature. Eur Urol 2000;38(1):2–19.

26. Mishra VC, Browne J, Emberton M. Role of alpha-blockers in type III prostatitis: a systematic review of the literature. J Urol 2007;177(1):25–30.

27. Yaycioglu O, Altan-Yaycioglu R. Intraoperative floppy iris syndrome: facts for the urologist. Urology 2010;76:272–6.

28. Storr-Paulsen A, Norregaard JC, Borme KK, et al. Intraoperative floppy iris syndrome (IFIS): a practical approach to medical and surgical considerations in cataract extractions. Acta Ophthalmol 2009;87(7):704–8.

29. Dorsam J, Altwein J. 5alpha-Reductase inhibitor treatment of prostatic diseases: background and practical implications. Prostate Cancer Prostatic Dis 2009;12(2):130–6.

30. Lepor H, Williford WO, Barry MJ, et al. The efficacy of terazosin, finasteride, or both in benign prostatic hyperplasia. Veterans Affairs Cooperative Studies Benign Prostatic Hyperplasia Study Group. N Engl J Med 1996;335(8):533–9.

31. Kirby RS, Roehrborn C, Boyle P, et al. Efficacy and tolerability of doxazosin and finasteride, alone or in combination, in treatment of symptomatic benign prostatic hyperplasia: the Prospective European Doxazosin and Combination Therapy (PREDICT) trial. Urology 2003;61(1):119–26.

32. McConnell JD, Roehrborn CG, Bautista OM, et al. The long-term effect of doxazosin, finasteride, and combination therapy on the clinical progression of benign prostatic hyperplasia. N Engl J Med 2003;349(25):2387–98.

33. Roehrborn CG, Siami P, Barkin J, et al. The effects of combination therapy with dutasteride and tamsulosin on clinical outcomes in men with symptomatic benign prostatic hyperplasia: 4-year results from the CombAT study. Eur Urol 2010;57(1): 123–31.

34. Kaplan SA, Wein AJ, Staskin DR, et al. Urinary retention and post-void residual urine in men: separating truth from tradition. J Urol 2008;180(1):47–54.

35. Abrams P, Kaplan S, De Koning Gans HJ, et al. Safety and tolerability of tolterodine for the treatment of overactive bladder in men with bladder outlet obstruction. J Urol 2006;175(3 Pt 1):999–1004 [discussion: 1004].

36. Chapple CR, Roehrborn CG. A shifted paradigm for the further understanding, evaluation, and treatment of lower urinary tract symptoms in men: focus on the bladder. Eur Urol 2006;49(4):651–8.

37. Martin-Merino E, Garcia-Rodriguez LA, Masso-Gonzalez EL, et al. Do oral antimuscarinic drugs carry an increased risk of acute urinary retention? J Urol 2009;182(4):1442–8.

38. Chapple CR, Khullar V, Gabriel Z, et al. The effects of antimuscarinic treatments in overactive bladder: an update of a systematic review and meta-analysis. Eur Urol 2008;54(3):543–62.

39. Lee JY, Kim HW, Lee SJ, et al. Comparison of doxazosin with or without tolterodine in men with symptomatic bladder outlet obstruction and an overactive bladder. BJU Int 2004;94(6):817–20.

40. Kaplan SA, Walmsley K, Te AE. Tolterodine extended release attenuates lower urinary tract symptoms in men with benign prostatic hyperplasia. J Urol 2005; 174(6):2273–5 [discussion: 2275–6].

41. Athanasopoulos AA, Perimenis PS. Comparison of doxazosin with or without tolterodine in men with symptomatic bladder outlet obstruction and an overactive bladder. BJU Int 2005;95(7):1117–8.

42. Novara G, Galfano A, Ficarra V, et al. Anticholinergic drugs in patients with bladder outlet obstruction and lower urinary tract symptoms: a systematic review. Eur Urol 2006;50(4):675–83.

43. Crawford ED, Wilson SS, McConnell JD, et al. Baseline factors as predictors of clinical progression of benign prostatic hyperplasia in men treated with placebo. J Urol 2006;175(4):1422–6 [discussion: 1426–7].

44. Roehrborn CG, Siami P, Barkin J, et al. The effects of dutasteride, tamsulosin and combination therapy on lower urinary tract symptoms in men with benign prostatic hyperplasia and prostatic enlargement: 2-year results from the CombAT study. J Urol 2008;179(2):616–21 [discussion: 621].

45. Siami P, Roehrborn CG, Barkin J, et al. Combination therapy with dutasteride and tamsulosin in men with moderate-to-severe benign prostatic hyperplasia and prostate enlargement: the CombAT (Combination of Avodart and Tamsulosin) trial rationale and study design. Contemp Clin Trials 2007;28(6):770–9.

46. Roehrborn CG, Kaplan SA, Jones JS, et al. Tolterodine extended release with or without tamsulosin in men with lower urinary tract symptoms including overactive bladder symptoms: effects of prostate size. Eur Urol 2009;55(2):472–9.

47. Roehrborn CG, Kaplan SA, Kraus SR, et al. Effects of serum PSA on efficacy of tolterodine extended release with or without tamsulosin in men with LUTS, including OAB. Urology 2008;72(5):1061–7 [discussion: 1067].

48. Kaplan SA, Roehrborn CG, Rovner ES, et al. Tolterodine and tamsulosin for treatment of men with lower urinary tract symptoms and overactive bladder: a randomized controlled trial. JAMA 2006;296(19):2319–28.

Urinary Incontinence in Women

Donna Y. Deng, MD

KEYWORDS

- Stress incontinence • Urge incontinence • Overactive bladder
- Urinary frequency • Urgency

Urinary incontinence (UI) is a significant problem that affects the quality of life of millions of Americans. It is a common problem at all ages but is most prevalent in the elderly, especially among those living in an institution. Patients may not report incontinence to their primary care providers because of embarrassment or misconceptions regarding treatment. Most of those who eventually seek help do so only after an average of 4 years of enduring the symptoms and unhappiness this condition causes. Inadequate information and training have been major obstacles to the improved management of urinary incontinence. Yet this common and costly problem is eminently treatable in the community setting. It therefore behooves the health care professional to identify patients who might benefit from treatment.

DEFINITION AND CLASSIFICATION OF UI

Incontinence is the involuntary loss of urine. The lower urinary tract is composed of the urinary bladder as reservoir and the bladder outlet as sphincteric mechanism. Micturition is a complex series of finely tuned and integrated neuromuscular events that involve anatomic and neurologic mechanisms. Alterations in any of these components may result in dysfunctional voiding or UI. Urine leakage occurs when the pressure in the bladder exceeds that within the urethra.

The main types of UI in women are stress incontinence, urge incontinence, and mixed incontinence.

Stress UI (SUI) is involuntary leakage on effort or exertion or any sudden increase in abdominal pressure. This includes coughing, sneezing, sport activities, sudden changes of position, and the like. For those with severe incontinence, minimal exertion can cause leakage. SUI occurs as a result of the variable combination of intrinsic urethral sphincter muscle weakness and an anatomic defect in the urethral support, leading to insufficient closure pressure in the urethra during physical effort. The etiology is multifactorial and includes pregnancy, vaginal delivery, pelvic surgery,

The author has no financial interests to disclose.
Department of Urology, University of California San Francisco, 400 Parnassus Avenue A633, Box 0738, San Francisco, CA 94143-0738, USA
E-mail address: ddeng@urology.ucsf.edu

Med Clin N Am 95 (2011) 101–109
doi:10.1016/j.mcna.2010.08.022
0025-7125/11/$ – see front matter © 2011 Elsevier Inc. All rights reserved.

neurologic causes, active lifestyle, and synergistic causes that are mainly due to aging and comorbidities.

Urge UI (UUI) is the involuntary loss of urine accompanied by or immediately preceded by a sudden, strong desire to void (urgency). This can be caused by an involuntary bladder contraction that overcomes the sphincter mechanism or poor bladder compliance that results from loss of the viscoelastic features of the bladder. UUI is a part of the spectrum of overactive bladder (OAB). OAB is defined as urgency, with or without urge incontinence, usually with frequency and nocturia.[1] Detrusor overactivity is a urodynamic observation characterized by involuntary detrusor contractions found in some patients with OAB. Detrusor overactivity may be idiopathic, or it may be associated with a neurologic condition.

Mixed urinary incontinence is the symptom complex of involuntary leakage associated with both urgency and effort and exertion.

PREVALENCE AND RISK FACTORS

UI is a common symptom that affects women at all ages, and there is a wide range of severity and nature of symptoms. Mixed and urge incontinence predominate in older women, while young and middle-aged women predominantly suffer from stress incontinence. UI in long-term institution residents tends to be more severe, costly, and have a greater burden on caregivers. There is a lower prevalence of UI in black, Hispanic, and Asian women compared with white women. The prevalence of OAB is approximately 16% in the general population (men and women), affecting 33 million adults in America, with equal weight between men and women.[2] However, more women than men have incontinence associated with OAB, referred to as wet OAB.

Risk factors for UI can be classified as predisposing, obstetric and gynecologic, and promoting. Predisposing factors include race (eg, Caucasian women are more susceptible), genetics, congenital defects, and neurologic abnormalities such as Parkinson disease, multiple sclerosis, stroke, or herpes zoster infection. Obstetric and gynecologic factors include pregnancy/childbirth/parity, effects of pelvic surgery and radiation, and pelvic organ prolapse. Promoting factors include age, comorbidities (eg, diabetes, vascular disease, and changes in mobility), obesity, conditions associated with increased abdominal pressure, urinary tract infection (UTI), cognitive impairment, menopause, and medications such as diuretics, angiotensin-converting enzyme (ACE) inhibitors causing chronic cough, or anticholinergic agents causing urinary retention and overflow incontinence. **Table 1** shows the main risk factors with more detailed explanations and examples.

In the geriatric population, causes of transient incontinence should be ruled out. These causes can be remembered with the mnemonic DIAPPERS[3]: delirium, infection, atrophic vaginitis or urethritis, pharmaceuticals, psychological problems, excess urine output, restricted mobility, and stool impaction.

EVALUATION

Although the history may define the patient's problem, it may be misleading. Urge incontinence may be triggered by activities such as coughing, so according to the patient's history, she seems to have stress incontinence. A patient who complains only of urge incontinence may also have stress incontinence. Mixed incontinence is very common; at least 65% of patients with stress incontinence have associated urgency or urge incontinence. The evaluation of the incontinent patient includes a history, physical examination, laboratory tests, and possibly urodynamic testing.

Table 1
Risk factors of urinary incontinence

Predisposing	Obstetric/Gynecologic	Promoting
Race Caucasian women are more susceptible to SUI than African American or Asian women Genetics Increased risk of incontinence if other female family member is incontinent Congenital Congenital defects (eg, ectopic ureter) of the urinary tract can cause UI. Neurologic Spina bifida Spinal cord injury Brain injury Parkinson disease Multiple sclerosis Stroke Dementia Transverse myelitis Guillaine-Barre syndrome Herpes zoster Pelvic surgery	Pregnancy/Childbirth/Parity Questionable whether pregnancy itself contributes to UI later in life or whether factors of childbirth do. Women incontinent during pregnancy may be predisposed to develop UI later. Vaginal delivery, episiotomy, and instrumental delivery may increase likelihood of UI Large infant birth weight over 4 kg may predispose to UI Number of children increases risk of UI. Association strongest with over 4 children but decreases with mother's age. Side effects of pelvic surgery and radiotherapy Associated nerve/muscle damage may be implicated Pelvic organ prolapse Pelvic organ prolapse is commonly found together with UI and may be a possible cause of the UI	Age Predisposition to UI is associated with increased age Comorbidities Diabetes, vascular disease, and congestive heart failure may result in UI Changes in patient mobility and accessibility of toilets may contribute to UI Obesity Obesity is an established contributing factor to UI and SUI. Weight reduction correlates to a reduction in UI Increased intra-abdominal pressure Constipation Lung disease Occupational and recreational activities Activities that cause intra-abdominal pressure increase risk of UI. Higher impact activities have higher correlation. Cognitive impairment Dementia and cognitive impairment as well as associated changes in mobility are correlated with UI Menopause Changes during menopause are associated with UTIs but not clear if they are independent risk factors for UI. Medications Many drugs have side effects that influence continence

Abbreviations: UI, urinary incontinence; UTI, urinary tract infection.

History

The onset, frequency, severity, and pattern of incontinence should be sought, as well as any associated symptoms such as frequency, dysuria, urgency, and nocturia. Incontinence may be quantified by asking the patient if she wears a pad and how often the pad is changed. Obstructive symptoms, such as a feeling of incomplete emptying, hesitancy, straining, or weak stream, may coexist with incontinence, particularly in patients with previous incontinence corrective procedures, cystoceles, or poor detrusor contractility. Patients should be asked about symptoms of pelvic prolapse, such as recurrent UTI, a sensation of vaginal fullness or pressure, or the observation of a bulge in the vagina. The patient should be queried specifically about neurologic conditions that are known to affect bladder and sphincteric function, such as multiple sclerosis, spinal cord injury, diabetes, myelodysplasia, stroke, and Parkinson disease. In this regard, it is important to ask about double vision, muscular weakness, paralysis or poor coordination, tremor, numbness, and tingling sensation. A history of vaginal surgery or previous surgical repair of incontinence should suggest the possibility of sphincteric injury. Abdominoperineal resection of the rectum or radical hysterectomy may be associated with neurologic injury to the bladder and sphincter. Radiation therapy may adversely affect bladder capacity or compliance. A list of the patient's current medications (specifically sedatives, diuretics, and anticholinergics, among others) and over-the-counter medications should be obtained.

Physical Examination

A complete physical examination should be performed, with emphasis on neurologic assessment and on abdominal, pelvic, and rectal examinations. The general examination should include height and weight, which will allow for objective assessment of body mass index, as obesity is an established risk factor of UI. The abdominal examination will allow evaluation of scars and palpation for possible distended bladder. The neurologic examination should concentrate on the sacral segments. This should include testing of lower limb movement and innervation and perineal sensation to exclude a neurologic cause for UI. In the elderly, a mini-mental status assessment and cognitive function state assessment and evaluation of mobility are useful.

The genital/perineal examination should begin with a description of the skin condition around the genitals (such as excoriation or erythema due to incontinence). The condition of the vaginal mucosa (well-estrogenized or atrophic) should be noted. A stress test will allow observation of leakage of urine through the urethra when the patient is asked to cough or strain in the supine or upright position. The presence of associated pelvic organ prolapse should be noted, because it can contribute to the patient's voiding problems and may have an impact on diagnosis and treatment. A rectal examination should include the evaluation of anal sphincter tone and perineal sensation.

Studies

A urinalysis is performed to determine if there is any evidence of hematuria, pyuria, glucosuria, or proteinuria. A urine specimen is sent for cytologic examination for urothelial cancer if there is hematuria or irritative voiding symptoms. The urine is cultured if there is pyuria or bacteriuria. Infection should be treated before further investigations or interventions. Hematuria consisting of more than three red cells per high-power field warrants further investigation by imaging and cystoscopy.

A postvoid residual (PVR) should be measured either with a bladder scan, pelvic ultrasound, or directly with a catheter. A PVR less than 50 mL is not usually significant;

one between 50 and 200 mL can be equivocal, and a PVR greater than 200 mL should be referred for specialist evaluation. A significant PVR volume may reflect either bladder outlet obstruction or poor bladder contractility. The only way to distinguish outlet obstruction from poor contractility is with urodynamic testing. A single number may not provide the answer to the etiology of a patient's incontinence; the PVR value needs to be taken into consideration as a part of the entire workup.

Urodynamic testing is used to delineate more precisely the etiology of a patient's incontinence; however, many patients can be successfully treated without urodynamic testing. This involves placement of a small catheter (7Fr) into the bladder, which can provide pressure readings of the bladder while the bladder is slowly filled (via the same catheter). Typically another small catheter is placed in the rectum to allow recording of intra-abdominal pressure at the same time. The purpose of urodynamic testing is to examine compliance, assess for the presence of stress incontinence or detrusor overactivity, and rule out obstruction as a cause of either overflow or urge incontinence. Urodynamic testing ideally should be performed before invasive therapies, certainly in patients who are undergoing repeat procedures, and in all patients with known neurologic disease, since progression of disease can often be silent.

TREATMENT FOR STRESS INCONTINENCE

All treatment interventions for incontinence are based on the information gathered during the assessment and investigations conducted on the individual. For most incontinence sufferers, cure or improvement is possible. As a general rule, the first choice should be the least-invasive treatment with the fewest potential adverse complications. Treatment options can be divided into conservative measures, pharmacotherapy, and surgical intervention (**Table 2**).

Conservative

Various lifestyle factors may play a role in either the pathogenesis or subsequent resolution of incontinence. Most published studies about lifestyle, however, only report associations and do not assess the actual effect of applying or eliminating the behavior involved in incontinence. Relatively few randomized trials have been performed to assess the effect of specific lifestyle factors on incontinence. Conservative therapies are useful for both stress and urge incontinence.

Weight loss has been shown to decrease UI. The data on caffeine and incontinence are conflicting. Decreasing fluid intake should be reserved for patients with high fluid intakes. Often, patients already limit their fluid intake and may dehydrate themselves in an attempt to prevent leakage. Constipation should be treated, as the chronic straining may be a risk factor for pelvic organ prolapse and UI. Any conditions that result in chronic coughing increase the severity of incontinence. Patients should be encouraged to stop smoking; in addition to the chronic cough causing both SUI and UUI, nicotine may have a direct role by inducing bladder muscle contraction. The objective of timed voiding is to empty the bladder before it exceeds its maximum capacity.

Pelvic floor muscle exercises (PFME), also known as Kegel exercises, work by increasing the strength and tone of the pelvic floor muscles. This increases the urethral closure force, preventing stress incontinence during an abrupt increase in intra-abdominal pressure. It also can be used in the management of urge incontinence, because detrusor contractions can be reflexively or voluntarily inhibited by tightening the pelvic floor. The success of PFME depends on the patient's ability to perform this correctly and the motivation to actually practice this regularly. There is level 1 evidence that for all women with UI (stress, urge, and mixed); PFME is better than no treatment

Table 2
Treatments of urinary incontinence

	Stress Incontinence	Urge Incontinence
Conservative	Weight loss Fluid management Treat constipation Treat chronic cough PFME External compression devices	Weight loss Fluid management Timed voiding Bladder training PFME

Pharmacologic	α agonists
	   Phenylpropanolamine
	   Pseudoephedrine
	Mixed
	   Imipramine
		Antimuscarinic/Anticholinergic
		   Oxybutynin
		   Tolterodine
		   Solifenacin
		   Darifenacin
		   Trospium
		   Hyoscyamine
		Mixed
		   Imipramine

Surgical	Urethral injection with bulking agents Urethral sling Retropubic suspensions	Intravesical Botox injection Percutaneous nerve stimulation Sacral nerve stimulation Bladder augmentation

Abbreviation: PFME, pelvic floor muscle exercises.

and should be offered as a first-line therapy.[4] PFME supervised by a physiotherapist plus the addition of biofeedback may be more effective than home-based practice if the patient is not noticing any improvement. Biofeedback includes either digital feedback, visual feedback using a perineometer or vaginal probe, or sensory feedback with weighted vaginal cones.

Continence depends on the harmonious interaction of anatomic and neuromuscular mechanisms as well as appropriate incorporation of learned behavior. Behavioral strategies are designed to reduce the frequency of incontinence episodes. These interventions can be used before or in addition to pharmacotherapy, or in some cases surgery. Bladder training is designed to help the patient regain control of her bladder by teaching her to resist and suppress the desire to pass urine. This will help increase bladder capacity and reduce the episodes of incontinence. The patient is instructed to void every hour during the day. A shorter initial voiding interval may be necessary if her baseline voiding interval is less than 1 hour. When a 1-hour interval is achieved, increasing intervals by 15–30 minutes/week, depending on tolerance of the schedule, until a 2 to 3 hour voiding interval is achieved may be curative. This needs to be personalized, as many patients can only increase in intervals of a few minutes each time.

Timed voiding is comprised of a fixed voiding schedule aimed to prevent incontinence by providing regular opportunities for emptying before leakage. Timed voiding can be used for women who have infrequent or irregular voiding patterns in an outpatient setting, and can be used for those in institutional settings where passive toileting assistance is available every 2 to 3 hours.

External devices to treat stress incontinence are available but not often used. The aim is to mechanically occlude the urethra. The intraurethral devices (plugs) have demonstrated high levels of efficacy but have been associated with UTI, hematuria, and discomfort. The patient needs to have good manual dexterity, and the device has to be replaced after each use. External devices may be most appropriate for intermittent and occasional use, such as during vigorous exercise. The intravaginal devices include traditional tampons, pessaries, diaphragms, and those specifically designed to support the bladder neck. The success and use of these devices depend on availability of product, patient ability (manual dexterity), patient acceptance, and cost.

Pharmacotherapy

Action on the smooth muscle sphincter tone is mediated by stimulation of alpha-adrenoceptors. The bladder neck and proximal urethra have abundant α receptors. Alpha-agonists such as phenylpropanolamine and pseudoephedrine (Sudafed) have been used to treat stress incontinence. However, efficacy has been limited and side effects have restricted their clinical use. Tricyclic antidepressants, such as imipramine (Tofranil), have both α-agonist and anticholinergic properties.

Action on the striated muscle sphincter tone is mediated by stimulation of nicotinic receptors by acetylcholine. Duloxetine (Cymbalta) is a combined serotonin and norepinephrine reuptake inhibitor, which has been shown to significantly increase sphincteric muscle activity. Although there was significant decrease in incontinence episodes compared with placebo, duloxetine failed to obtain US approval for stress incontinence amidst concerns for liver toxicity and suicidal events. It is approved for this indication in Europe. There is no medication available in the United States that is significantly effective for pure stress urinary incontinence.

Surgical Treatment

Surgical therapy for stress incontinence is indicated when a patient does not wish to pursue nonsurgical therapy, or if such therapy has failed.

Urethral bulking procedures are designed to treat stress incontinence by artificially inflating the submucosal tissues of the proximal urethra/bladder neck. These procedures involve injecting synthetic or autologous fillers (eg, bovine collagen, carbon bead particles, calcium hydroxylapatite, polydimethylsiloxane) into the wall of the urethra to make it fuller, improving the urethral coaptation and restoring the mucosal seal mechanism of continence. Continence depends in part on a leak-proof mucosal seal that is provided by the supple urothelium and the vascularity of the submucosal vessels of the urethra. Injection of bulking agents has low morbidity and minor complications of UTI and short-term voiding dysfunction. However, its efficacy is only 40% or less in well-selected patients, and these results quickly deteriorate with time, necessitating reinjections.

Synthetic midurethral slings are now the mainstay treatment for women with stress incontinence. It is not appropriate for those with predominantly urge incontinence. It is a minimally invasive outpatient procedure involving placement of a piece of synthetic mesh around the urethra. The mechanism of action is thought to be the prevention of the posterior and inferior descent of the bladder neck when intra-abdominal pressure rises, as well as the reinforcement of the suburethral vaginal support. Reported patient satisfaction rates are 80% to 90%, with durable results out to 10 years (the synthetic sling was first introduced in 1998). The sling can be placed via a retropubic or transobturator approach and should be determined based on the individual history and findings of the patient.

Slings using other materials, such as autologous or cadaveric fascia, have been used with very good results for decades, but have become more second-line therapies given the ease and minimal morbidity using the synthetic sling. Similarly, retropubic cystourethropexy (Burch suspension) is an effective procedure with proven long-term success for stress incontinence, but its use has decreased significantly because of the reduced surgical morbidity and shorter hospital stay associated with the synthetic slings.

TREATMENT FOR URGE INCONTINENCE
Conservative

Noninvasive therapies for urge incontinence are similar to those mentioned in the section under conservative treatments for stress incontinence. These include lifestyle and behavior changes such as fluid management, avoidance of bladder irritants, bladder training and timed voiding, and pelvic floor muscle exercises with or without biofeedback.

Pharmacotherapy

Pharmacotherapy is the mainstay of treatment for urgency and urge incontinence (OAB), and antimuscarinics are still the most widely used agents. The mechanism of action is to block acetylcholine from binding to the muscarinic receptors on the detrusor muscle to decrease the contraction of the bladder. Currently used antimuscarinics are associated with a good efficacy (30% over placebo) and tolerability profile. Despite the many available antimuscarinics on the market, there is little difference in efficacy between them.

The side effect profile of this class of drugs is as important a consideration as the efficacy when treating patients. The side effects are due to the inhibition of muscarinic receptors in organs other than the bladder. The class-related adverse effects of M3 receptors include dry mouth, constipation, and blurred vision. These are most common but mostly tolerated by patients with low safety concerns. The adverse effects of M1 and M2 receptors include cognitive dysfunction, memory loss, attention deficit, cardiovascular effects, palpitations, and tachycardia. These are less common but of greater safety concern.

Antimuscarinic use is contraindicated in untreated narrow-angle glaucoma.

Surgical Treatment

Patients who have failed medical treatment do have several minimally invasive surgical options. Neuromodulation by stimulation of the S3 sacral nerve root by an implanted nerve stimulator can provide effective relief of overactive bladder symptoms and neurogenic retention. This was first developed in 1981 and has been US Food and Drug Administration (FDA)-approved since 1997. Percutaneous stimulation of the tibial nerve using an acupuncture needle attached to an electrical stimulator is an even less invasive procedure. This typically involves 30-minute weekly session in the clinic over 2 to 3 months to show effect.

International studies using botulinum toxin over the past decade are proving the efficacy of local intravesical injections.[5] The toxin blocks the release of acetylcholine and results in decreased bladder muscle contractility. New nerve terminals regenerate in about 3 to 6 months, and reinjection is required to sustain effect. A good response is obtained within 1 week and can last from 6 to 9 months before reinjection is necessary. The safety of these products appears to be satisfactory; however, they are not yet FDA-approved.

For patients who have failed the conservative, medical, and less invasive surgical therapies, bladder augmentation is an effective management option. This is major reconstructive surgery using a piece of small bowel sewn onto a bisected bladder to increase the size of the bladder. Positive results have been obtained in up to 90% of patients with neurogenic lower urinary tract dysfunction. Significant potential complications require life-long follow-up. Such complications include the need for intermittent self-catheterization (although by the time this point in the treatment menu has been reached, urinary retention is not an unreasonable result, and the main issue is one of patient informed consent), recurrent UTI and calculi, electrolyte imbalance, delayed bladder perforation, and increased risk for tumor formation.

SUMMARY

UI is a common and disruptive problem for many. This will only amplify as the population ages. Although there is no miracle cure for the patient, small adjustments or improvements can have a significant impact on the quality of life. The management pathway begins with the diagnosis, because the treatment options for the two main types of incontinence are quite different. The key is to encourage patients to adopt conservative measures as much as possible. If behavioral modifications and pharmacotherapy fail, then there are minimally invasive procedures that can be of further benefit. Incontinence can be controlled, but it takes patience and partnership.

REFERENCES

1. Abrams P, Cardozo L, Fall M, et al. The standardization of terminology of lower urinary tract function: report from the Standadisation Subcommittee of the International Continence Society. Neurourol Urodyn 2002;21:167–78.
2. Stewart WF, Van Rooyen JB, Cundiff GW, et al. Prevalence and burden of overactive bladder in the United States. World J Urol 2003;20(6):327–36.
3. Resnick NM. Geriatric incontinence. Urol Clin North Am 1996;23(1):55–75.
4. Burgio KL, Locher JL, Goode PS, et al. Behavioral vs drug treatment for urge urinary incontinence in older women: a randomized controlled trial. JAMA 1998; 280:1995–2000.
5. Karsenty G, Denys P, Amarenco G, et al. Botulinum toxin A (Botox) intradetrusor injections in adults with neurogenic detrusor overactivity/neurogenic overactive bladder: a systematic literature review. Eur Urol 2008;53(2):275–87.

The Neurogenic Bladder: An Update with Management Strategies for Primary Care Physicians

Adam P. Klausner, MD[a],*, William D. Steers, MD[b]

KEYWORDS

- Neurogenic bladder • Urodynamics
- Bladder outlet obstruction

INTRODUCTION: THE MICTURITION REFLEX AND NORMAL VOIDING

To void in an efficient manner, there must be a finely coordinated reciprocal functionality of the urinary bladder and urinary sphincter. When the bladder contracts, the external urethral sphincter must relax. Conversely, when the urinary bladder is relaxed, the urinary sphincter contracts and maintains tone. The reciprocal coordination of these 2 functional units within the lower urinary tract is mediated by a specialized control center in the brain stem called the pontine micturition center.[1]

It is important to emphasize a few key concepts of urine storage. As the bladder fills with urine, the intravesical pressure remains low until the threshold for micturition is reached. This progressive increase in volumes with minimal increase in pressure is termed compliance and is defined by the equation ΔVolume/ΔPressure.[2] In a normal 50-year-old man, the typical cystometric bladder capacity is approximately 400 mL.[3] During the increase in volume from 0 to 400 mL, it is expected that the pressure within the bladder will increase to only about 10 cm H_2O, resulting in a compliance of 40 mL/cm H_2O. The compliance of the bladder is a function of its inherent viscoelasticity, the ability of detrusor muscle cells to elongate while still maintaining efficient contractility, and the neurally mediated suppression of signals that promote detrusor contraction.[4] A normally complaint bladder is essential for proper functioning of the lower urinary tract.

[a] Division of Urology, Department of Surgery, Virginia Commonwealth University School of Medicine, PO Box 980118, Richmond, VA 23298-0118, USA
[b] Department of Urology, University of Virginia School of Medicine, VA, USA
* Corresponding author.
E-mail address: apklausner@vcu.edu

Med Clin N Am 95 (2011) 111–120
doi:10.1016/j.mcna.2010.08.027
0025-7125/11/$ – see front matter © 2011 Published by Elsevier Inc.

A patient with symptoms of or proven dysfunction of the lower urinary tract and neurologic findings (or a known neurologic disorder) is said to have a neurogenic bladder. Poor compliance is one consequence of neurogenic bladder dysfunction, but compliance can only be determined during a formal urodynamic evaluation, in which filling pressures and volumes are recorded simultaneously. Therefore, one of the most important pieces of information that is obtained from a urodynamic evaluation is a determination of the bladder compliance.

The micturition reflex is an autonomic process under voluntary control. In other words, the reflex can be aborted midstream by inhibitory neural inputs from higher cortical brain centers. Conversely, the reflex can be accelerated by neurologic processes that affect or damage these areas that produce inhibitory inputs. Damage to the cerebral cortex reduces inhibitory input to the pontine micturition center and might cause urinary frequency, urgency, or even urge incontinence. Patients with this type of reduced inhibitory control are those with Parkinson disease, cortical strokes, brain tumors, normal pressure hydrocephalus, traumatic brain injury, or Alzheimer type dementia.[5] Alternatively, patients with diseases such as multiple sclerosis, degenerative disk disease, or spinal cord pathology have neurologic lesions caudal to the pontine micturition center but rostral to the sacral spinal cord. Typically, lesions in this location result in a loss of coordination between the bladder and its outlet, creating obstruction.[5] In addition to often demonstrating detrusor overactivity, these patients may exhibit either slowed external sphincter relaxation (eg, Parkinson disease) or complete loss of coordination (eg, suprasacral spinal cord injury [SCI]). Whether overactive bladder symptoms are merely caused by detrusor overactivity or are the result of bladder outlet obstruction requires special physiologic testing of the lower urinary tract termed urodynamics.

URODYNAMICS: INDICATIONS AND TECHNIQUE
Indications for Urodynamics

Multichannel pressure-flow urodynamics offers the most complete and useful evaluation of neurogenic bladder dysfunction. Urodynamic evaluation consists of several tests used alone or in combination (multichannel). Tests include voiding flow rate, cystometry, sphincter electromyography (EMG), and urethral pressure profilometry. The goal of a urodynamic evaluation is to reproduce the patient's typical micturition cycle and associated urinary symptoms. It is crucial for the urodynamicist to take a comprehensive history and be aware of the patient's underlying neurologic status.

Urodynamic Technique

The cystometry portion of urodynamics is accomplished by infusing saline at room temperature at the rate of 40 to 60 mL/min. Although faster than physiologic filling, these rates have been chosen because of time constraints and to help unmask detrusor overactivity. During the filling phase, the urodynamicist asks the patient to identify various sensory thresholds including the volumes at which the patient has the first sensation of filling, the first desire to void, and a strong desire to void. The diagnosis of increased bladder sensation is made when patients achieve sensory thresholds at lower-than-expected volumes. Reduced or absent sensation is diagnosed when patients achieve sensory thresholds at lower-than-expected volumes or not at all.

During the filling phase, any involuntary bladder contractions should be noted. Although involuntary detrusor contractions (IDCs) are identified in up to 20% of asymptomatic patients during cystometry,[6,7] their presence is considered abnormal.

Thus, the presence of one or more IDCs during the filling phase allows the urodynamicist to diagnose detrusor overactivity. In the setting of known neurogenic bladder dysfunction, the diagnosis is neurogenic detrusor overactivity as opposed to idiopathic detrusor overactivity. In addition, at a volume equal to about 50% of the known or expected bladder capacity, filling is temporarily stopped and provocative maneuvers are sometimes performed to evaluate for the possibility of an incompetent urethral sphincter closure mechanism, which is commonly found in patients with stress incontinence.

Once the patient reaches cystometric capacity, the filling is discontinued and the patient is given permission to void. Oftentimes, the patient is unable to wait and voids involuntarily, which leads to the urodynamic diagnosis of detrusor overactivity incontinence. During the voiding phase, the voiding flow rate is obtained using a flowmeter that collects urine while calculating a urinary flow rate. Multichannel capability allows flow and intravesical pressure to be graphed at the same time. This simultaneous measurement of bladder pressure and urine flow is also called a pressure-flow study. The pressure-flow study is the only test that can accurately determine whether physiologic bladder outlet obstruction exists. A low peak voiding flow rate (<12 mL/s) may suggest obstruction but cannot, in itself, exclude impaired detrusor contractility. The diagnosis of bladder outlet obstruction is made only when elevated bladder pressures and low urinary flow rates (ie, high pressure, low flow) are seen simultaneously. The urodynamic criteria for obstruction in men has been clearly defined and can be graphed on a standardized nomogram,[8] whereas such a measure in women is somewhat controversial. Fluoroscopy performed simultaneously with multichannel urodynamic evaluation (termed videourodynamics) allows the operator to note the level of obstruction, such as the bladder neck, prostate, external sphincter, or distal urethra.

EMG activity of the urinary sphincter is used to determine if the bladder and sphincter are acting in a coordinated manner. In the setting of neurogenic bladder dysfunction, obstruction often occurs because of a lack of neurally mediated coordination of the sphincter and bladder, a process termed detrusor-sphincter dyssynergia (DSD). It is crucial that the urodynamicist differentiate true dyssynergia from dysfunctional voiding, a learned behavior or an artifact. The following cases illustrate how urodynamics is used to diagnosis and treat patients with neurogenic voiding dysfunction:

URODYNAMIC INTERPRETATION AND PATIENT MANAGEMENT
Case 1: Neurogenic Bladder Dysfunction Caused by Injury Above the Level of the Pontine Micturition Center

An 82-year-old man complains of persistent urinary frequency and urgency with some urge incontinence after having an ischemic cerebrovascular injury. His neurologic examination reveals hemiparesis of the left side, and he has an enlarged prostate on digital rectal examination. Are his symptoms caused by stroke or bladder outlet obstruction from prostatic enlargement? Although empiric therapy can be attempted, urodynamic testing is needed to exclude obstruction and document whether detrusor overactivity exists.

During the filling phase of cystometry, he reports a strong desire to void at an infused volume of 125 mL, associated with an IDC and involuntary leakage. His urinary sphincter and bladder are reported to act in a coordinated manner based on the EMG data, and he has no definitive evidence of bladder outlet obstruction. In this case, the urodynamic diagnosis is neurogenic detrusor overactivity incontinence. The cause is likely stroke-induced damage to inhibitory cortical inputs to the pontine micturition center, which clinically presents as a reduced warning time associated with urinary urgency and urge incontinence.

This patient should first be treated with timed or prompted voiding, fluid management, and urge suppression maneuvers. Diuretics should be avoided because these will exacerbate his symptoms. Patients who do not fully respond to behavioral modification may be managed with antimuscarinic medications. However, many of these medications have inconvenient side effects such as dry mouth and constipation, which limit their long-term efficacy, and some are associated with short-term memory impairment, making them more risky for use in the elderly.[9] Certainly, patients should be counseled that symptoms may improve spontaneously in parallel with recovery of other motor and cognitive functions after an acute stroke. Chronic symptoms that are severe, bothersome, and refractory to behavioral modifications and medical therapy can be treated by sacral or tibial nerve neuromodulation or even with off-label usage of botulinum toxin injected into the bladder muscle.[10,11]

Case 2: Neurogenic Bladder Dysfunction Caused by Suprasacral SCI

One year after a motor vehicle crash, a 26-year-old woman is paraplegic as a result of an incomplete SCI at the T5 level. She complains of the need to urinate coinciding with increased spasticity in her legs and associated with profuse sweating and facial flushing. She wears adult diapers. During a urodynamic evaluation, she is noted to have absent sensation of bladder filling but has a relatively normal cystometric capacity (350 mL). At an infused volume of 300 mL, she develops a high-pressure sustained IDC, with a maximum pressure of 110 cm H_2O. She empties about 50% of her cystometric capacity, but voiding is prolonged (4 minutes duration), comes in interrupted spurts, and is associated with an increased EMG activity of the urinary sphincter. Provocative maneuvers demonstrate no evidence of stress incontinence.

Based on the history and the data obtained from the urodynamic evaluation, it is noted that this patient is not properly managing her bladder and is at high risk for renal deterioration. Because her injury is below the pontine micturition center, the coordinated reciprocal functionality of the urinary bladder and urinary sphincter is absent. Clinically, the patient has DSD. DSD causes bladder outlet obstruction and inefficient emptying. As a direct result of the obstruction, the patient's voiding pressures are very high. Typical unobstructed voiding pressures are at or less than 40 cm H_2O; however, this patient's pressures are well above 100 cm H_2O. The high pressures may overwhelm the intrinsic valve mechanism of the ureters as they course through the bladder wall and create reflux of high-pressure urine that is likely colonized by multiple bacterial pathogens. This combination places the patient at significant risk for kidney damage and other complications.

Treatment includes limiting fluid intake to less than 2 L/d to increase the time interval between voiding events. In addition, antimuscarinic medications should be prescribed and may need to be used at much higher doses than are typically recommended.[12] Finally, the patient should be trained to perform intermittent catheterization using a clean or sterile technique. The timing of catheterization should be adjusted to keep the urine volumes less than the value at which high-pressure bladder contractions developed (<300 mL in this patient). A voiding diary or daily voiding log can be used to help keep track of residual volumes. Because urodynamic evaluation indicates a high detrusor leak point pressure, renal function should be monitored at 3- to 6-month intervals using serum creatinine levels and renal ultrasonographys. The inability to perform catheterization or lack of compliance with catheterization should prompt discussion of more aggressive treatment options, including urinary diversion using segments of bowel or botulinum toxin injections into the detrusor. Primary care providers should recognize that patients such as these require lifelong urologic management and should be referred to a urologist or other providers with training in neurourology and urodynamics.

URODYNAMIC RISK FACTORS FOR KIDNEY DAMAGE AND OTHER UROLOGIC COMPLICATIONS

The preceding cases illustrate many of the urodynamic risk factors for kidney damage or upper urinary tract deterioration in patients with neurogenic bladder obstruction or dysfunction. These risk factors include poor bladder compliance, bladder pressures greater than 40 cm H_2O, and the presence of DSD. Data supporting these risk factors are discussed in the following sections.

Poor Bladder Compliance

Exact criteria to categorize bladder compliance in patients with neurogenic bladder dysfunction do not exist. In a study by Hackler and colleagues,[13] a compliance less than 20 mL/cm H_2O on urodynamic studies was considered as low. In their study, 69% of patients with low compliance were found to have renal damage on imaging studies as compared with 21% of patients with normal compliance. In other investigations, cutoff value for poor compliance was set even lower at 12.5 mL/cm H_2O and high rates for renal damage and other urologic complications was demonstrated in patients with values below this threshold.[14]

DSD

DSD is defined as the involuntary contraction or lack of relaxation of the striated sphincter during a bladder contraction.[5] DSD should exist only in patients who have a neurologic abnormality below the brain stem and above the sacral spinal cord where motor outflow to the bladder originates. In fact, nearly 75% of patients with suprasacral SCI[15] will have DSD, and patients with this type of neurologic injury should be considered to have DSD until proven otherwise.

DSD is considered a risk factor for the development of renal damage. In a study of male patients with SCI, Linsenmeyer and colleagues[16] found that patients with prolonged voiding had the greatest risk of developing hydronephrosis. Patients with prolonged voiding, like the patient in case 2, may have both DSD and poorly compliant bladders. Untreated DSD is clearly associated with the development of renal damage,[17] and 50% of patients with untreated DSD will develop significant urologic complications, including vesicoureteral reflux, renal damage, urolithiasis, urosepsis, and ureterovesical obstruction.[18] Pharmacologic treatment with α-blockers may be considered because these drugs work by reducing outlet resistance at the level of the bladder neck; however, there is limited evidence that these agents actually improve outcomes or decrease risk of complications in patients with DSD.[19–22]

Because of α-blockers and other types of pharmacotherapy lack efficacy, the mainstay of treatment of DSD is performance of intermittent catheterization. Patients should be counseled to time the catheterizations to keep the volumes of urine below the threshold for the development of involuntary bladder contractions and/or below the volume at which a detrusor leak point pressure of 40 cm H_2O develops. In conjunction with fluid restriction, catheterization can often be accomplished every 4 to 6 hours. However, some patients may need to catheterize far more frequently or may not be willing or able to catheterize at all. In these more challenging situations, patients can be offered botulinum toxin injection to paralyze the urinary sphincter, formal surgical sphincterotomy, or placement of a urethral stent (UroLume, American Medical Systems Inc, Minnetonka, MN, USA) across the sphincter. All these methods are designed to render the sphincter nonfunctional, leaving the patient safe but totally incontinent. This option may be acceptable in men in whom urine leakage can be effectively collected using a condom or Texas Catheter. However, in women, lack of an effective external collecting device necessitates the need to use diapers or an indwelling catheter. Studies have demonstrated the efficacy of botulinum toxin for the treatment of DSD. However, at present, the therapy is not approved by the Food and Drug Administration and requires repeat cystoscopic injections on every 6- to 9-month basis.[23,24] In addition, sphincterotomy and urethral stenting have high complication and/or failure rates.[25] For these reasons, many individuals with DSD and inability to perform self-catheterization are managed with urinary diversion using sections of bowel or are maintained with indwelling urethral catheters.

Detrusor Pressures Greater Than 40 cm H₂O

The value of urodynamic evaluations for patients with neurogenic bladder dysfunction was demonstrated in studies by McGuire and colleagues[26] in which more than 80% of patients with myelodysplasia experiencing urine leakage at bladder pressures greater than 40 cm H_2O were found to have ureteral or renal dilation (hydronephrosis). This cutoff value was dramatic in that only 10% of patients who had leakage at pressures lower than 40 cm H_2O had similar findings. Kim and colleagues[27] followed up 55 patients with SCI managed with at least 1 sphincterotomy. These investigators found that patients with bladder pressures greater than 40 cm H_2O had the greatest risk of renal damage and development of recurrent DSD. These studies were mainly performed on patients with detrusor acontractility. However, studies in patients with SCI and detrusor overactivity have found, similarly, that sustained bladder pressures greater than 40 cm H_2O are associated with greater risk of upper urinary tract deterioration.[28] Based on this, primary care physicians caring for patients with neurologic diseases need to question whether the bladder pressures in their patients are safe. The answer is provided by urodynamic studies demonstrating filling pressures less than the critical threshold of 40 cm H_2O.

SPECIAL SITUATIONS FOR THE MANAGEMENT OF NEUROGENIC BLADDER DYSFUNCTION
The Indwelling Urinary Catheter

The long-term use of indwelling urethral (Foley) or suprapubic catheters is associated with severe complications,[29–31] including development of frequent urinary tract infections or sepsis,[32] predisposition to renal failure and dialysis,[33,34] formation of kidney or bladder stones,[35] shrinkage of the bladder with potential obstruction of the kidneys or reflux of contaminated urine, and extremely high rates of invasive and potentially lethal bladder cancer.[36] If an indwelling catheter is to be used long-term, a suprapubic tube is preferred to avoid creation of fistulous tracts from the urethra or the bladder to the skin, damage to the sphincter muscles resulting in total incontinence, dilation of the urethra with leakage around the catheter, urethral carcinoma, and erosion and splitting of the penis called traumatic hypospadias.[37] Serial upsizing of a urethral catheter to prevent urine leakage in women is to be condemned.

Because of these severe complications, use of chronic indwelling catheters is discouraged by urologists and other providers involved in the care of individuals with neurogenic bladder dysfunction. In 1972, the treatment of individuals with neurogenic bladder dysfunction was revolutionized by the institution of a technique known as clean intermittent self-catheterization (CISC) by Lapides and colleagues.[38] CISC involves placing a new or clean catheter into the bladder to drain urine at defined times or at times when the individual feels a need to urinate. This method is much safer than the use of indwelling catheters.[39–41] Despite this advice, a large percentage of patients with retention or incontinence caused by a neurogenic bladder are managed with catheters. With close monitoring and aggressive treatment of symptomatic infections and calculi, some think that chronic catheters can be more safely used. Review of recent series on patients managed with suprapubic catheters demonstrates reduced morbidity and risk of renal deterioration when compared with more historic reports.[42]

Urinary Tract Infections: to Treat or Not to Treat

Primary care physicians are encouraged to differentiate between chronic bacterial colonization and symptomatic bacterial infection. In patients with neurogenic bladders, only symptomatic infections (eg, worsening dysreflexia, malaise, fever, spasms) or colonization with *Proteus* sp should be treated. Colonization with bacterial organisms occurs universally within 30 days of catheterization,[43] and attempts at eradication of asymptomatic bacteria are generally contraindicated. These practices contribute to high rates of multidrug-resistant pathogens in patients with neurogenic bladder dysfunction and a lack of effective antimicrobial agents in the case of truly symptomatic infections or urosepsis. In addition, antibiotic prophylaxis is not indicated before routine catheter changes, and studies demonstrate that low-dose prophylaxis in patients with neurogenic bladder dysfunction does not reduce the risk of symptomatic infection.[44] Furthermore, there is no evidence that the use of cranberry tablets or oral methenamine reduces the incidence of complex urinary tract infections in patients with neurogenic bladder dysfunction.[45] Based on these data, primary care physicians are encouraged to avoid obtaining routine urine cultures and should avoid antimicrobial treatment in asymptomatic patients with neurogenic bladders.

The Role of Fluid Restriction

Certainly, the blanket recommendation to "drink more water" to prevent urinary tract infections or promote urinary health does not apply to many patients with neurogenic bladder dysfunction. In fact, patients who experience high-pressure IDCs are often managed with a combination of fluid restriction and antimuscarinic medications. Patients are frequently told to limit fluids to less than 2 L/d. In theory, this recommendation allows patients to empty their bladders using intermittent catheterization at less-frequent and potentially safer, time intervals. However, there are limited data to support the use of this fluid volume in the prevention of urologic complications. Therefore, fluid management in patients with neurogenic bladder dysfunction needs to be tailored to individual patient factors and should be considered after review of urodynamic and other objective data.

The Role of Autonomic Dysreflexia

In patients with neurogenic bladder dysfunction caused by SCI, it is important to recognize autonomic dysreflexia (AD). This condition is seen in patients with SCIs above the T6 level, with much higher rates seen in patients with complete injuries than in those with incomplete injuries. AD is a medical emergency associated with acute elevations of blood pressure and a reflex bradycardia. Clinically, the disorder may be asymptomatic or may be associated with symptoms including flushing, sweating, and headache as displayed in case 2. Severe elevations in blood pressure can lead to cardiovascular complications, cerebrovascular accidents, or even death. The pathophysiology is associated with unchecked sympathetic outflow triggered by noxious stimuli below the level of injury. The bladder is the most common source of AD, and primary care physicians who care for patients with neurologic conditions must be aware of this condition and be ready to treat it aggressively. The first step is to eliminate the noxious stimulus. In patients with SCI, this elimination can often be accomplished by emptying a distended bladder through catheterization or irrigation of an obstructed catheter. Short-term treatment of hypertension using nitroglycerine paste or sublingual nifedipine is often required, and prevention with the use of oral α-blockers can be effective. In recurrent episodes, a search for an occult urologic cause, such as a calculus or an improper bladder management, should be initiated.[46]

SUMMARY

Patients with lesions of the central nervous system often have neurogenic bladder dysfunction. Lifelong bladder monitoring and management in these patients is necessary to prevent severe complications, including renal damage. The urodynamic test, performed by neurourologists or other specially trained providers, is the definitive test for diagnosis and management of neurogenic bladder dysfunction. This test can help determine if a patient has a safe or an unsafe bladder, and primary care physicians should refer patients for urodynamic testing as soon as neurogenic bladder dysfunction in known or suspected.

REFERENCES

1. Mallory BS, Roppolo JR, de Groat WC. Pharmacological modulation of the pontine micturition center. Brain Res 1991;546(2):310–20.
2. Abrams P, Cardozo L, Fall M, et al. The standardisation of terminology of lower urinary tract function: report from the Standardisation Sub-committee of the International Continence Society. Neurourol Urodyn 2002;21(2):167–78.
3. Blanker MH, Groeneveld FP, Bohnen AM, et al. Voided volumes: normal values and relation to lower urinary tract symptoms in elderly men, a community-based study. Urology 2001;57(6):1093–8 [discussion: 1098–9].
4. Damaser MS. Whole bladder mechanics during filling. Scand J Urol Nephrol Suppl 1999;201:51–8 [discussion: 76–102].
5. Wein AJ. Lower urinary tract dysfunction in neurologic injury and disease. In: Wein AJ, Partin A, Peters C, et al, editors. Campbell-Walsh urology. 9th edition. Philadelphia: Saunders Elsevier; 2007. p. 2014–7, 2037.
6. Heslington K, Hilton P. Ambulatory monitoring and conventional cystometry in asymptomatic female volunteers. Br J Obstet Gynaecol 1996;103(5):434–41.
7. Robertson AS, Griffiths CJ, Ramsden PD, et al. Bladder function in healthy volunteers: ambulatory monitoring and conventional urodynamic studies. Br J Urol 1994;73(3):242–9.
8. Griffiths D, Höfner K, van Mastrigt R, et al. Standardization of terminology of lower urinary tract function: pressure-flow studies of voiding, urethral resistance, and urethral obstruction. International Continence Society Subcommittee on Standardization of Terminology of Pressure-Flow Studies. Neurourol Urodyn 1997;16(1):1–18.
9. Klausner AP, Steers WD. Antimuscarinics for the treatment of overactive bladder: a review of central nervous system effects. Curr Urol Rep 2007;8(6):441–7.

10. Campbell JD, Gries KS, Watanabe JH, et al. Treatment success for overactive bladder with urinary urge incontinence refractory to oral antimuscarinics: a review of published evidence. BMC Urol 2009;9:18.

11. Peters KM, Carrico DJ, Perez-Marrero RA, et al. Randomized trial of percutaneous tibial nerve stimulation versus Sham efficacy in the treatment of overactive bladder syndrome: results from the SUmiT trial. J Urol 2010;183(4): 1438–43.

12. Bennett N, O'Leary M, Patel AS, et al. Can higher doses of oxybutynin improve efficacy in neurogenic bladder? J Urol 2004;171(2 Pt 1):749–51.

13. Hackler RH, Hall MK, Zampieri TA. Bladder hypocompliance in the spinal cord injury population. J Urol 1989;141(6):1390–3.

14. Weld KJ, Graney MJ, Dmochowski RR. Differences in bladder compliance with time and associations of bladder management with compliance in spinal cord injured patients. J Urol 2000;163(4):1228–33.

15. Wyndaele JJ. Correlation between clinical neurological data and urodynamic function in spinal cord injured patients. Spinal Cord 1997;35(4): 213–6.

16. Linsenmeyer TA, Bagaria SP, Gendron B. The impact of urodynamic parameters on the upper tracts of spinal cord injured men who void reflexly. J Spinal Cord Med 1998;21(1):15–20.

17. Buczynski AZ. Urodynamic studies in evaluating detrusor sphincter dyssynergia and their effects on the treatment. Paraplegia 1984;22(3):168–72.

18. Rivas DA, Chancellor MB. Neurogenic vesical dysfunction. Urol Clin North Am 1995;22(3):579–91.

19. Bennett JK, Foote J, El-Leithy TR, et al. Terazosin for vesicosphincter dyssynergia in spinal cord-injured male patients. Mol Urol 2000;4(4):415–20.

20. Chancellor MB, Erhard MJ, Rivas DA. Clinical effect of alpha-1 antagonism by terazosin on external and internal urinary sphincter function. J Am Paraplegia Soc 1993;16(4):207–14.

21. Perkash I. Efficacy and safety of terazosin to improve voiding in spinal cord injury patients. J Spinal Cord Med 1995;18(4):236–9.

22. Swierzewski SJ 3rd, Gormley EA, Belville WD, et al. The effect of terazosin on bladder function in the spinal cord injured patient. J Urol 1994;151(4):951–4.

23. Smith CP, Nishiguchi J, O'Leary M, et al. Single-institution experience in 110 patients with botulinum toxin A injection into bladder or urethra. Urology 2005; 65(1):37–41.

24. Kuo HC. Botulinum A toxin urethral injection for the treatment of lower urinary tract dysfunction. J Urol 2003;170(5):1908–12.

25. Chancellor MB, Gajewski J, Ackman CF, et al. Long-term followup of the North American multicenter UroLume trial for the treatment of external detrusor-sphincter dyssynergia. J Urol 1999;161(5):1545–50.

26. McGuire EJ, Woodside JR, Borden TA, et al. Prognostic value of urodynamic testing in myelodysplastic patients. J Urol 1981;126(2):205–9.

27. Kim YH, Kattan MW, Boone TB. Bladder leak point pressure: the measure for sphincterotomy success in spinal cord injured patients with external detrusor-sphincter dyssynergia. J Urol 1998;159(2):493–6 [discussion: 496–7].

28. Shingleton WB, Bodner DR. The development of urologic complications in relationship to bladder pressure in spinal cord injured patients. J Am Paraplegia Soc 1993;16(1):14–7.

29. Jacobs SC, Kaufman JM. Complications of permanent bladder catheter drainage in spinal cord injury patients. J Urol 1978;119(6):740–1.

30. Selzman AA, Hampel N. Urologic complications of spinal cord injury. Urol Clin North Am 1993;20(3):453–64.

31. Vaidyanathan S, Mansour P, Soni BM, et al. The method of bladder drainage in spinal cord injury patients may influence the histological changes in the mucosa of neuropathic bladder - a hypothesis. BMC Urol 2002;2:5.

32. Cardenas DD, Hooton TM. Urinary tract infection in persons with spinal cord injury. Arch Phys Med Rehabil 1995;76(3):272–80.

33. Wall BM, Huch KM, Mangold TA, et al. Risk factors for development of proteinuria in chronic spinal cord injury. Am J Kidney Dis 1999;33(5):899–903.

34. Chao R, Clowers D, Mayo ME. Fate of upper urinary tracts in patients with indwelling catheters after spinal cord injury. Urology 1993;42(3):259–62.

35. Donnellan SM, Bolton DM. The impact of contemporary bladder management techniques on struvite calculi associated with spinal cord injury. BJU Int 1999; 84(3):280–5.

36. Hess MJ, Zhan EH, Foo DK, et al. Bladder cancer in patients with spinal cord injury. J Spinal Cord Med 2003;26(4):335–8.

37. Andrews HO, Nauth-Misir R, Shah PJ. Iatrogenic hypospadias–a preventable injury? Spinal Cord 1998;36(3):177–80.

38. Lapides J, Diokno AC, Silber SJ, et al. Clean, intermittent self-catheterization in the treatment of urinary tract disease. J Urol 1972;107(3):458–61.

39. Kovindha A, Mai WN, Madersbacher H. Reused silicone catheter for clean intermittent catheterization (CIC): is it safe for spinal cord-injured (SCI) men? Spinal Cord 2004;42(11):638–42.

40. Kuhn W, Rist M, Zaech GA. Intermittent urethral self-catheterisation: long term results (bacteriological evolution, continence, acceptance, complications). Paraplegia 1991;29(4):222–32.

41. Perrouin-Verbe B, Labat JJ, Richard I, et al. Clean intermittent catheterisation from the acute period in spinal cord injury patients. Long term evaluation of urethral and genital tolerance. Paraplegia 1995;33(11):619–24.

42. Feifer A, Corcos J. Contemporary role of suprapubic cystostomy in treatment of neuropathic bladder dysfunction in spinal cord injured patients. Neurourol Urodyn 2008;27(6):475–9.

43. Liedl B. Catheter-associated urinary tract infections. Curr Opin Urol 2001;11(1): 75–9.

44. Morton SC, Shekelle PG, Adams JL, et al. Antimicrobial prophylaxis for urinary tract infection in persons with spinal cord dysfunction. Arch Phys Med Rehabil 2002;83(1):129–38.

45. Lee BB, Haran MJ, Hunt LM, et al. Spinal-injured neuropathic bladder antisepsis (SINBA) trial. Spinal Cord 2007;45(8):542–50.

46. Krassioukov A, Warburton DE, Teasell R, et al. A systematic review of the management of autonomic dysreflexia after spinal cord injury. Arch Phys Med Rehabil 2009;90(4):682–95.

Assessment and Management of Irritative Voiding Symptoms

Michael L. Guralnick, MD, FRCS(C)[*,1], R. Corey O'Connor, MD[1],
William A. See, MD

KEYWORDS

• LUTS • Irritative voiding symptoms • Evaluation

Irritative voiding symptoms are to the urinary tract much as a cough is to the pulmonary system, that is, a nonspecific manifestation of multiple potential underlying causes. Similar to the lungs, the urinary bladder responds to a spectrum of pathologic processes with a limited repertoire of symptoms. Irrespective of whether the underlying disease is neoplastic, inflammatory, infectious, obstructive, iatrogenic, or neurogenic, irritative voiding constitutes the bladder's symptomatic manifestation of the disease.

Irritative symptoms of the lower urinary tract generally refer to urinary urgency, frequency, nocturia, painful voiding, bladder discomfort, or stranguria (**Box 1**). Although severity may vary over time, symptoms typically occur throughout the day and night. It is particularly important to recognize that the absence of nighttime symptoms are often less suggestive of significant abnormality. Given the association of irritative voiding symptoms with both common and uncommon urologic diseases, practitioners in the primary care setting frequently encounter patients with these symptoms as their chief complaint. Key to the evaluation and management of these patients is a clear understanding of the differential diagnosis, the diagnostic tests required for evaluation, and the role of specialists in diagnosis and treatment.

Lower urinary tract symptoms (LUTS) are common and increase with age. Two recent population-based survey studies demonstrated that 60% to 70% of men and women admit to some degree of LUTS.[4,5] Irritative or storage LUTS were noted in 59% of women and 51% of men in an international, cross-sectional telephone survey.[4]

---

[1]These authors contributed equally to the preparation of this article and as such are co-first authors.

Department of Urology, Medical College of Wisconsin, 9200 West Wisconsin Avenue, Milwaukee, WI 53226, USA

* Corresponding author.

E-mail address: mguralni@mcw.edu

Med Clin N Am 95 (2011) 121–127
doi:10.1016/j.mcna.2010.08.025
0025-7125/11/$ – see front matter © 2011 Elsevier Inc. All rights reserved.

Box 1
Irritative voiding symptom components and definitions

Urinary urgency: sudden desire to empty the bladder, which is difficult to defer[1]

Urinary frequency: eight or more voids in a 24-hour period[2]

Nocturia: waking up one or more times from nighttime sleep to void[3]

Painful urination (formerly dysuria): burning or stinging of the urethra and meatus associated with voiding[1]

Bladder discomfort: suprapubic or retropubic pain, pressure, or discomfort that usually increase with increased bladder volumes[1]

Stranguria: constant and penetrating sensation of needing to void, with the inability to produce urine

---

A similar Internet-based questionnaire found that 20% to 30% of adults older than 40 years reported symptoms of urgency, frequency, nocturia, or urge incontinence. The study also noted that 5% of men and 8% of women reported bladder pain; painful urination was found in 3% of adults. In addition, patients with the most severe LUTS had the greatest degree of bother, highest rates of clinical anxiety or depression, and the lowest quality of life.[5]

Other medical comorbidities are also commonly associated with LUTS. Obesity, alcohol consumption, smoking, diabetes, osteoarthritis, heart disease, and hypertension are just some of the medical conditions that have been positively associated with increased LUTS.[6,7] There is some evidence that chronic inflammation as measured using the levels of C-reactive protein may be associated with LUTS in men and women.[8]

A complete list of differential diagnoses for irritative voiding symptoms is listed in **Box 2**. Many of these diseases are addressed in detail in other articles in this issue. This article outlines a general diagnostic approach for patients with irritative voiding symptoms. Treatment approaches for the diseases, as well as the initial management that may be performed in the primary care setting, are also discussed.

EVALUATION AND MANAGEMENT

The initial evaluation of irritative voiding symptoms begins with a complete history and physical assessment, including abdominal and pelvic/rectal examination. Urinalysis, urine microscopy, and urine culture should also be performed to rule out bacteruria, pyuria, glucosuria, or microscopic hematuria. Significant microscopic hematuria in the absence of bacteruria can be defined as 3 or more red blood cells per high-powered microscopic field from 2 of 3 properly collected, centrifuged midstream urine specimens.[9] Findings that warrant referral for further investigation include hematuria without bacteruria, a past history of urothelial cancer now presenting with LUTS, or persistent pyuria on urinalysis despite negative urine culture (sterile pyuria).

Gonorrhea/chlamydia cultures or postprostatic massage urine cultures should be considered if clinically indicated. A urine cytology specimen to test for the presence of malignant cells should generally be obtained for patients with irritative symptoms at risk for bladder malignancy (eg, smokers) and for those with hematuria without bacteruria.

A postvoid residual urine measurement by either bladder ultrasonography or straight catheterization should be considered to exclude urinary retention as a cause of irritative voiding symptoms. A 24- or 48-hour fluid intake and voiding diary can provide an objective measure of fluid intake, voiding frequency, and voided volume and is an important part of the evaluation to rule out polydipsia or polyuria as a cause of irritative voiding.[10] Upper-tract imaging with and without intravenous contrast may be indicated to rule out a renal source of bleeding in patients with hematuria.[9] However, in general, all patients with gross hematuria and those with microscopic hematuria in the absence of infection should be referred for specialist evaluation. Cystoscopy is performed in select patients with irritative voiding symptoms to evaluate for foreign bodies within the bladder and rule out urothelial disease, especially in patients with associated hematuria. Urodynamics, with or without concomitant fluoroscopy, may be helpful to determine storage and emptying characteristics of the bladder, but these specialized tests are done at the discretion of a urologist. A more detailed description of the evaluation of LUTS is presented in another article by Claus G. Roehrborn; Donna Y. Deng elsewhere in this issue.

Primary care physicians should feel comfortable with the initial evaluation and management of patients with irritative voiding symptoms. The primary diagnosis that should be ruled out at the time of initial presentation of a patient with irritative LUTS is urinary tract infection (UTI). An infection causes a local inflammatory response, which can manifest as pyuria and/or hematuria and lead to the irritative symptoms. Although negative urinalysis and microscopy results do not always exclude a pathologic condition, a study that shows the absence of blood and leukocytes in the urine can generally be accepted as a good indicator of the absence of UTI. Urinalysis demonstrating pyuria with or without microscopic hematuria can initially be assumed to be the result of a bacterial UTI. A patient may empirically be treated with antibiotics; however, urine culture with antibiotic sensitivity testing should be performed before administering the first antibiotic dose to confirm or exclude UTI as the cause of the irritative symptoms.

If the result of a urine culture is negative despite a positive urinalysis result and LUTS persist despite antibiotics, a repeat urinalysis should be performed to evaluate for ongoing pyuria/hematuria. Such patients may have an infection that is not identified by routine laboratory culture techniques (eg, mycoplasmic or ureaplasmic infection, tuberculosis, schistosomiasis) or a noninfectious cause (eg, stone or foreign body, urothelial tumor). Mycoplasmic or ureaplasmic organisms are notoriously difficult to culture. Some investigators suggest treating women with chronic irritative LUTS (and their sexual partners) with a tetracycline antibiotic.[11] Genitourinary tuberculosis or schistosomiasis should be suspected based on a history of travel to an endemic area or known contact exposure. Testing and treatment of these entities can be difficult and warrant infectious disease specialist referral. Similarly, patients with a history of bladder cancer treated with intravesical therapy who present with irritative LUTS in the absence of bacteriuria should be referred to a urologist for further evaluation to exclude recurrent disease.

Prior treatment of lower urinary tract cancer (bladder, prostate, or urethra) using modalities such as surgery, irradiation, cryotherapy, high-intensity focused ultrasound, or chemotherapy may result in local inflammation and subsequent irritative LUTS. Urinalysis may show pyuria and/or hematuria. Culture should be obtained to ensure that UTI is not the primary cause of symptoms. A negative culture result should warrant a urologic referral to evaluate further for recurrent cancer. Cyclophosphamide, often used to treat hematologic malignancies, is a known urothelial carcinogen as well as a potential bladder irritant and cause of hematuria. Patients with a history of cyclophosphamide exposure who present with irritative LUTS (especially if associated with hematuria) should be referred to a urologist for further investigation. Another possible

Box 2
Differential diagnoses of irritative voiding symptoms

Infectious

    Bacterial

    Parasitic

    Tuberculosis

    Viral

Iatrogenic

    Bladder or prostate surgery

    Pelvic radiotherapy

    Indwelling bladder catheter

Congenital

    Bladder exstrophy

    Epispadias

    Posterior urethral valves

Drugs

    Cyclophosphamide

    Intravesical chemotherapy or immunotherapy

    Diuretics

Obstruction

    Urethral stricture

    Prostatic hyperplasia

    Dysfunctional voiding

    Prior urethral surgery

Inflammation

    Foreign body (bladder calculus, ureteral stent)

    Vesicoenteric fistula

Metabolic

    Hyperglycemia

    Postobstructive diuresis

Neoplastic

    Urothelial carcinoma

    Locally advanced prostatic cancer

    Extrinsic pelvic mass

    Metastatic disease

Neurologic

    Myelomeningocele

    Cerebrovascular accident

    Multiple sclerosis

    Spinal cord injury

Spinal surgery

Parkinson disease

Pelvic surgery

Behavioral /Psychogenic

Hinman syndrome[a]

Chronic constipation

Water intoxication

Acquired/other

Idiopathic detrusor overactivity or hypersensate bladder

Pelvic organ prolapse

Estrogen deficiency

Dementia

Sleep apnea

Diabetes insipidus

Painful bladder syndrome

Fluid shifts

Postsurgical

Peripheral edema

[a] Hinman syndrome: nonneurogenic, neurogenic voiding dysfunction, essentially dysfunctional voiding (failure to relax sphincter while trying to urinate) associated with volitional avoidance of voiding or infrequent bladder emptying that can ultimately result in severe bladder and renal dysfunction.

inflammatory cause is a foreign body within the bladder. Prior pelvic surgery can result in the inadvertent placement or erosion of suture material or clip into the bladder, with resultant irritative LUTS. Self-insertion of foreign bodies into the urinary tract by the patient has also been widely reported. Urinary tract calculi, especially within the distal ureter or bladder, often result in irritative LUTS. Patients presenting with irritative LUTS in the absence of UTI, especially if associated with abdominal or flank pain, may be evaluated with a noncontrast computed tomography of the abdomen and pelvis to rule out calculi or other foreign bodies within the urinary tract.

Patients with neurologic diseases often have associated LUTS. As with other patients, it is important to rule out infection, hematuria, and incomplete bladder emptying as possible causes of symptoms. In the absence of infection, urologic referral is generally warranted for further neurourologic evaluation. Treatment, although tailored to the individual patient, often involves a combination of anticholinergics, α-blockers, and clean intermittent catheterization.

Vaginal prolapse and pelvic floor disorders (eg, pelvic floor myalgia) are also associated with irritative LUTS. Physical examination is needed to establish the diagnosis. Patients with pelvic floor dysfunction may report the sensation of urinary urgency during pelvic examination with palpation of the levator muscles. Pelvic floor (Kegel) exercises or pelvic floor physical therapy and other behavioral modification approaches (fluid management, bladder retraining) are the mainstays in the initial management of these symptoms, as discussed in the article by Donna Y. Deng elsewhere in this issue. Biofeedback is often used in patients with poor control of their pelvic floor muscles to teach proper contraction of the pelvic floor musculature. Anticholinergic medications (eg, oxybutynin, 2.5–5 mg 2–4 times a day; tolterodine, 4 mg every day; solifenacin, 5–10 mg every day; darifenacin, 7.5–15 mg every day; fesoterodine, 4–8 mg every day) may provide beneficial symptomatic improvement. Pelvic organ prolapse up to or beyond the hymen (stage 2 or greater) warrants specialist referral for possible pessary fitting or surgical correction. Urogenital atrophy, which develops postmenopausally, is known to affect sensory thresholds in the lower urinary tract, resulting in irritative LUTS.[12] Vaginal reestrogenization using cream or vaginal suppositories can improve urinary symptoms. A subset of young, healthy women may begin to experience irritative LUTS after taking oral contraceptives. Vaginal reestrogenization with low-dose topical estrogen (cream or suppository) can often dramatically improve their voiding symptoms within a month.[13]

Central to the management of any patient with irritative LUTS is the appropriate management of fluid intake. A reasonable daily fluid intake ranges from 40 to 60 fl oz. Thus, the popular concept of the need to consume eight 8-ounce glasses of water each day (64 fl oz) is acceptable provided that not much more fluid is consumed through food or other beverages. However, many patients consume 8 glasses of water in addition to other liquids such as coffee and tea. The end result is invariably polyuria. Furthermore, some fluids are notorious for their irritant effect on the bladder: caffeine, soda (particularly diet soda), alcohol, and citrus beverages. Patients with irritative LUTS should minimize intake of or avoid these fluids if it has been demonstrated that their consumption aggravates urinary symptoms. Iatrogenic polyuria related to the use of diuretic medication to treat hypertension, edema, or *congestive heart failure* is another common cause of urinary frequency. In addition, taking diuretics before going to bed is a preventable cause of nocturia. Proper education as to the need for the medication and the anticipated effects on urine output and urinary frequency is crucial in the management of this issue and patients' expectations.

Constipation is a well-recognized bladder irritant. The rectum and bladder lie in close proximity. Constipation causes the rectum to distend and compress the posterior bladder surface. The end result is worsening irritative voiding symptoms. Aggressive management of constipation is crucial in the treatment of patients with irritative or storage LUTS.

SUMMARY

Irritative voiding symptoms occur with a high prevalence in the general population. Many of these individuals present to their primary caretaker for the initial evaluation of their symptoms. As such, it is important that general practitioners and internists have a clear understanding of the causes of irritative voiding symptoms and the appropriate initial evaluation. By distinguishing patients with common, readily treatable causes from those requiring a more complex evaluation, the treating physician can optimize patient care and maximize the efficient use of resources.

REFERENCES

1. Haylen BT, de Ridder D, Freeman RM, et al. An International Urogynecological Association (IUGA)/International Continence Society (ICS) joint report on the terminology for female pelvic floor dysfunction. Neurourol Urodyn 2010;29:4–20.
2. Warren JW, Meyer WA, Greenberg P, et al. Using the International Continence Society's definition of painful bladder syndrome. Urology 2006;67:1138–42 [discussion: 1142–3].

3. Van Kerrebroeck P, Abrams P, Chaikin D, et al. The standardization of terminology in nocturia: report from the standardization subcommittee of the International Continence Society. BJU Int 2002;90(Suppl 3):11–5.

4. Irwin DE, Milsom I, Hunskaar S, et al. Population-based survey of urinary incontinence, overactive bladder, and other lower urinary tract symptoms in five countries: results of the epic study. Eur Urol 2006;50:1306–14 [discussion: 1314–5].

5. Coyne KS, Sexton CC, Thompson CL, et al. The prevalence of lower urinary tract symptoms (LUTS) in the USA, the UK and Sweden: results from the Epidemiology of LUTS (EPILUTS) Study. BJU Int 2009;104:352–60.

6. Seim A, Hoyo C, Ostbye T, et al. The prevalence and correlates of urinary tract symptoms in Norwegian men: the HUNT study. BJU Int 2005;96:88–92.

7. Kupelian V, McVary KT, Kaplan SA, et al. Association of lower urinary tract symptoms and the metabolic syndrome: results from the Boston Area Community Health Survey. J Urol 2009;182:616–24 [discussion: 624–5].

8. Kupelian V, McVary KT, Barry MJ, et al. Association of C-reactive protein and lower urinary tract symptoms in men and women: results from Boston Area Community Health Survey. Urology 2009;73:950–7.

9. Grossfeld GD, Wolf JS Jr, Litwan MS, et al. Asymptomatic microscopic hematuria in adults: summary of the AUA best practice policy recommendations. Am Fam Physician 2001;63:1145–54.

10. Weiss JP. Nocturia: "do the math". J Urol 2006;175:S16–8.

11. Burkhard FC, Blick N, Hochreiter WW, et al. Urinary urgency and frequency, and chronic urethral and/or pelvic pain in females. Can doxycycline help? J Urol 2004; 172:232–5.

12. Klutke JJ, Bergman A. Hormonal influence on the urinary tract. Urol Clin North Am 1995;22:629–39.

13. Pinggera GM, Feuchtner G, Frauscher F, et al. Effects of local estrogen therapy on recurrent urinary tract infections in young females under oral contraceptives. Eur Urol 2005;47:243–9.

Urologic Aspects of HIV Infection

Alan W. Shindel, MD[a,b], Ardavan Akhavan, MD[c],
Ira D. Sharlip, MD[a],*

KEYWORDS

- Human immunodeficiency virus • Genitourinary infection
- Genitourinary tumors • Erectile dysfunction
- Male circumcision

In 2008, UNAIDS (Joint United Nations Program on HIV/AIDS) and the World Health Organization estimated that approximately 33.4 million people worldwide were infected with human immunodeficiency virus (HIV), the pathogen that causes acquired immune deficiency syndrome (AIDS).[1] About 1.4 million of these people were living in North America.[1] It is estimated that there were 55,000 new cases of HIV infection in the United States in 2008.[1]

Urologic manifestations of HIV/AIDS play an important role in the overall morbidity of this disease state; familiarity with these conditions is critical for physicians caring for the HIV/AIDS patient. In this review, the authors highlight some of the most common urologic manifestations of HIV infection with respect to both evaluation and treatment. Management suggestions for the primary care physician are included as well as advice on when urologic consultation should be considered. The authors also briefly consider the role of circumcision in prevention of HIV in sub-Saharan Africa, a region where the virus is endemic.

INFECTIONS

Genito-urinary infections are one of the most important defining characteristics of HIV infection and AIDS. HIV binds to CD4 immune cells and replicates rapidly, leading to progressive decline in CD4 lymphocyte count and subsequent loss of immune system function. Loss of immune function increases the risk of urinary tract infection (UTI) with *Escherichia coli* and other common uropathogens. In addition to greater susceptibility

[a] Department of Urology, University of California at San Francisco, 400 Parnassus Avenue, Suite A-660, San Francisco, CA 94143-0738, USA
[b] Department of Urology, University of California at Davis, 4860 Y Street, Suite 3500, Sacramento, CA 95817, USA
[c] Department of Urology, Mount Sinai Medical Center, One Gustave L. Levy Place, New York, NY 10029, USA
* Corresponding author. Department of Urology, University of California at San Francisco, 2100 Webster Street, Suite 222, San Francisco, CA 94115.
E-mail address: isharlip@aol.com

Med Clin N Am 95 (2011) 129–151
doi:10.1016/j.mcna.2010.08.017   medical.theclinics.com

to common uropathogens, HIV-positive (HIV+) people with CD4 counts below 500/mm^3 are at increased risk for opportunistic infections; this risk increases dramatically when the CD4 count falls to less than 200/mm^3.[2]

Bladder Infections

Bacterial UTI is more common in HIV+ individuals relative to HIV-negative (HIV−) people, although the difference is driven in large part by those HIV+ patients with CD4 counts less than 500.[3,4] Immunosuppression is the principal factor driving the increased incidence of UTI in this population. Voiding dysfunction (more common in the HIV+ population and addressed later in this article) may also predispose HIV+ patients to poorer clearance of pathogens from the urinary tract.[3] Given differences in perineal anatomy, women are much more likely to contract bladder level infections than men; men who are uncircumcised are more likely than circumcised men to develop a UTI but the increase in risk is not great.

Cystitis in the HIV+ population is associated with typical uropathogens (*E coli*, *Enterobacter*, *Proteus*, *Klebsiella*, and other gram-negative bacteria).[3,5,6] *Salmonella* UTI is of particular concern; this infection needs to be aggressively managed with lifelong prophylactic suppression, as this pathogen carries a high risk of fatal recurrence.[7]

Patients with bladder infections may present to their primary care physicians with complaints of urinary urgency, frequency, dysuria, hematuria, and/or malodorous urine. In HIV+ patients with CD4 counts above 500, workup and treatment of these symptoms should be similar to what is done for HIV− patients, namely history and physical examination (H&P), urinalysis, and routine urine bacterial culture. The H&P should focus on localizing the infection, ruling out any underlying voiding dysfunction or potential nidus for recurrent infection, and assessment for signs of systemic disease. HIV+ patients should be treated initially with broad-spectrum antibiotics after a urine culture is obtained; antibiotics should be continued until sensitivities are available. A prolonged course (at least 7–10 days) of antibiotics should be given because of the increased risk of UTI recurrence.[3,5,6] If there are systemic symptoms or signs of urosepsis, consideration should be given to imaging of the upper tracts to rule out pyelonephritis or urinary obstruction.

HIV+ patients who do not respond after a few days of empiric antibiotics and those with CD4 counts less than 500 should be screened for atypical and opportunistic infections; suspicion should be particularly high in those with CD4 counts less than 250.[5] Organisms of particular concern include: fungi such as *Candida*, *Aspergillus*, *Blastomyces*, *Cryptococcus*, *Cryptosporidia*, and *Histoplasma*; parasites such as *Toxoplasma* and *Pneumocystis*; *Mycobacterium tuberculosis*; and viruses such as cytomegalovirus (CMV) and adenovirus.[5] In general, culture is sufficient for diagnosis of these pathogens although diagnosis of viral infection may require urologic consultation for tissue biopsy.[2,5] Prolonged therapy with appropriately selected agents is the rule to prevent recurrence or upper tract progression.

Kidney Infections

HIV patients are more prone to infections of the upper urinary tract.[5] HIV+ patients who present with signs of cystitis and systemic symptoms such as fever, flank pain, and/or hemodynamic instability should be given a provisional diagnosis of pyelonephritis. All HIV+ patients with suspected pyelonephritis and CD4 counts less than 500 should be cultured for opportunistic pathogens, started empirically on broad-spectrum antibiotics, and imaged with either ultrasonography or computed tomography (CT).[2,8] Evidence of nephrocalcinosis or hypoechoic mass lesions on ultrasonography or cross-sectional imaging may indicate infection with opportunistic pathogens. Imaging may also reveal hydronephrosis, nephrolithiasis, or fluid collection within the kidney or the perirenal space. Any of these findings should prompt immediate urologic consultation for consideration of management options, including ureteral stent placement and open versus percutaneous drainage of fluid collections.[9] Placement of a Foley catheter to decompress the urinary system may help to clear infected urine in this context.

Gram-negative bacteria are the most common cause of pyelonephritis in general, including the HIV+ population. The most common opportunistic renal pathogens in the HIV+ population are *Pneumocystis carinii*, *Mycobaterium* species, *Candida*, and *Histoplasmosis*. A urologist should be consulted in all diagnosed cases of opportunistic infection of the kidney to help determine whether a nephrectomy, either immediate or delayed, is necessary; this may be more often the case in cases of mycobacterial infections.

Mycobacterial infection of the kidney is detected at autopsy in 6% to 23% of AIDS patients; a significant proportion of these had not experienced symptoms of infection prior to death.[2,10,11] The most common mycobacterial organism is *M tuberculosis*, followed by *M avium* and *M intracellulare*. Mycobacterial infection of the genitourinary tract typically presents in a descending fashion, with renal involvement preceding lower tract disease. After initial infection, the disease can remain latent for years until a single focus reactivates. If renal tuberculosis is suspected, Ziehl-Nielsen stain of a urine specimen may be performed, with high specificity (96.7%), but poor sensitivity (42.1%–52.1%). Urine culture for acid-fast bacilli (AFB) has higher sensitivity, but given the fastidious nature of bacilli in urine, 3 to 6 early morning cultures must be drawn separately and results may take up to 6 weeks.[12] The polymerase chain reaction may be useful as a rapid assay to detect *M tuberculosis*–specific DNA or RNA materials in the urine.[13,14]

When mycobacterial infection of the urinary tract is diagnosed, treatment with long-term antimycobacterial agents is standard. Of note, in HIV+ patients rifampin induces cytochrome P450, which lowers concentrations of protease inhibitors and nonnucleoside reverse transcriptase inhibitors; drug levels should be monitored and adjusted accordingly.[15] On follow-up, viable bacilli can be detected in urine after up to 9 months of treatment in HIV– patients; relapse rate in HIV– individuals is 6.3%,[16] and HIV+ patients are known to have 10 times the risk of reactivation of latent mycobacterial disease relative to HIV– patients.[17,18] Primary care doctors should follow these patients with annual urine culture for AFB up to 10 years after treatment to screen for reactivation of disease.

Prostate Infections

Prostatitis is diagnosed in 3% of men with HIV and in 14% of those with AIDS, compared with rates of 1% to 2% in the general population.[19] Typical symptoms of prostatitis include chronic pelvic pain, dysuria, frequency, urgency, and other lower urinary tract symptoms. This diagnosis should be considered in cases where symptoms persist after a 1- to 2-week course of antibiotic therapy and/or there is concomitant perineal or pelvic pain. Prostatitis can be diagnosed by gentle digital rectal examination of the prostate, which may be revealing of fluctuance and extreme tenderness. Culture of expressed prostatic secretions or post-prostate massage urine may be useful in some cases, but the diagnostic yield of this procedure in definitively isolating a pathogenic organism is unclear.[20] In cases where there are concomitant signs of urosepsis, CT scan of the pelvis or transrectal ultrasound imaging of the prostate should be performed to rule out prostatic abscess, which is common in HIV+ patients with CD4 counts 3500/mm^3.[21,22]

Prolonged treatment with antibiotics that have a good capacity for penetration into the prostate (typically 4–6 weeks of fluoroquinolone or sulfa antibiotic) are a frequent first-line therapy. Even after antibiotic treatment of bacterial prostatitis, up to 70% of HIV+ patients have relapsing symptoms, so retreatment is common.[5,6,19] Special consideration must be given to cryptococcal prostatitis, which may persist after treatment in up to 29% of cases, and may serve as a reservoir for relapsing meningitis; these patients require long-term or even lifelong antifungals depending on immune status.[2]

Urologic consultation is warranted in cases of prostatitis that is refractory or recurrent after a 4- to 6-week course of appropriate antibiotics or when prostate abscess is present, as this may necessitate transurethral unroofing, transperineal aspiration, or transrectal aspiration.[3,21]

Testicular and Epididymal Infections

Infection of the epididymis and/or testicle is a common finding in men with HIV; indeed, epididymo-orchitis has been reported as a common "presenting" manifestation of HIV infection.[23] These infections tend to be chronic and recurrent; it has been observed that obstructive changes within the tubular structures of the epididymis are common in AIDS patients. These changes are likely due to persistent inflammation, and may predispose patients to recurrent infections from inadequate clearance of tubular secretions.[24]

Autopsy studies of AIDS patients who succumbed to systemic opportunistic infections demonstrated that 25 to 39% of men had identical organisms harvested from their testes, suggesting that the testes and epididymes may be a reservoir for delayed and potentially life-threatening opportunistic infection. The most common organisms isolated from the testes in these cases were *Gonococcus*, *Salmonella*, CMV, *Mycobacterium avium intracellulare*, *Toxoplasma*, *Histoplasma*, and *Candida*.[5,25] Again, *Salmonella* infection in the urinary tract is difficult to eradicate and can result in overwhelming sepsis, so lifelong prophylaxis is the rule after this entity has been identified.[6,7]

The most common symptom of epididymo-orchitis is severe pain posterior to the testicle, although many men localize the pain to the testicle itself. Men with epididymo-orchitis may have concomitant symptoms of bladder level infection; like prostatitis, epididymo-orchitis should be considered when antibiotics fail to clear symptoms of UTI. Physical examination is typically revealing of unilateral swelling and exquisite tenderness of the testis and/or epididymis, which can be severe. Ultrasound evaluation may be considered to rule out abscess or other causes of scrotal pain such as testicular tumor and spermatic cord torsion.

Standard management is with urine culture-specific antibiotics for 4 to 6 weeks. If cultures are not available or are negative, doxycycline and a fluoroquinolone may be administered for 2 to 4 weeks.[5] Urgent urologic consultation is warranted when evaluation reveals testicular tumor, spermatic cord torsion, or abscess. In cases where infection fails to resolve or when pain is intractable to analgesic management, urologic intervention may also be considered for epididymectomy or orchiectomy. This approach is more often necessary in men with HIV infection as compared with men without HIV infection.[23]

Urethritis

Urethritis in HIV+ patients often manifests with dysuria and urethral discharge. Urethritis is usually presumed to be secondary to infection with *Chlamydia* and/or gonorrhea. Gonorrhea is of particular importance, as it has been demonstrated to increase the infectivity of HIV.

Appropriate culture swabs of the urethra should be obtained and treatment initiated with ciprofloxacin 500 mg, cefixime 400 mg, or ofloxacin 400 g as a single dose, AND azithromycin 1 g as a single dose or doxycycline 100 mg twice daily for 7 days.[5] Patients with urethritis should be re-educated on safer sex practices, and use of barriers and partner screening is warranted. If symptoms of urethral irritation and pain persist after appropriate antibiotic therapy, urologic referral for cystoscopy should be considered.

Ulcerating Skin Infections

The most common cause of genital ulcers in the HIV patient is sexually transmitted infections (STI) such as herpes (painful grouped vesicles on an erythematous base from infection with herpes simplex virus), syphilis (painless ulcer in the primary phase of the disease from infection with *Treponema pallidum*), and chancroid (painful genital ulceration from infection with *Haemophilus ducreyi*). Systemic viral illnesses such as shingles and CMV are additional considerations as risk factors for genital ulcer disease in HIV+ individuals.[5] Certain medications that may be used more frequently in the HIV+ population may also lead to cutaneous genital manifestations. Urinary excretion of the antiviral drug foscarnet may lead to genital ulceration. Treatment with sulfa-based antibiotics has also been associated with new onset of a maculopapular, morbiliform rash that may involved the genitals.[2,26–28]

Genital ulcers in HIV+ patients should be swabbed and assessed with Tzanck smear to rule out herpes simplex and CMV infection. If positive, treatment with acyclovir and/or foscarnet should be initiated to resolve the symptoms. Suppressive therapy with famciclovir may help to reduce future outbreaks. Syphilis is typically treated with intravenous penicillin G, although doxycycline and ceftriaxone may be considered in patients allergic to penicillin.[29] Chancroid responds well to treatment with azithromycin or triamphenicol.[30]

Nonulcerating Skin Infections

Genital warts (condyloma acuminata) are present in 20% of HIV patients compared with 0.1% of the general population, and are caused by the human papilloma virus (HPV); HPV 6 and 11 are the most common. These lesions are typically raised, flesh-colored lesions that may have a "cauliflower-like" appearance. Treatment is via topical preparations including podophyllotoxin, trichloroacetic acid, interferon, or imiquimod. In cases with extensive or recurrent disease, dermatologic or urologic consultation for biopsy and further management may be indicated. Management in these specialized cases may be by surgical resection using laser vaporization, cryotherapy, electrocauterization, or excision.[5]

Molluscum contagiosum are raised, papular lesions that typically occur in clusters and are caused by a pox virus. These lesions may be self-limited in healthy individuals but this may not occur in patients with HIV. Approximately 5% to 18% of HIV patients have evidence of molluscum contagiosum. Treatment of these entities is similar to that of genital warts. Molluscum infection increases the risk of secondary bacterial infections and should therefore be managed as more than a cosmetic issue.[5,31]

HIV patients are at greater risk of cellulitis of the perineum, which presents with erythema and pain. Management is with antibiotics having gram-positive activity; consideration should also be given to treatment using drugs having activity against methicillin-resistant *Staphylococcus aureus* (MRSA). It is of particular importance to consider the diagnosis of Fournier gangrene, a form of necrotizing fasciitis involving the perineum and genitalia. Fournier typically presents with rapidly progressing erythema and necrosis of the perineal or genital skin, and is often associated with signs of systemic sepsis. Physical examination should include digital rectal examination, and may be revealing of erythema, crepitus, and even frank necrosis. Emergent urologic and surgical consultation for wide debridement is necessary in this setting; even with prompt management, mortality rates are very high.[5]

HEMATURIA

Microscopic hematuria occurs in 20% to 35% of HIV patients; the likelihood of blood in the urine is greater in patients with more advanced disease and lower CD4 counts. Hematuria may be a sign of other disease processes within the genitourinary tract: an infectious cause can be detected in 35% of cases, HIV-associated nephropathy (HIVAN) in 13%, and urolithiasis in 13%.[32] In a 2-year follow-up study of young (mean age 32 years for men and 30 for women) HIV patients with microscopic hematuria, none of 67 fully evaluated were diagnosed with malignancy. Etiology for hematuria was determined in 31 (46%) cases; in just 3 of these cases was treatment beyond antibiotics required and all 3 of these cases presented with additional urologic symptoms. Hence, it has been recommended that assessment of creatinine and urine culture are the only tests routinely indicated for young patients with asymptomatic microscopic hematuria and no other risk factors for urinary tract malignancy.[32] The decision on whether to pursue upper tract imaging, cystoscopy, and/or urinary cytology should be based on other signs/symptoms and risk factors, including patient age. Consultation with a urologist may help to guide decision making in these patients.

VOIDING DYSFUNCTION

Lower urinary tract symptoms (LUTS) are a common source of morbidity in the HIV+ population and tend to worsen as the disease progresses. LUTS, including acute urinary retention and sacral sensory loss, may also be the sentinel event that presages HIV seroconversion; this is likely secondary to transient neurologic symptoms, which may occur with acute HIV infection.[2,5,33]

LUTS may be loosely categorized as irritative (including urgency, dysuria, frequency, incontinence) or obstructive (hesitancy, nocturia, stranguria, urinary retention, intermittency), although there tends to be a great deal of overlap between the 2 categories. It is often difficult to definitively diagnose the cause of LUTS based on symptoms alone. A basic evaluation, including history and physical examination, may rule out several common causes of this troublesome condition. Patients who drink copious amounts of fluid, particularly caffeinated or alcoholic beverages, may be prone to LUTS; lifestyle changes may mitigate against this. Evaluation of the genitals (including the prostate in men) may reveal anatomic variants that predispose to urinary difficulty, such as meatal stenosis or an enlarged prostate. LUTS are often related to UTI in HIV+ individuals, and for this reason urine culture is always indicated in the HIV+ patient with new-onset urinary symptoms.[2,5,34] Assessment of postvoid residual urine by ultrasonography or postvoid catheterization may determine if there is an element of urinary retention.

Neurologic conditions that may lead to voiding dysfunction include cerebral toxoplasmosis, HIV encephalitis, HIV demyelination disorders, CMV polyradiculopathy, central nervous system neoplasms, AIDS-related dementia, peripheral neuropathies, and side effects of highly active antiretroviral treatment (HAART) or other medications.[2,5–7,22,35–38] Awareness of CMV infection is of particular importance in the HIV+ patient. Indolent CMV infection is present in the majority (90%) of the adult population. With HIV infection and low CD4 counts, there is a greater than 40% rate of virus reactivation with subsequent risk of bladder end-organ damage and life-threatening infection.[39] In situations where there is combined bladder dysfunction, bowel dysfunction, and back or sciatic pain, the diagnosis of CMV polyradiculopathy should be considered and lumbar puncture performed immediately for diagnosis; this condition may be reversible if detected early.[40]

Treatment of urinary symptoms in the HIV patient should be individualized to the patient's specific symptom complex. Empiric treatment with an oral medication may be initiated before referral to a urologist.[41] Anticholinergics (oxybutinin, tolterodine, and others) are the first-line therapy of choice for irritative urinary symptoms in women, and are available as oral pills and transdermal patches or gels. These medications are generally well tolerated but carry the risk of anticholinergic effects such as dry mouth and constipation. Older-generation anticholinergics may also impair central nervous system cholinergic function, so caution should be used when prescribing to HIV+ patients with neurologic diseases; in these situations a newer and more selective agent should be considered. α-Blockers (including terazosin, doxazosin, tamsulosin, and alfuzozsin) and/or 5α-reductase inhibitors (finasteride, dutasteride) should be considered in men with obstructive symptoms and may be of benefit for men with irritative symptoms. α-Blocker medications tend to produce a more rapid onset of symptomatic relief, although 5α-reductase inhibitors are superior at preventing progression of disease.[42] Anticholinergics are another option in the management of irritative urinary symptoms in men, although in most cases α-blockers are considered first-line treatment. Theoretically, anticholinergic drugs may precipitate urinary retention in men with prostatic enlargement, but the actual incidence of this adverse event appears to be very low.[43] A simplified algorithm for management of LUTS is presented in **Fig. 1**.

If first-line oral therapy for LUTS fails, referral to a urologist should be considered. Urologists may perform cystoscopy for direct visual assessment of the urethra, prostate, and bladder and/or urodynamic testing as a functional test of lower urinary tract function. Urodynamics, including cystometry, are particularly useful in the setting of recurrent failure of treatment or when surgical options are being considered.[37] Objective cystometric abnormalities are very frequent in the HIV+ population. The most common findings include detrusor-sphincter dyssnergia (loss of coordinated activity between the detrusor muscle and the urethral sphincter), acontractile bladder (leading to poor bladder emptying), bladder overactivity (leading to urgency and other bladder symptoms), and bladder outlet obstruction (leading to poor emptying).[37,40] In some of these cases a cause unrelated to HIV infection (such as prostate enlargement) can be identified, but more often a neurologic cause is implicated.[40]

Most urologists will initiate management with a change in medical therapies for LUTS. In cases where medications fail, second-line therapies for LUTS include intravesical botulinum toxin, transurethral resection of the prostate, and neuromodulatory therapies including sacral afferent nerve stimulation and Interstim. For patients with bladder atony or urinary retention, clean intermittent catheterization is the preferred management for urinary retention in this population if corrective therapy is not possible. Indwelling urethral catheters should be avoided unless absolutely necessary, due to the risk of iatrogenic infection.[2]

Of note, neurogenic voiding dysfunction in the AIDS patient may be a sign of end-stage disease; over the course of a 2-year study, 17 of 35 (44%) patients with new-onset neuro-urologic dysfunction died at a mean of 8 months of onset of voiding symptoms.[37] However, this study was published in 1996, before the widespread use of HAART therapy; whether neurogenic voiding dysfunction remains as powerful a predictor of mortality in the modern era is unclear.

UROLITHIASIS

Up to 40% of AIDS patients have urinary stones on autopsy.[44] Metabolic derangements secondary to malnutrition and/or diarrhea are common in HIV+ patients and can contribute to urinary stone formation.[45] Specific defects may include dehydration,

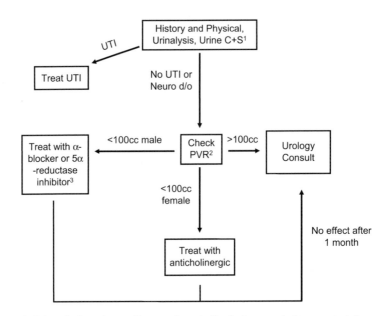

1- Culture for bacteria as well as mycobacteria, fungi, viruses, and other opportunistic
   infections if CD4 count <500
2- Determine by either bladder ultrasound or straight catheterization
3- α- blocker typically produces results in 1-2 weeks. 5α-reductase inhibitor most
   effective in patients with "large" prostates (> 4cm wide or ~40 mL estimated volume)
   and may decrease odds of disease progression but take 3-12 months for effect.

C+S: culture and sensitivity
PVR: postvoid residual

Fig. 1. Recommended treatment algorithm for voiding dysfunction in HIV+ patients. C + S, culture and sensitivity test; d/o, disorder; PVR, postvoid residual; UTI, urinary tract infection.

urinary acidification, and hypocitraturia.[5,45] Uric acid stones may also be more common in the HIV+ population secondary to cell lysis after chemotherapy for AIDS-associated lymphoma or treatment with sulfadiazine or acyclovir.[2,46,47]

One unique cause of urinary stones in this population is protease inhibitor therapy. Indinavir, an early-generation protease inhibitor, has been reported to cause renal stone disease in anywhere from 3% to 22% of patients on this medication, with significant dose-dependent effect for development of stone disease.[5,45,48] This agent is metabolized and renally excreted with a tendency to precipitate in alkaline urine.[49] These stones are radiolucent and may not be detected on plain film or CT scan; however, they may also serve as a nidus for precipitation of calcium or other salts and therefore may be visualized in some cases.[2] Indinavir is less often used in the modern era secondary to its stone-producing proclivities.[49,50] Newer protease inhibitors such as lopinavir, atanazavir, amprinavir, and nelfinavir have been also been associated with the development of stone disease, but their rate of stone formation appears to be much lower relative to indinavir.[51,52]

Renal stones typically present with renal colic, often in association with nausea.[3] Acute management of urinary stones in HIV+ patients should follow standard recommendations. Stones 4 mm or less in diameter are likely to pass spontaneously. Some evidence suggests that therapy with a daily-dose α-blocker (most commonly tamsulosin) may help speed passage of urinary stones as large as 10 mm.[53] Hence, α-blocker therapy should be considered for patients attempting spontaneous stone passage. For stones larger than 4 mm or in the setting of severe pain and/or nausea, prompt urologic consultation and management with ureteroscopy and lithotripsy (smaller stones) or percutaneous nephrolithotomy (larger stones) should be considered. In the setting of worsening renal function, fever, or other signs of systemic infection, emergent urologic consultation should be obtained for immediate decompression via ureteral stent or nephrostomy tube.[5] Stenting may be slightly preferred because protease inhibitor stones tend to consist of a sludge of precipitate in a gelatinous matrix and often pass with simple ureteral cannulation, although cystoscopy and ureteral stent does require greater manipulation of the urinary tract and is not preferred in cases of infection.[5,45]

Patients who have experienced a single episode of urinary stone formation should have a serum metabolic panel that must include uric acid assay. A 24-hour urine collection should be performed to determine if there is an overabundance of stone promoters (calcium, oxalate, uric acid, and so forth) or lack of stone inhibitors (citrate, magnesium) in the urine. Thiazide diuretics may be useful in patients with hypercalciuria and allopurinol in patients with hyperuricosuria.[54] Supplementation with potassium or sodium citrate may be useful in patients with uric acid stones and/or those with hypocitraturia.[54] Calcium restriction is not standard for stone patients except in very rare cases because it is thought that calcium is needed in the gut to complex with oxalate. Calcium oxalate is then excreted in the stool, reducing oxaluria as well as calciuria. General advice given to all stone-forming patients is: (1) increase fluid intake to 2 L or greater per day (preferably water or water with freshly squeezed lemon juice), (2) limit intake of salt, and (3) limit intake of red meat.[55]

It is unclear whether routine radiographic surveillance for new stone formation is required; this may permit early detection of stone disease but carries some expense and the risk of radiation exposure. Clinical judgment should be used to determine the frequency of such surveillance, based on the patient's general state of health as well as the severity and frequency of stone episodes.

SEXUAL FUNCTION

Sexual problems appear more commonly in HIV+ patients relative to population norms, with prevalence even higher in patients with AIDS or depressed CD4 counts.[56] As sexual problems are associated with age and older adults represent a growing segment of the HIV+ population (both as new diagnoses and from increased longevity), these concerns are of increasing relevance to physicians caring for HIV+ patients.[57,58]

The numerous organic comorbidities associated with HIV infection may affect the neurologic, vascular, and hormonal systems responsible for sexual desire and arousal in both men and women.[5,56,59–62] In addition, psychological stress from HIV infection may be considerable and is likely to affect sexual function.[56,58,60] Finally, HAART, particularly protease inhibitors, may be a risk factor for sexual problems,[56,63,64] although the association is controversial and by no means universally accepted.[58,65]

Evaluation and management of sexual problems in the HIV+ men may be accomplished in a fashion similar to what is done for the HIV− men.[66] Making an accurate diagnosis of the precise nature of the sexual concern (erectile dysfunction [ED], premature ejaculation, orgasmic disorder, and so forth) will help to appropriately target therapy. Attention to lifestyle factors (diet, exercise, changes in medication regimen, stress management) may be useful in improving sexual function or at minimum slowing further deterioration.[67] Given the high rate of hypogonadism in the HIV+ male population (see later discussion), morning serum testosterone concentration should be determined in men complaining of decreased libido. Testosterone levels peak at around 10 AM, so levels should always be measured in the morning. If a symptomatic patient has evidence from 2 separate testosterone assays of hypogonadism (concentrations <300 ng/dL), testosterone supplementation may be considered. Testosterone is reasonably effective at boosting sexual desire but the true utility of testosterone supplementation for ED remains controversial.[68–71] Indeed, several reports have failed to demonstrate an association between hypogonadism and sexual dysfunction in HIV+ men,[56,58] although some HIV+ men do report nonsexuality-specific improvements in quality of life with testosterone supplementation.[58]

Management options for men with ED are presented in **Table 1**. Prescription of phosphodiesterase type 5 inhibitors (PDE5I) or any other treatment for management of ED in HIV+ individuals has been controversial secondary to concerns about "sanctioning" the spread of HIV infection.[72] Several studies have indicated that PDE5I use is associated with higher risk of HIV seroconversion, likely due in most cases to concomitant high-risk sexual behavior in men who may not always meet criteria for ED despite use of PDE5I.[73–75] Other studies have suggested no difference in HIV risk behaviors between men given medical treatments for ED,[76] and it has been argued that PDE5I may help to minimize condom-associated ED and thereby encourage safer sex practices.[77]

In general, there is no legal precedent by which a provider can be held responsible for predicting with certainty whether an HIV+ patient will behave responsibly after prescription of a PDE5I; hence, a provider who declines to provide such a prescription must be able to clearly document and defend a decision not to provide such a treatment, preferably based on the principles of nonmalfeasance or social (as opposed to individual) justice.[72] Moreover, it may be illegal to discriminate against HIV+ persons by withholding treatment for a medical condition such as ED. It is the authors' opinion that prescribers should provide PDE5I to HIV+ patients in whom these medications are appropriate medical therapy; however, it is mandated that patients receive instruction on safer sex practices when such prescriptions are given.

PDE5I are generally safe for use in the HIV population as long as guidelines regarding hepatic and renal dosing are followed. Patients with moderate or severe hepatic dysfunction or severe renal dysfunction should be started on the lowest dose of PDE5I medication (25 mg for sildenafil, 5 mg for tadalafil and vardenafil on demand, and 2.5 mg for tadalafil daily dose) and dosage should not be more than doubled. Many protease inhibitors (including ritonavir and saquinavir) block activity of the CYP3A cytochrome[5]; therefore, patients on protease inhibitors should also start at the lowest possible dose for PDE5I and not advance beyond 50 mg for sildenafil, 10 mg for vardenafil and tadalafil on demand, and 2.5 mg daily for tadalafil. PDE5I are not for use in patients taking nitrates and should be taken at least 4 hours separate from α-blocking medications.

In men who fail treatment with oral PDE5I, additional management options (sexual counseling/therapy, intracavernous injection therapy, vacuum tumescence device, penile implants) mirror similar algorithms for use in the HIV− population.[78] Urologic consultation typically should be initiated to discuss these second-line therapies, although certain interested primary care physicians may choose to manage patients with these treatment options.

Evaluation for common sources of sexual distress in HIV+ women (hypoactive sexual desire disorder, arousal disorder, inadequate lubrication, pain with sex, and anorgasmia) should include inquiry into the nature and duration of the problem.[66,79]

Table 1
Management options for men with erectile dysfunction

Treatment	Examples	Pro	Con
Lifestyle modification	Stress reduction, diet, exercise, medication modification	Low cost, may convey other health benefits, lack of medication-related side effects	May take months or years until effects seen; adherence to therapy problematic, benefit may be slight
Psychosocial therapy	Sexual therapy, couples counseling, sexual education	May improve relationship, lack of medication-related side effects	Expensive in terms of time and money, objective data on treatment outcome lacking. Recidivism not known but expected to be significant
Vacuum therapy device	Various manufacturers	Lack of medication-related side effects	Barotrauma, penile pain, ejaculatory obstruction; some patients do not like use of mechanical device
Hormone supplementation	Testosterone (intramuscular injections, transdermal gels, subcutaneous pellets, and so forth)	May improve libido, has been shown to improve efficacy of phosphodiesterase-5 inhibitors in hypogonadal men	Need for monitoring of mixed efficacy for improvement in erectile function, clear benefit only in hypogonadal men, risk of polycythemia, theoretical risk of worsening sleep apnea or prostate-related urinary symptoms
Phosphodiesterase-5 inhibitors	Vardenafil, Tadalafil, Sildenafil	Well tolerated, convenient, favorable side effect profile	Expensive if paid for out-of-pocket. Risk of headache, flushing, rhinitis; special dosing for those on protease inhibitors or those with renal or hepatic insufficiency; cannot be used in patients on nitrates
Urethral suppositories	Medicated Urethral Suppository for Erections (MUSE)	Low risk of systemic side effects	Slight risk of priapism, local discomfort, marginal efficacy
Intracavernosal injection	Prostaglandin E1, papaverine + phentolamine (bimix), papaverine/phentolamine/prostaglandin (trimix)	Effective in cases of phosphodiesterase-5 inhibitor failure, low risk of systemic side effects	Risk of priapism, penile pain
Penile implant	Two- or 3-piece inflatable penile prosthesis, semirigid or malleable prosthesis	Reliable, no risk of systemic side effects, permits erection of any duration	Requires surgery and hospitalization; risk of infection, mechanical failure (typically ~10% per 5-year period)

Physical examination may reveal genital abnormalities that can predispose to sexual problems such as dyspareunia. Assessment of serum sex hormones (estrogen, testosterone, and so forth) may indicate hormonal imbalances that can contribute to problems with libido or genital tissue health. Given the dearth of therapies for women with sexual concerns approved by the Food and Drug Administration, there are currently no clear contraindications to such therapies as are available for women with HIV. Counseling, off-label use of medications such as testosterone and PDE5I, and attention to relationship factors are of great importance in the current management schema for HIV+ women with sexual concerns.[79]

Regardless of the decision whether or not to prescribe treatment for sexual problems, education on safer sex practices should be routine when counseling men and women with HIV infection.[5] This advice is of particular importance for older heterosexuals, who have been largely neglected by HIV education campaigns and may be more likely to engage in unsafe sexual practices due to a perception that they are at minimal risk of HIV infection.[57,80,81]

FERTILITY

With increases in life expectancy, both men and women with HIV are considering options for fertility treatment.[82] Although management of complex fertility concerns are typically not the province of the primary care provider, referral to a specialist is appropriate even in the setting of HIV. Options are available for HIV+ individuals wishing to have children, and information on the approach to these issues is included for general informational purposes.

New protocols and algorithms have reduced the risk of mother-to-child transmission of HIV infection to less than 1%.[83] Although mother-child transmission of HIV may be minimized, the fact that HIV is present in vaginal secretions and semen[84] mandates that some form of ex vivo gamete manipulation should occur to minimize the risk of HIV transfer.[85] This protocol applies principally to serodiscordant couples, but is of importance even in dyads in which both partners have HIV due to concerns about potentially different drug resistance profiles between partners. Protocols such as sperm washing (separation of sperm cells, which do not carry HIV, from seminal fluid and other cells that harbor viral particles) may eliminate the virus in 94% to 95% of cases.[82] Additional options may include in vitro fertilization with intracytoplasmic sperm injection so as to further minimize the risk of virus transfer. Separate laboratory areas for handling of potentially infected gametes/embryos have been advanced as considerations to reduce the risk of viral transmission. To date, more than 3000 children have been born to HIV+ fathers without any seroconversions noted in the literature.[82]

Most men with AIDS have grossly abnormal sperm and leukocytospermia.[86] A 1998 study indicated that mean semen volume, sperm concentration, percent motility, percent rapid and linear motility, and normal morphology was greater in 38 healthy fertile men relative to 250 men with HIV infection. The trend in sperm abnormalities was associated with decreasing CD4 count.[87] Infertility and suppression of semen parameters in men with HIV may be due in large part to testicular atrophy. Testicular atrophy itself may be secondary to several causes in the HIV+ population, including direct involvement of the testicle with HIV infection, opportunistic infection, perturbation of the hypothalamic-pituitary gonadal axis, and systemic illness.[68] Hypogonadism in HIV+ men tends to be associated with lower luteinizing hormone and follicle-stimulating hormone values, suggesting a central etiology in many cases.[58] HIV+ men who are on chronic testosterone therapy are highly likely to have suppressed hypothalamic-pituitary-testicular axes resulting in azoospermia.

A generalized decline in fertility status has been reported in women with HIV infection; it is speculated that some of this effect may be secondary to lower conception rates and greater pregnancy loss.[88] Up to a 40% incidence of tubal factor infertility has been reported in women with HIV presenting for infertility care to a center in the United Kingdom.[82] The cause of this is not immediately clear, but it may be speculated that a history of other STI and pelvic inflammatory disease may be at fault.

CANCER

Malignancy is a common source of morbidity and mortality in the HIV population and occurs more frequently than in age-matched HIV− people.[89] Fifteen percent of HIV patients and 30% to 50% of AIDS patients develop malignancy of some kind, with Kaposi sarcoma (KS), lymphoma (Hodgkin and non-Hodgkin), cervical, liver, testicular, and melanoma being the most prevalent cancers in the HIV+ population. Renal cell carcinoma is 8.5 times more common in HIV+ individuals and presents at an earlier age than it does in HIV− patients.[90] Of note, there have been reports that prostate cancer incidence is lower in HIV patients, but this may be due in large part to diagnostic bias.[91]

One of the more common indications for urologic consultation in the cancer patient is retroperitoneal adenopathy or fibrosis leading to ureteral obstruction, hydronephrosis, and potential kidney failure. Lymphoma may present with ureteral obstruction and hydronephrosis in this fashion. If patients present with flank pain or evidence of worsening renal function, ultrasound or CT evaluation of the abdomen and pelvis is indicated to assess for hydronephrosis. Moderate to severe hydronephrosis is often but not always indicative of ureteral obstruction; in equivocal cases a nuclear medicine renal scan with furosemide washout may clarify if true obstruction is present. In situations of ureteral obstruction, urologic consultation is indicated for placement of a ureteral stent or percutaneous nephrostomy.[3]

Kaposi Sarcoma

This sarcoma is the most common HIV-related malignancy, with a prevalence 7000 times higher than in the non-HIV population. The disease is transmitted by the KS herpes virus (also known as HHV8).[5,22] KS typically manifests as cutaneous lesions, which may be red, black, purple, or brown nodules, macules, or patches that can be ulcerated and painful.[5-7] KS of the penis may occur in up to 20% of cases but involvement of any urologic organ is possible. Genitourinary KS may present as penile edema, meatal stenosis, urinary tract symptoms including urinary retention, and even gangrene of the penis. Diagnosis is confirmed by biopsy, followed by staging by CT. The condition may go into remission with HAART; surgical resection, cryotherapy, laser vaporization radiotherapy, or topical steroids may also be used to shrink symptomatic lesions.[2,6] In the case of disseminated or visceral disease chemotherapy may be used, with a response rate of greater than 80%; however, relapse is common and death from opportunistic infections is the primary cause of mortality.[5]

Non-Hodgkin Lymphoma

Non-Hodgkin lymphoma (NHL) is 60 to 200 times more common in HIV patients than in the general population, with patients having CD4 counts less than 50 at greatest risk. NHL in the HIV+ patient is typically of the aggressive undifferentiated B-cell type.[92] Management of lymphoma in HIV+ patients is with HAART and radiation/chemotherapy. Complete response rates of 50% to 75% have been obtained, with 40% to 60% of patients having overall survival of 2 to 3 years.[93]

Renal involvement is present in 6% to 12% of lymphoma patients, typically present-ing as bilateral, multifocal, or diffuse involvement of the renal parenchyma.[94] Testicular lymphoma is also more common in the HIV+ population; the disease is typically bilat-eral and aggressive.[5] Treatment is with orchiectomy, which on rare occasions of completely isolated involvement may be curative. However, disseminated disease is the norm and systemic chemotherapy is usually required. Relapse rates are high.[95]

Testicular Germ Cell Tumors

Germ cell tumors of the testis are the third most common AIDS-related malignancy, occurring at a rate 25 to 50 times higher in the immunocompromised man.[96,97] These tumors typically present as painless nodules within the parenchyma of the testicle, although they may also present with scrotal pain, swelling, or distant metastases. Any patient with a nodule of the testicle should undergo scrotal sonogram with urgent referral to urology if an intratesticular mass is identified.

Of note, response rates and tumor-free survival are similar between HIV+ and HIV− men[98,99] although it has been suggested that the chances of false understaging of disease may be higher in the HIV+ population.[46] Furthermore, patients with prior bone marrow suppression or severely depressed immunity from advanced HIV disease do not tolerate chemotherapy well and often have worse outcomes for these reasons.[97]

Penile Cancer

Penile cancer, as well as precursor lesions such as Bowen disease and penile carci-noma in situ (CIS), are more common in HIV+ men.[5] Squamous cell carcinoma (SCC) and verrucous carcinoma are also more common and typically follow a more aggres-sive course in HIV patients. Part of the increase in susceptibility to these cancers may be related to the generally increased risk of sexually transmitted disease in HIV patients, including infection with the HPV subtypes (HPV 16 and 18) commonly asso-ciated with CIS and SCC of the penis.[3] Management of penile cancer is via partial or complete penectomy, although in less advanced cases penis sparing approaches such as Moh micrographic surgery, laser ablation, and minimally invasive surgical approaches may be considered.[5]

Prostate Cancer

Increased risk of prostate cancer and higher serum prostate-specific antigen (PSA) have not been conclusively linked to HIV infection,[100] although some investigators have suggested that the disease is more common in older HIV+ men than in HIV− men of similar age.[101] Regardless of any direct association, prostate cancer is becoming increasingly relevant to HIV+ men as life expectancy with HIV infection continues to increase.[89,100]

Although published data are scant, peritreatment morbidity appears to be similar or only slightly higher in HIV+ men after treatment for prostate cancer using radiation or surgical therapy.[102,103] Hence, it is recommended that HIV+ men be screened as per the HIV− population.[89] While PSA screening for prostate cancer is itself controversial, the American Urological Association recommends that if life expectancy is greater than 10 years, screening by serum PSA and digital rectal examination should be dis-cussed and offered to men beginning at age 40. Men who have less than 10 years of life expectancy (due to HIV or non-HIV related causes) generally do not benefit from prostate cancer screening. Subsequent rectal examination and PSA assessment as well as referral for discussion of prostate biopsy can be provided as indicated by base-line PSA levels and other risk factors, including family history and race (men of African descent are at higher risk of the disease).[104] Prostate biopsy has generally been found to be safe in appropriately selected immunosuppressed patients, and there have been no reports of increased morbidity after biopsy in HIV+ patients relative to HIV− patients.[89,105]

URINARY FISTULAE

Fistula formation between the urinary bladder and the bowel may occur in HIV patients due to bladder cryptosporidiosis, KS, NHL, or other malignant processes.[5] The most common presenting symptom for vesicoenteric fistula is recurrent UTI. Pneumaturia is another important and nearly pathognomonic sign, although it does not occur in every case. Patients who report pneumaturia should undergo cystography and/or contrast study of the colon and be referred for urology and general surgery consultations.[5] Urologic evaluation for fistulae of the urogenital system should include cystoscopy and biopsy. Management of the underlying causes of the condition is critical. Diversion of urine and/or stool may in some cases improve the clinical situation, but surgical repair of fistulae is often required.

RENAL INSUFFICIENCY/FAILURE

Kidney disease occurs in 25% to 35% of HIV patients,[106–108] and renal failure is the fourth leading cause of death in this population.[3] The most common source of renal failure in HIV patients is HIVAN. This entity is related to advanced disease and occurs much more frequently in HIV patients of African descent relative to HIV patients of Caucasian ancestry.[3] The syndrome presents as severe proteinuria (>3.5 g/day), rising creatinine, hypoalbuminemia, edema of the extremities, and hypertension.[109] Imaging typically demonstrates renal enlargement with increased echogenicity and loss of corticomedullary differentiation. At the histologic level, HIVAN is characterized by focal and segmental glomerulosclerosis, proliferation of podocytes, interstitial fibrosis, and leukocyte infiltration.[109]

HIVAN is an indicator that HAART should be initiated immediately if it has not been already started. Supportive management of electrolytes and volume should be instituted; angiotensin-converting enzyme inhibitors may help to delay disease progression.[3] Unfortunately, the rate of disease progression in the setting of HIVAN is very high, with median progression to end-stage renal disease within 10 months and 50% mortality at 1 year.[3,110]

In addition to HIVAN, renal failure in this population may be secondary to hypovolemia from diarrhea/emesis, kidney infections, urinary obstruction (stones or lymphoma), and nephrotoxic medications (antiretrovirals; antivirals such as foscarnet and acyclovir; antifungals such as amphotericin; anti–Pneumocystis pneumonia medications such as trimethoprim-sulfamethoxazole, pentamidine, and dapsone; and antibacterial agents such as aminoglycosides, sulfadiazine, and rifampicin).[5]

MALE CIRCUMCISION AND HIV

In the United States, it is rare to use the term male circumcision (MC) rather than just circumcision, but for international application male circumcision must be differentiated from female circumcision, which remains prevalent in some parts of the world. The term MC is the standard one used by the World Health Organization.

As early as the 1980s, HIV prevalence and population data as well as observations of AIDS workers in Africa led to speculation that circumcision might be protective against HIV infection.[111] Prior to 2005, almost all studies of the relationship of HIV disease and MC were observational and could not account for potentially important confounding factors such as differences in sexual practices, religious beliefs, and cultural norms.[112,113] A Cochrane database review in 2003 suggested that there was insufficient evidence to recommend MC as a means to prevent HIV.[112]

In 2005 and 2007 3 large, prospective, randomized clinical trials of circumcision versus no circumcision were published. The trials included a total of over 11,000 men from South Africa, Uganda, and Kenya. In each trial, one half of the HIV− men were circumcised at trial entry and one half of HIV− men were to be offered circumcision at the end of the trial. Over a 1- to 2-year period, the rates of HIV seroconversion were measured. Each of the trials showed that MC reduced the risk of HIV infection by 50% to 60%.[114–117] These 3 landmark clinical trials have provided unassailable evidence that MC is a strong protector against HIV infection in heterosexual men in sub-Saharan Africa. The effects of MC were consistent irrespective of the number of sexual partners and other variations in sexual practices.[115,116] In one subset analysis, sexual dysfunctions were no more prevalent in the circumcised versus uncircumcised group at follow-up.[118] Adverse events in these clinical trials occurred in 1.5% to 3.6% of circumcised men and were generally mild and self-limited.[114–117]

While the benefit of MC in heterosexual men has been well supported by these reports, the role of MC for HIV prevention among men who have sex with men (MSM) is less clear. A recent meta-analysis suggested that MC offered a protective effect against HIV in MSM but strict statistical significance was not confirmed.[119] Retrospective data from a recent HIV vaccine trial enrolling over 4800 MSM has suggested that MC status was not protective against HIV; the most rational explanation for these findings is the much higher incidence of anal insertive and receptive intercourse among MSM relative to heterosexual men.[120] It may be conjectured that anal intercourse minimizes the protective effect of circumcision, but this is by no means certain. It is clear that additional studies of circumcision in MSM are indicated to determine the efficacy of this intervention in this population.[113] Furthermore, MC in a man who already has HIV infection has not been shown to reduce the transmission of HIV to female sexual partners.[121]

The most plausible explanation for how MC reduces the risk of HIV transmission is based on studies that show numerous HIV target cells under the dermis of the foreskin.[122] Other studies have demonstrated that the inner surface of the foreskin is poorly keratinized and potentially prone to abrasions and lacerations during sexual activity.[123,124] Trauma to the foreskin with subsequent ingress of HIV to areas with a high density of HIV target cells may set the stage for easier transmission of the infection. Hence, removal of this vulnerable skin is thought to reduce the risk of HIV infection. Other theories for MC's protective effects against HIV have been proposed, including greater density of anaerobic bacteria in the uncircumcised preputial skin. This condition may lead to inflammation and infiltration of Langerhans cells, which in turn present HIV to CD4 cells and initiate the process of HIV infection.[125]

Although MC is a powerful medical intervention for prevention of HIV infection, it does not obviate the need for many other very important elements of HIV prevention programs such as sex and AIDS education, safe sex practices, education on proper use of barrier contraception, and reduction of the number of sexual partners and use of prostitutes, points emphasized in the original clinical trial publications and follow-up editorials.

SUMMARY

HIV infection and its treatment may lead to several urologic manifestations and conditions. Attention to these issues is an important aspect of primary care for the HIV patient, particularly because HIV infection of the genitourinary system may have serious implications for prevention of transmission of the virus. In collaboration with specialists in infectious disease and urology, the primary care provider can contribute substantially to both quality and length of life in the HIV+ population.

REFERENCES

1. UNAIDS. AIDS epidemic update: 2009. Geneva (Switzerland): Joint United Nations Programme on HIV/AIDS (UNAIDS) and World Health Organization (WHO); 2009.
2. Lee LK, Dinneen MD, Ahmad S. The urologist and the patient infected with human immunodeficiency virus or with acquired immunodeficiency syndrome. BJU Int 2001;88(6):500–10.
3. Lebovitch S, Mydlo JH. HIV-AIDS: urologic considerations. Urol Clin North Am 2008;35(1):59–68, vi.
4. Hoepelman AI, van Buren M, van den Broek J, et al. Bacteriuria in men infected with HIV-1 is related to their immune status (CD4+ cell count). AIDS 1992;6(2): 179–84.
5. Heyns CF, Fisher M. The urological management of the patient with acquired immunodeficiency syndrome. BJU Int 2005;95(5):709–16.
6. Kwan DJ, Lowe FC. Genitourinary manifestations of the acquired immunodeficiency syndrome. Urology 1995;45(1):13–27.
7. Kwan DJ, Lowe FC. Acquired immunodeficiency syndrome. A venereal disease. Urol Clin North Am 1992;19(1):13–24.
8. Gokalp A, Gultekin EY, Ozdamar S. Genito-urinary tuberculosis: a review of 83 cases. Br J Clin Pract 1990;44(12):599–600.
9. Brandeis JM, Baskin LS, Kogan BA, et al. Recurrent *Staphylococcus aureus* renal abscess in a child positive for the human immunodeficiency virus. Urology 1995;46(2):246–8.
10. Marques LP, Rioja LS, Oliveira CA, et al. AIDS-associated renal tuberculosis. Nephron 1996;74(4):701–4.
11. van der Reijden HJ, Schipper ME, Danner SA, et al. Glomerular lesions and opportunistic infections of the kidney in AIDS: an autopsy study of 47 cases. Adv Exp Med Biol 1989;252:181–8.
12. Figueiredo AA, Lucon AM, Ikejiri DS, et al. Urogenital tuberculosis in a patient with AIDS: an unusual presentation. Nat Clin Pract Urol 2008;5(8):455–60.
13. Dinnes J, Deeks J, Kunst H, et al. A systematic review of rapid diagnostic tests for the detection of tuberculosis infection. Health Technol Assess 2007;11(3): 1–196.
14. Moussa OM, Eraky I, El-Far MA, et al. Rapid diagnosis of genitourinary tuberculosis by polymerase chain reaction and non-radioactive DNA hybridization. J Urol 2000;164(2):584–8.
15. Havlir DV, Barnes PF. Tuberculosis in patients with human immunodeficiency virus infection. N Engl J Med 1999;340(5):367–73.
16. Butler MR, O'Flynn JD. Reactivation of genito-urinary tuberculosis: a retrospective review of 838 cases. Eur Urol 1975;1(1):14–7.
17. Henn L, Nagel F, Dal Pizzol F. Comparison between human immunodeficiency virus positive and negative patients with tuberculosis in Southern Brazil. Mem Inst Oswaldo Cruz 1999;94(3):377–81.
18. Control CfD. Reported HIV status of tuberculosis patients—United States, 1993–2005. MMWR Morb Mortal Wkly Rep 2007;56(42):1103–6.

19. Leport C, Rousseau F, Perronne C, et al. Bacterial prostatitis in patients infected with the human immunodeficiency virus. J Urol 1989;141(2):334–6.

20. Nickel JC, Shoskes D, Wang Y, et al. How does the pre-massage and post-massage 2-glass test compare to the Meares-Stamey 4-glass test in men with chronic prostatitis/chronic pelvic pain syndrome? J Urol 2006;176(1):119–24.

21. Trauzzi SJ, Kay CJ, Kaufman DG, et al. Management of prostatic abscess in patients with human immunodeficiency syndrome. Urology 1994;43(5):629–33.

22. Hyun G, Lowe FC. AIDS and the urologist. Urol Clin North Am 2003;30(1):101–9.

23. Coburn M. Urological manifestations of HIV infection. AIDS Res Hum Retroviruses 1998;14(Suppl 1):S23–5.

24. Dalton AD, Harcourt-Webster JN. The histopathology of the testis and epididymis in AIDS—a post-mortem study. J Pathol 1991;163(1):47–52.

25. De Paepe ME, Waxman M. Testicular atrophy in AIDS: a study of 57 autopsy cases. Hum Pathol 1989;20(3):210–4.

26. Kaplan MH, Sadick N, McNutt NS, et al. Dermatologic findings and manifestations of acquired immunodeficiency syndrome (AIDS). J Am Acad Dermatol 1987;16(3 Pt 1):485–506.

27. Cockerell CJ. Cutaneous manifestations of HIV infection other than Kaposi's sarcoma: clinical and histologic aspects. J Am Acad Dermatol 1990;22(6 Pt 2):1260–9.

28. Coopman SA, Johnson RA, Platt R, et al. Cutaneous disease and drug reactions in HIV infection. N Engl J Med 1993;328(23):1670–4.

29. Workowski KA, Berman SM. Sexually transmitted diseases treatment guidelines, 2006. MMWR Recomm Rep 2006;55(RR–11):1–94.

30. Belda W Jr, Di Chiacchio NG, Di Chiacchio N, et al. A comparative study of single-dose treatment of chancroid using thiamphenicol versus Azithromycin. Braz J Infect Dis 2009;13(3):218–20.

31. Tyring SK. Molluscum contagiosum: the importance of early diagnosis and treatment. Am J Obstet Gynecol 2003;189(Suppl 3):S12–6.

32. Cespedes RD, Peretsman SJ, Blatt SP. The significance of hematuria in patients infected with the human immunodeficiency virus. J Urol 1995;154(4):1455–6.

33. Zeman A, Donaghy M. Acute infection with human immunodeficiency virus presenting with neurogenic urinary retention. Genitourin Med 1991;67(4):345–7.

34. Gyrtrup HJ, Kristiansen VB, Zachariae CO, et al. Voiding problems in patients with HIV infection and AIDS. Scand J Urol Nephrol 1995;29(3):295–8.

35. Khan Z, Singh VK, Yang WC. Neurogenic bladder in acquired immune deficiency syndrome (AIDS). Urology 1992;40(3):289–91.

36. Levy RM, Bredesen DE, Rosenblum ML. Neurological manifestations of the acquired immunodeficiency syndrome (AIDS): experience at UCSF and review of the literature. J Neurosurg 1985;62(4):475–95.

37. Hermieu JF, Delmas V, Boccon-Gibod L. Micturition disturbances and human immunodeficiency virus infection. J Urol 1996;156(1):157–9.

38. Snider WD, Simpson DM, Nielsen S, et al. Neurological complications of acquired immune deficiency syndrome: analysis of 50 patients. Ann Neurol 1983;14(4):403–18.

39. Collier AC, Meyers JD, Corey L, et al. Cytomegalovirus infection in homosexual men. Relationship to sexual practices, antibody to human immunodeficiency virus, and cell-mediated immunity. Am J Med 1987;82(3):593–601.

40. Kane CJ, Bolton DM, Connolly JA, et al. Voiding dysfunction in human immunodeficiency virus infections. J Urol 1996;155(2):523–6.

41. McGuire BB, O'Brien MF, McLoughlin S, et al. Should patients with symptomatic BPH have a trial of medical therapy by their general practitioner prior to referral for urological assessment? Ir Med J 2007;100(4):428–9.
42. Madersbacher S, Marszalek M, Lackner J, et al. The long-term outcome of medical therapy for BPH. Eur Urol 2007;51(6):1522–33.
43. Chapple C. Antimuscarinics in men with lower urinary tract symptoms suggestive of bladder outlet obstruction due to benign prostatic hyperplasia. Curr Opin Urol 2010;20(1):43–8.
44. Seney FD Jr, Burns DK, Silva FG. Acquired immunodeficiency syndrome and the kidney. Am J Kidney Dis 1990;16(1):1–13.
45. Nadler RB, Rubenstein JN, Eggener SE, et al. The etiology of urolithiasis in HIV infected patients. J Urol 2003;169(2):475–7.
46. Christin S, Baumelou A, Bahri S, et al. Acute renal failure due to sulfadiazine in patients with AIDS. Nephron 1990;55(2):233–4.
47. Sawyer MH, Webb DE, Balow JE, et al. Acyclovir-induced renal failure. Clinical course and histology. Am J Med 1988;84(6):1067–71.
48. Collin F, Chene G, Retout S, et al. Indinavir trough concentration as a determinant of early nephrolithiasis in HIV-1-infected adults. Ther Drug Monit 2007; 29(2):164–70.
49. Kopp JB, Miller KD, Mican JA, et al. Crystalluria and urinary tract abnormalities associated with indinavir. Ann Intern Med 1997;127(2):119–25.
50. Itani S, Bartlett JA. Strategies of antiretroviral therapy in adults. Urol Clin North Am 1999;26(4):809–20, ix–x.
51. Masarani M, Dinneen M, Coyne KM, et al. The genitourinary complications of HIV infection in men. Br J Hosp Med (Lond) 2008;69(3):141–6.
52. Feicke A, Rentsch KM, Oertle D, et al. Same patient, new stone composition: amprenavir urinary stone. Antivir Ther 2008;13(5):733–4.
53. Al-Ansari A, Al-Naimi A, Alobaidy A, et al. Efficacy of tamsulosin in the management of lower ureteral stones: a randomized double-blind placebo-controlled study of 100 patients. Urology 2010;75(1):4–7.
54. Worcester EM, Coe FL. Nephrolithiasis. Prim Care 2008;35(2):369–91, vii.
55. Taylor EN, Curhan GC. Diet and fluid prescription in stone disease. Kidney Int 2006;70(5):835–9.
56. Collazos J, Martinez E, Mayo J, et al. Sexual dysfunction in HIV-infected patients treated with highly active antiretroviral therapy. J Acquir Immune Defic Syndr 2002;31(3):322–6.
57. Karlovsky M, Lebed B, Mydlo JH. Increasing incidence and importance of HIV/AIDS and gonorrhea among men aged >/= 50 years in the US in the era of erectile dysfunction therapy. Scand J Urol Nephrol 2004;38(3):247–52.
58. Crum-Cianflone NF, Bavaro M, Hale B, et al. Erectile dysfunction and hypogonadism among men with HIV. AIDS Patient Care STDS 2007;21(1):9–19.
59. Mao L, Newman CE, Kidd MR, et al. Self-reported sexual difficulties and their association with depression and other factors among gay men attending high HIV-caseload general practices in Australia. J Sex Med 2009;6(5):1378–85.
60. Bancroft J, Carnes L, Janssen E. Unprotected anal intercourse in HIV-positive and HIV-negative gay men: the relevance of sexual arousability, mood, sensation seeking, and erectile problems. Arch Sex Behav 2005;34(3):299–305.
61. Keegan A, Lambert S, Petrak J. Sex and relationships for HIV-positive women since HAART: a qualitative study. AIDS Patient Care STDS 2005;19(10):645–54.
62. Wilson TE, Jean-Louis G, Schwartz R, et al. HIV infection and women's sexual functioning. J Acquir Immune Defic Syndr 2010;54(4):360–7.

63. Colson AE, Keller MJ, Sax PE, et al. Male sexual dysfunction associated with antiretroviral therapy. J Acquir Immune Defic Syndr 2002;30(1):27–32.

64. Collazos J. Sexual dysfunction in the highly active antiretroviral therapy era. AIDS Rev 2007;9(4):237–45.

65. Lallemand F, Salhi Y, Linard F, et al. Sexual dysfunction in 156 ambulatory HIV-infected men receiving highly active antiretroviral therapy combinations with and without protease inhibitors. J Acquir Immune Defic Syndr 2002;30(2):187–90.

66. Hatzichristou D, Rosen RC, Derogatis LR, et al. Recommendations for the clinical evaluation of men and women with sexual dysfunction. J Sex Med 2010;7(1 Pt 2):337–48.

67. Esposito K, Ciotola M, Giugliano F, et al. Effects of intensive lifestyle changes on erectile dysfunction in men. J Sex Med 2009;6(1):243–50.

68. Poretsky L, Can S, Zumoff B. Testicular dysfunction in human immunodeficiency virus-infected men. Metabolism 1995;44(7):946–53.

69. Cohan GR. HIV-associated hypogonadism. AIDS Read 2006;16(7):341–5, 348, 352–4.

70. Wunder DM, Bersinger NA, Fux CA, et al. Hypogonadism in HIV-1-infected men is common and does not resolve during antiretroviral therapy. Antivir Ther 2007; 12(2):261–5.

71. Guaraldi G, Luzi K, Murri R, et al. Sexual dysfunction in HIV-infected men: role of antiretroviral therapy, hypogonadism and lipodystrophy. Antivir Ther 2007;12(7): 1059–65.

72. Kell P, Sadeghi-Nejad H, Price D. An ethical dilemma: erectile dysfunction in the HIV-positive patient: to treat or not to treat. Int J STD AIDS 2002;13(6):355–7.

73. Nettles CD, Benotsch EG, Uban KA. Sexual risk behaviors among men who have sex with men using erectile dysfunction medications. AIDS Patient Care STDS 2009;23(12):1017–23.

74. Ostrow DG, Plankey MW, Cox C, et al. Specific sex drug combinations contribute to the majority of recent HIV seroconversions among MSM in the MACS. J Acquir Immune Defic Syndr 2009;51(3):349–55.

75. Prestage G, Jin F, Kippax S, et al. Use of illicit drugs and erectile dysfunction medications and subsequent HIV infection among gay men in Sydney, Australia. J Sex Med 2009;6(8):2311–20.

76. Cook RL, McGinnis KA, Samet JH, et al. Erectile dysfunction drug receipt, risky sexual behavior and sexually transmitted diseases in HIV-infected and HIV-uninfected men. J Gen Intern Med 2010;25(2):115–21.

77. Sanders SA, Milhausen RR, Crosby RA, et al. Do phosphodiesterase type 5 inhibitors protect against condom-associated erection loss and condom slippage? J Sex Med 2009;6(5):1451–6.

78. Hijazi L, Nandwani R, Kell P. Medical management of sexual difficulties in HIV-positive individuals. Int J STD AIDS 2002;13(9):587–92.

79. Basson R, Wierman ME, van Lankveld J, et al. Summary of the recommendations on sexual dysfunctions in women. J Sex Med 2010;7(1 Pt 2):314–26.

80. Wallace JI, Paauw DS, Spach DH. HIV infection in older patients: when to suspect the unexpected. Geriatrics 1993;48(6):61–4, 69–70.

81. Skiest DJ, Keiser P. Human immunodeficiency virus infection in patients older than 50 years. A survey of primary care physicians' beliefs, practices, and knowledge. Arch Fam Med 1997;6(3):289–94.

82. Frodsham LC, Boag F, Barton S, et al. Human immunodeficiency virus infection and fertility care in the United Kingdom: demand and supply. Fertil Steril 2006; 85(2):285–9.

83. Lyall EG, Blott M, de Ruiter A, et al. Guidelines for the management of HIV infection in pregnant women and the prevention of mother-to-child transmission. HIV Med 2001;2(4):314–34.
84. Krieger JN, Coombs RW, Collier AC, et al. Intermittent shedding of human immunodeficiency virus in semen: implications for sexual transmission. J Urol 1995; 154(3):1035–40.
85. Honeck P, Weigel M, Kwon ST, et al. Assisted procreation in cases of hepatitis B, hepatitis C or human immunodeficiency virus infection of the male partner. Hum Reprod 2006;21(5):1117–21.
86. Krieger JN, Coombs RW, Collier AC, et al. Fertility parameters in men infected with human immunodeficiency virus. J Infect Dis 1991;164(3):464–9.
87. Muller CH, Coombs RW, Krieger JN. Effects of clinical stage and immunological status on semen analysis results in human immunodeficiency virus type 1-seropositive men. Andrologia 1998;30(Suppl 1):15–22.
88. Gray RH, Wawer MJ, Serwadda D, et al. Population-based study of fertility in women with HIV-1 infection in Uganda. Lancet 1998;351(9096):98–103.
89. Silberstein J, Downs T, Lakin C, et al. HIV and prostate cancer: a systematic review of the literature. Prostate Cancer Prostatic Dis 2009;12(1):6–12.
90. Baynham SA, Katner HP, Cleveland KB. Increased prevalence of renal cell carcinoma in patients with HIV infection. AIDS Patient Care STDS 1997;11(3):161–5.
91. Patel P, Hanson DL, Sullivan PS, et al. Incidence of types of cancer among HIV-infected persons compared with the general population in the United States, 1992–2003. Ann Intern Med 2008;148(10):728–36.
92. Stebbing J, Gazzard B, Mandalia S, et al. Antiretroviral treatment regimens and immune parameters in the prevention of systemic AIDS-related non-Hodgkin's lymphoma. J Clin Oncol 2004;22(11):2177–83.
93. Behler CM, Kaplan LD. Advances in the management of HIV-related non-Hodgkin lymphoma. Curr Opin Oncol 2006;18(5):437–43.
94. D'Agati V, Appel GB. Renal pathology of human immunodeficiency virus infection. Semin Nephrol 1998;18(4):406–21.
95. Sokovich RS, Bormes TP, McKiel CF. Acquired immunodeficiency syndrome presenting as testicular lymphoma. J Urol 1992;147(4):1110–1.
96. Wilson WT, Frenkel E, Vuitch F, et al. Testicular tumors in men with human immunodeficiency virus. J Urol 1992;147(4):1038–40.
97. Leibovitch I, Baniel J, Rowland RG, et al. Malignant testicular neoplasms in immunosuppressed patients. J Urol 1996;155(6):1938–42.
98. Krain J, Dieckmann KP. Treatment of testicular seminoma in patients with HIV infection. Report of two cases. Eur Urol 1994;26(2):184–6.
99. Powles T, Bower M, Shamash J, et al. Outcome of patients with HIV-related germ cell tumours: a case-control study. Br J Cancer 2004;90(8):1526–30.
100. Vianna LE, Lo Y, Klein RS. Serum prostate-specific antigen levels in older men with or at risk of HIV infection. HIV Med 2006;7(7):471–6.
101. Crum NF, Spencer CR, Amling CL. Prostate carcinoma among men with human immunodeficiency virus infection. Cancer 2004;101(2):294–9.
102. Huang SP, Huang CY, Wu WJ, et al. Association of vitamin D receptor FokI polymorphism with prostate cancer risk, clinicopathological features and recurrence of prostate specific antigen after radical prostatectomy. Int J Cancer 2006; 119(8):1902–7.
103. Ng T, Stein NF, Kaminetsky J, et al. Preliminary results of radiation therapy for prostate cancer in human immunodeficiency virus-positive patients. Urology 2008;72(5):1135–8 [discussion: 1138].

104. Greene KL, Albertsen PC, Babaian RJ, American Urologic Association. Prostate-specific antigen (PSA) best practice statement: 2009 update. J Urol 2009;182(5):2232–41.
105. Wammack R, Djavan B, Remzi M, et al. Morbidity of transrectal ultrasound-guided prostate needle biopsy in patients receiving immunosuppression. Urology 2001;58(6):1004–7.
106. Rao TK, Filippone EJ, Nicastri AD, et al. Associated focal and segmental glomerulosclerosis in the acquired immunodeficiency syndrome. N Engl J Med 1984;310(11):669–73.
107. Gardenswartz MH, Lerner CW, Seligson GR, et al. Renal disease in patients with AIDS: a clinicopathologic study. Clin Nephrol 1984;21(4):197–204.
108. Coleburn NH, Scholes JV, Lowe FC. Renal failure in patients with AIDS-related complex. Urology 1991;37(6):523–7.
109. Shah SN, He CJ, Klotman P. Update on HIV-associated nephropathy. Curr Opin Nephrol Hypertens 2006;15(4):450–5.
110. Rao TK. Acute renal failure syndromes in human immunodeficiency virus infection. Semin Nephrol 1998;18(4):378–95.
111. Bongaarts J, Reining P, Way P, et al. The relationship between male circumcision and HIV infection in African populations. AIDS 1989;3(6):373–7.
112. Siegfried N, Muller M, Volmink J, et al. Male circumcision for prevention of heterosexual acquisition of HIV in men. Cochrane Database Syst Rev 2003;3: CD003362.
113. Vermund SH, Qian HZ. Circumcision and HIV prevention among men who have sex with men: no final word. JAMA 2008;300(14):1698–700.
114. Auvert B, Taljaard D, Lagarde E, et al. Randomized, controlled intervention trial of male circumcision for reduction of HIV infection risk: the ANRS 1265 Trial. PLoS Med 2005;2(11):e298.
115. Gray RH, Kigozi G, Serwadda D, et al. Male circumcision for HIV prevention in men in Rakai, Uganda: a randomised trial. Lancet 2007;369(9562):657–66.
116. Bailey RC, Moses S, Parker CB, et al. Male circumcision for HIV prevention in young men in Kisumu, Kenya: a randomised controlled trial. Lancet 2007; 369(9562):643–56.
117. Siegfried N, Muller M, Deeks JJ, et al. Male circumcision for prevention of heterosexual acquisition of HIV in men. Cochrane Database Syst Rev 2009;2: CD003362.
118. Krieger JN, Mehta SD, Bailey RC, et al. Adult male circumcision: effects on sexual function and sexual satisfaction in Kisumu, Kenya. J Sex Med 2008; 5(11):2610–22.
119. Millett GA, Flores SA, Marks G, et al. Circumcision status and risk of HIV and sexually transmitted infections among men who have sex with men: a meta-analysis. JAMA 2008;300(14):1674–84.
120. Gust DA, Wiegand RE, Kretsinger K, et al. Circumcision status and HIV infection among MSM: reanalysis of a Phase III HIV vaccine clinical trial. AIDS 2010; 24(8):1135–43.
121. Wawer MJ, Makumbi F, Kigozi G, et al. Circumcision in HIV-infected men and its effect on HIV transmission to female partners in Rakai, Uganda: a randomised controlled trial. Lancet 2009;374(9685):229–37.
122. McCoombe SG, Short RV. Potential HIV-1 target cells in the human penis. AIDS 2006;20(11):1491–5.
123. Dinh MH, McRaven MD, Kelley Z, et al. Keratinization of the adult male foreskin and implications for male circumcision. AIDS 2010;24(6):899–906.

124. Patterson BK, Landay A, Siegel JN, et al. Susceptibility to human immunodeficiency virus-1 infection of human foreskin and cervical tissue grown in explant culture. Am J Pathol 2002;161(3):867–73.
125. Price LB, Liu CM, Johnson KE, et al. The effects of circumcision on the penis microbiome. PLoS One 2010;5(1):e8422.

Assessment of Hematuria

Vitaly Margulis, MD*, Arthur I. Sagalowsky, MD

KEYWORDS

- Microscopic hematuria • Gross hematuria
- Differential diagnosis • Evaluation

Hematuria is a common clinical finding in the adult population, with a prevalence ranging from 2.5% to 20.0%.[1,2] Although gross hematuria is defined simply as visible urine discoloration because of the presence of blood, there is controversy regarding the exact definition of microscopic hematuria. The American Urological Association (AUA) guidelines define clinically significant microscopic hematuria as more than 3 red blood cells (RBCs) per high-power field on 2 of 3 properly collected urine specimens over a period of 2 to 3 weeks.[3] However, patients at high risk for significant urologic disease (see later discussion) should be evaluated for hematuria if a single urinalysis demonstrates 2 or more RBCs per high-power field.[4] Appropriate and timely evaluation is imperative, because any degree of hematuria can be a sign of a serious genitourinary disease.[4,5] The focus of this article is on the logical and cost-effective evaluation of hematuria in adults, with specific attention directed to the indications and practice patterns for performing laboratory tests, imaging studies, and cystoscopy.

CAUSE

The most common causes of hematuria in adult populations include urinary tract infections, urolithiasis, benign prostatic enlargement, and urologic malignancy.[1,2,4] However, the complete differential is extensive (**Box 1**). The incidence of specific conditions associated with hematuria varies with patient age, type of hematuria (gross or microscopic, symptomatic or asymptomatic), and existence of risk factors for urologic malignancy. Overall, approximately 5% of patients with microscopic hematuria and up to 40% of patients with gross hematuria are found to harbor a neoplasm of the genitourinary tract.[3,5,6] Conversely, in up to 40% of patients with asymptomatic microhematuria, no identifiable source is found.[1] As a result, a clinician should consider otherwise unexplained hematuria of any degree to be of a possible malignant origin, until proven otherwise.

The authors have nothing to disclose.

Department of Urology, The University of Texas Southwestern Medical Center, 5339 Harry Hines Boulevard, Dallas, TX 75390-9110, USA

* Corresponding author.

E-mail address: Vitaly.margulis@utsouthwestern.edu

Med Clin N Am 95 (2011) 153–159

doi:10.1016/j.mcna.2010.08.028

Box 1
Causes of hematuria

Urinary tract infection

Urinary calculi

Urinary tract malignancy

    Urothelial cancer

    Renal cancer

    Prostate cancer

Benign prostatic hyperplasia

Radiation cystitis and/or nephritis

Endometriosis

Anatomic abnormalities

    Arteriovenous malformation

    Urothelial stricture disease

    Ureteropelvic junction obstruction

    Vesicoureteral reflux

    Nutcracker syndrome

Medical or renal disease

    Glomerulonephritis

    Interstitial nephritis

    Papillary necrosis

    Alport syndrome

    Renal artery stenosis

Metabolic disorders

    Hypercalciuria

    Hyperuricosuria

    Coagulation abnormalities

Miscellaneous

    Trauma

    Exercise-induced hematuria

    Benign familial hematuria

    Loin pain–hematuria syndrome

EVALUATION

Diagnosis

The urinary dipstick test is the most common test used to evaluate urine and provides a semiquantitative analysis of the number of RBCs. Dipsticks detect 1 to 2 RBCs per high-power field and are therefore at least as sensitive as microscopic examination of the urine sediment.[7] False-positive findings can be seen with hemoglobinuria, myoglobinuria, and urine contaminants; consequently, a positive test result (whether trace or 3+) should immediately be followed by a microscopic examination of the urinary sediment to confirm or exclude the presence of RBCs.[8] Correspondingly, gross discoloration of urine should not be presumed to be due to hematuria because a range of dietary, metabolic, and pharmacologic factors such as beets, blackberries, melanin, bile, porphyrin, iron, and various medications can also be responsible.

History and Physical Examination

Detailed and systematic patient history and physical examination should aim to elicit potential glomerular and extraglomerular causes of hematuria and to stratify patients according to their risk for urologic malignancy.

Risk factors for urothelial cancer in patients with microscopic hematuria
  Smoking history
  Occupational exposure to chemicals or dyes (benzenes or aromatic amines)
  History of gross hematuria
  Age greater than 40 years
  History of urologic disorder or disease
  History of irritative voiding symptoms
  History of urinary tract infection
  Analgesic abuse
  History of pelvic irradiation.

A thorough health history includes medical and surgical history, family history, social history, occupational or radiation exposure, and medications taken. For example, increased frequency and dysuria may suggest urinary tract infection, whereas colicky pain suggests urolithiasis. Presence of prostatism-related lower urinary tract symptoms, such as hesitancy, intermittency, and decrease in the force of the urinary stream, are usually due to benign prostatic enlargement. Recent upper respiratory tract or skin infection may be associated with glomerulonephritis. Recent menstruation, vigorous exercise, or sexual activities may produce transient hematuria in otherwise healthy patients. A family history of polycystic kidney disease and other renal diseases, sickle cell anemia, and a history of travel to areas with endemic schistosomiasis, malaria, or tuberculosis may be additional important clues to the cause of hematuria.

The physical examination should focus on the detection of hypertension that is present along with nephritic syndrome and renal vascular disease, edema associated with nephrotic syndrome, palpable abdominal or flank mass suggesting a renal neoplasm, and costovertebral or suprapubic tenderness, common with urinary tract infection. A rectal examination in men may reveal prostatic nodularity or enlargement as a potential cause.

Laboratory Studies

Focused laboratory evaluation should be directed at the differentiation of glomerular and nonglomerular sources of hematuria and identification of potential associated systemic infections and inflammatory and immunologic conditions.[3,9] Initial tests should include urinalysis with examination of the urinary sediment, complete blood cell count, estimation of serum creatinine and electrolyte levels, and urine culture. Patients with urinary tract infection should be treated appropriately, and urinalysis should be repeated 2 to 6 weeks after treatment. Similarly, patients with documented urinary tract calculi and asymptomatic microscopic hematuria should have a repeat urinalysis after stone clearance. Additional laboratory investigation should be guided by specific findings of the history, physical examination, and urinalysis.

Formal urinalysis can aid in the identification of glomerular disease as the source of bleeding; this analysis being important for prognosis and optimization of subsequent evaluation. The presence of dysmorphic RBCs, RBC casts, or proteinuria (protein excretion exceeding 500 mg/d with no concomitant gross hematuria) supports a diagnosis of hematuria of glomerular origin, warranting nephrologic consultation.[10]

Urologic consultation and evaluation of the upper and lower urinary tracts is necessary in all patients with gross hematuria, and should be considered in high-risk individuals with microhematuria not associated with glomerular disease (**Fig. 1**).[3,9,11]

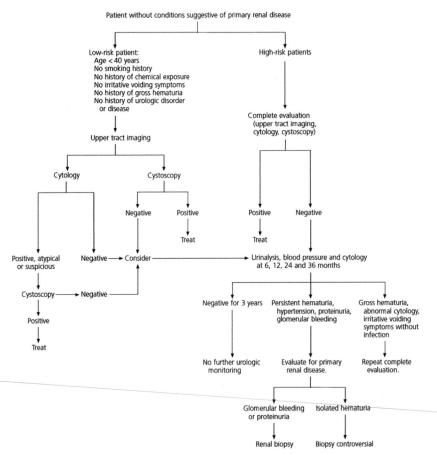

Fig. 1. Workup of hematuria in adults based on AUA best practice policy recommendations. (*Data from* Grossfeld GD, Wolf JS Jr, Litwan MS, et al. Asymptomatic microscopic hematuria in adults: summary of the AUA best practice policy recommendations. Am Fam Physician 2001;63(6):1148; and *Adapted from* Grossfeld GD, Wolf JS, Litwin MS, et al. Evaluation of asymptomatic microscopic hematuria in adults: the American Urological Association best practice policy recommendations. Part II: patient evaluation, cytology, voided markers, imaging, cystoscopy, nephrology evaluation, and follow-up. Urology 2001;57(4):607; with permission.)

Radiological Imaging of the Upper Urinary Tract

Several modalities are available to evaluate the upper genitourinary tract in patients with hematuria. These modalities include conventional radiography, intravenous pyelography, retrograde pyelography, ultrasonography, magnetic resonance imaging, magnetic resonance urography, conventional computed tomography (CT) scanning, and multidetector CT urography (CTU).[12–15] **Table 1** summarizes limitations associated with these radiological imaging modalities.

Because there are no data comparing the effect of various radiological modalities on the treatment of patients with hematuria, no formal guidelines for their use in the clinical setting have been established. However, most clinicians consider CTU to be the preferred initial imaging modality in most patients with unexplained hematuria.[14–17] CTU is a 3-phase CT scan with a noncontrast phase evaluating for urolithiasis, a contrast-enhanced phase for renal parenchymal abnormalities, and delayed images of the renal collecting system and ureters for pathologic conditions affecting the urothelial lining.[15] AUA guidelines suggest that patients with microscopic hematuria who are found to be at low risk for urologic malignancy and urolithiasis from noncontrast CT scan do not need further imaging and exposure to intravenous contrast.[3,9]

Patients in whom contraindications to the administration of intravenous contrast exist can be effectively imaged with the selective use of noncontrast CT, ultrasonography, magnetic resonance imaging, and retrograde pyelography, depending on clinical history and suspected causes within the differential diagnosis.[14] Urologic consultation may be of value.

Cystoscopy and Cytology

Even though the urinary bladder and its lumen can be visualized on radiological imaging, the lower urinary tract can only be adequately evaluated by cystoscopy. Consequently, direct visualization of the urothelium to determine the presence of lower urinary tract infection is mandatory in all patients at high risk for urologic disease. Modern cystoscopic equipment allows for well-tolerated, safe, and accurate assessment of the bladder and urethra in the outpatient setting.[18] Patients who are found to have a bladder tumor by cystoscopy should still undergo an initial imaging study of the upper urinary tract because of the multifocal nature of urothelial carcinoma.[3] Conversely, the identification of upper urinary tract infection does not preclude the need for cystoscopy.

Cytologic evaluation of the urine demonstrates excellent sensitivity and specificity for high-grade urothelial carcinoma, but has limited (45%–70%) sensitivity and specificity for low-grade disease, and requires an experienced cytopathologist for

Table 1	
Imaging modalities for evaluation of the upper urinary tract and their limitations.	
Imaging Modality	**Limitations**
Intravenous Urography	Poor sensitivity for and ability to characterize renal parenchymal masses, intravenous contrast exposure
Retrograde Pyelography	Poor sensitivity for and ability to characterize renal parenchymal masses, invasive
Ultrasonography	Limited ability to detect urolithiasis, small (<3 cm) renal mass, and urothelial abnormality
Magnetic Resonance Imaging	Expensive, time consuming, poor sensitivity for urolithiasis
CTU	Largest cumulative radiation exposure, expensive

interpretation of the results.[9] According to the AUA best practice guidelines, voided urinary cytology can be substituted for cystoscopy in patients without high-risk features for urologic disease (see **Fig. 1**).[11] Cystoscopy can then be performed if malignant or suspicious cells are identified. However, cytology may be used as an adjunct to cystoscopy in high-risk patients.

Because of the limitations of urinary cytology, several urine-based molecular tests for the detection of urothelial cancer have been developed (BTA stat, Polymedco Inc, Cortlandt, Manor, NY, USA; NMP-22, Matritech Inc, Newton, MA, USA; UroVysion, Vysis Inc, Downers Grove, IL, USA).[19] However, the role of these tests in the detection and follow-up of patients at risk for urothelial cancer is not defined at present. These costly urine markers are therefore not currently recommended in the initial evaluation of patients with hematuria.[9]

Follow-up

A small proportion of patients (≤1%) with a negative result in the initial hematuria evaluation are subsequently diagnosed with urologic malignancy. Consequently, periodic follow-up may be warranted.[6,20] AUA best practice guidelines suggest repeating urinalysis, voided urinary cytology, and blood pressure measurements at 6, 12, 24, and 36 months after the initial diagnosis of hematuria.[9] However, several recent studies question the cost-effectiveness of such a follow-up schedule in asymptomatic low-risk individuals owing to the very low incidence of positive findings.[1,21] Follow-up imaging studies and cystoscopy may be warranted in patients with persistent hematuria, in whom there is a high index of suspicion for significant underlying disease.

SUMMARY

Hematuria can be a sign of serious underlying genitourinary disease. Prompt and systematic evaluation of the genitourinary system should be initiated in the primary care setting and nephrologic or urologic consultations should be obtained, based on the suspected cause of hematuria. Methodical assessment of the upper and lower urinary tracts, as recommended by the AUA best practice guidelines (see **Fig. 1**), is paramount for the early detection and successful management of the underlying genitourinary disease.[11]

REFERENCES

1. Khadra MH, Pickard RS, Charlton M, et al. A prospective analysis of 1,930 patients with hematuria to evaluate current diagnostic practice. J Urol 2000; 163(2):524–7.
2. Mariani AJ, Mariani MC, Macchioni C, et al. The significance of adult hematuria: 1,000 hematuria evaluations including a risk-benefit and cost-effectiveness analysis. J Urol 1989;141(2):350–5.
3. Grossfeld GD, Litwin MS, Wolf JS, et al. Evaluation of asymptomatic microscopic hematuria in adults: the American Urological Association best practice policy– part I: definition, detection, prevalence, and etiology. Urology 2001;57(4): 599–603.
4. Sutton JM. Evaluation of hematuria in adults. JAMA 1990;263(18):2475–80.
5. Carter WC 3rd, Rous SN. Gross hematuria in 110 adult urologic hospital patients. Urology 1981;18(4):342–4.
6. Cohen RA, Brown RS. Clinical practice. Microscopic hematuria. N Engl J Med 2003;348(23):2330–8.

7. Mariani AJ, Luangphinith S, Loo S, et al. Dipstick chemical urinalysis: an accurate cost-effective screening test. J Urol 1984;132(1):64–6.

8. Yun EJ, Meng MV, Carroll PR. Evaluation of the patient with hematuria. Med Clin North Am 2004;88(2):329–43.

9. Grossfeld GD, Litwin MS, Wolf JS Jr, et al. Evaluation of asymptomatic microscopic hematuria in adults: the American Urological Association best practice policy–part II: patient evaluation, cytology, voided markers, imaging, cystoscopy, nephrology evaluation, and follow-up. Urology 2001;57(4):604–10.

10. Schramek P, Schuster FX, Georgopoulos M, et al. Value of urinary erythrocyte morphology in assessment of symptomless microhaematuria. Lancet 1989; 2(8675):1316–9.

11. Grossfeld GD, Wolf JS Jr, Litwan MS, et al. Asymptomatic microscopic hematuria in adults: summary of the AUA best practice policy recommendations. Am Fam Physician 2001;63(6):1145–54.

12. Warshauer DM, McCarthy SM, Street L, et al. Detection of renal masses: sensitivities and specificities of excretory urography/linear tomography, US, and CT. Radiology 1988;169(2):363–5.

13. Kawashima A, Glockner JF, King BF Jr. CT urography and MR urography. Radiol Clin North Am 2003;41(5):945–61.

14. O'Connor OJ, McSweeney SE, Maher MM. Imaging of hematuria. Radiol Clin North Am 2008;46(1):113–32, vii.

15. Sudakoff GS, Dunn DP, Guralnick ML, et al. Multidetector computerized tomography urography as the primary imaging modality for detecting urinary tract neoplasms in patients with asymptomatic hematuria. J Urol 2008;179(3):862–7 [discussion: 867].

16. Gray Sears CL, Ward JF, Sears ST, et al. Prospective comparison of computerized tomography and excretory urography in the initial evaluation of asymptomatic microhematuria. J Urol 2002;168(6):2457–60.

17. Choyke PL. Radiologic evaluation of hematuria: guidelines from the American College of Radiology's appropriateness criteria. Am Fam Physician 2008;78(3): 347–52.

18. Denholm SW, Conn IG, Newsam JE, et al. Morbidity following cystoscopy: comparison of flexible and rigid techniques. Br J Urol 1990;66(2):152–4.

19. Lotan Y, Roehrborn CG. Sensitivity and specificity of commonly available bladder tumor markers versus cytology: results of a comprehensive literature review and meta-analyses. Urology 2003;61(1):109–18 [discussion: 118].

20. Hiatt RA, Ordonez JD. Dipstick urinalysis screening, asymptomatic microhematuria, and subsequent urological cancers in a population-based sample. Cancer Epidemiol Biomarkers Prev 1994;3(5):439–43.

21. Madeb R, Golijanin D, Knopf J, et al. Long-term outcome of patients with a negative work-up for asymptomatic microhematuria. Urology 2010;75(1):20–5.

Urologic Assessment of Decreasing Renal Function

Mohummad Minhaj Siddiqui, MD*, W. Scott McDougal, MD

KEYWORDS

- Renal failure • Renal insufficiency • GFR
- Obstructive uropathy

The discussion of renal failure as it relates to urology is largely a discussion of obstructive uropathy. Obstructive uropathy has been identified in multiple series to account for approximately 10% of all cases of renal failure. On a total population scale, autopsy series have shown the prevalence of hydronephrosis in 3% of men and women who are younger than 65 years and 6% of men older than 65 years.[1] When benign prostatic hypertrophy (BPH) and renal stone disease are considered, obstructive uropathy is also one of the most common indications for surgery. In this review, the different causes of obstructive renal insufficiency and management options available are discussed.

ASSESSMENT OF RENAL FUNCTION

A variety of measures may be used by clinicians to help identify patients with renal failure. The gold standard is to measure the glomerular filtration rate (GFR). Normal GFR varies and generally decreases with age. On average, a patient's GFR decreases at a rate of 0.8 mL/min/1.73 m^2 per year from the age of 40 to 80 years.[2] The cause of this decrease is multifactorial, including microangiopathic changes, functional loss and atrophy of renal tubules and glomeruli, disintegration of tubular basement membranes, vacuole changes, and sclerosis of renal vasculature. Systemic diseases such as diabetes and hypertension can greatly accelerate this decrease. A decrease in renal mass is concurrently observed with decreasing GFR, with an average of 20% to 30% decrease in the mass noted in pathologic autopsy studies of patients aged 30 to 90 years and a 30% to 50% decrease in glomeruli in the cortex noted in histologic studies of patients aged 30 to 70 years.[3] Overall, a GFR greater than 90 mL/min/1.73 m^2 is considered to be normal renal function. A GFR between 60 and 90 mL/min/1.73 m^2 is considered mild chronic kidney disease, between 30 and 60 mL/min/1.73 m^2 moderate, and between 15 and 30 mL/min/1.73 m^2 severe. A GFR less than 15 mL/min/1.73 m^2 is considered renal failure.

Department of Urology, Massachusetts General Hospital, Harvard Medical School, 55 Fruit Street GRB 1102, Boston, MA 02114, USA
* Corresponding author.
E-mail address: mmsiddiqui@partners.org

Med Clin N Am 95 (2011) 161–168
doi:10.1016/j.mcna.2010.08.031
0025-7125/11/$ – see front matter © 2011 Elsevier Inc. All rights reserved.

The direct measurement of GFR can be tedious and impractical, hence the use of various proxy tests to estimate GFR. The most widespread measure of kidney function is the serum creatinine value. This measure remains imprecise at best because of its large degree of variability secondary to changes with age, gender, race and relationship with muscle mass. Therefore, although the creatinine value of 1.0 mg/dL may be generally considered normal, such a value may, in fact, signify renal insufficiency in children, the elderly, those with decreased muscle mass, and other individuals with various disorders.

Various equations have been devised to estimated GFR (eGFR) using easily gathered data. The Cockcroft-Gault equation includes the variables of serum creatinine value, age, mass, and gender.[4] The Modification of Diet in Renal Disease (MDRD) equation uses serum creatinine level, age, gender, and a correction factor for black patients. Of note, the MDRD equation does not account for body weight and tends to underestimate eGFR in heavy patients (and overestimate it in underweight patients). The MDRD equation was derived from patients with renal failure and performs best for low GFRs.[5] At higher GFRs, the newer Chronic Kidney Disease Epidemiology Collaboration equation has been found to be more valid.[6] This equation uses the same variables as the MDRD equation. Using these equations, eGFR is most appropriate for the practical ascertainment of renal insufficiency; however, the source population of the derivation of these equations is helpful in recognizing their limitations.

Of note, there are some patients specific to the urologic population, who have a falsely elevated serum creatinine level (ie, an elevated creatinine level in the setting of a normal GFR). Patients who have had urinary diversions, bladder augmentations, and neobladders constructed from a portion of the gastrointestinal tract reabsorb creatinine through the segments. These patients may have normally functioning kidneys; however, the resorption of creatinine results in a falsely elevated creatinine level.[7] Similarly, patients with urinary extravasation, such as those with a calyceal rupture from obstruction, resorb the urine and occasionally have a falsely elevated serum creatinine value.

DETERMINING THE CAUSE OF RENAL FAILURE

Acute renal failure is classified as prerenal, intrinsic, or postrenal. Information such as the clinical setting in which the renal failure took place is invaluable in determining the cause of the renal insufficiency. Information such as blood pressure, hemodynamic status, potential recent exposures to nephrotoxic insults, and concurrent systemic diseases all provide a critical insight as to the possible cause of the renal failure. The fractional excretion of sodium (FENa) is an often-used test to differentiate between the 3 causes of acute renal injury. An FENa less than 1% is considered consistent with a prerenal azotemia, whereas an FENa greater than 1% is observed more often with intrinsic and postrenal azotemia.

Urine studies are the foundation for the complete workup of renal insufficiency. Urinalysis with dipstick studies and microscopic analysis are both necessary tests for the complete workup of renal failure. They can provide immediate information such as pH, an approximation for osmolality, signs of infection, and sometimes, insight into the types of stones being formed because of crystals present on the smear. Different types of cellular casts give insight into causes such as acute tubular necrosis and nephritic syndrome. To gain further insight into any metabolic disorders, 24-hour urine analysis is necessary.

Renal ultrasonography is also a supplementary test that is helpful in determining obstructive uropathy. Hydronephrosis, hydroureteronephrosis, and renal parenchymal thickness can be observed on ultrasonography. These observations are helpful in narrowing the differential diagnosis as to the cause of obstructive uropathy. Any obstruction of the urinary tract associated with infection is a urologic emergency requiring immediate urologic consultation and intervention because sepsis and even death can be a consequence.

If these initial tests suggest the diagnosis of urinary tract obstruction, additional tests are helpful in further characterizing the nature of the obstruction. Noncontrast computed tomography (CT) can identify most stones and can be used to determine the hardness of the stone to provide an insight into its possible composition. CT can also be helpful in confirming obstruction secondary to malignancy; however, contrast CT and CT urography are best suited for identifying extrinsic and intrinsic sources of obstruction. Nuclear scans, such as the mercaptoacetyltriglycine (MAG3) with furosemide (Lasix) renal scan, are helpful in establishing the diagnosis of ureteropelvic junction (UPJ) obstruction and clinically significant ureteral stricture disease. Retrograde urography can be invaluable when the above-mentioned tests lead to unclear diagnosis. Antegrade urography and the Whitaker test, as well as an antegrade pressure-flow study to assess for obstruction, are less commonly used, given all the other less-invasive alternatives in practice at present, but these tests remain potentially useful studies under selected circumstances.

PHYSIOLOGIC CHANGES WITH OBSTRUCTION

There are significant differences between unilateral and bilateral ureteral obstructions. Many of these changes have been well characterized in animal models. Unilateral ureteral obstruction is characterized by an initial increase in pressure within the renal tubules and a decrease in GFR. In case of unilateral ureteral obstruction, the vasculature of the kidney attempts to compensate for the decreased GFR, with an increase in renal blood flow mediated by release of vasodilators from the affected kidney. A later-phase response with unilateral ureteral obstruction results in decreased blood flow secondary to increased release of vasoconstrictors, such as renin, resulting in the formation of angiotensin from the obstructed kidney.[8]

Bilateral ureteral obstruction (or equivalently unilateral obstruction in a uninephric system) is characterized by only a modest initial increase in renal blood flow followed by a more significant decrease in bilateral renal blood flow. Unlike unilateral ureteral obstruction, in which the ureteral urine pressure is initially elevated but quickly decreases, the ureteral pressure remains elevated for a longer period in bilateral obstruction. Because there is no second renal unit to compensate for the ureteral obstruction, the patient often has fluid accumulation and total body fluid overload. There is often an obliteration of the concentration gradient within the kidneys in the cases of bilateral ureteral obstruction.[9]

Of note, in cases of bilateral obstruction, release of the obstruction can lead to postobstructive diuresis. This diuresis is characterized by large volumes of urine production in the order of 200 mL per hour or more. However, much of this urine production is often a physiologic response to the fluid overload and electrolyte accumulation that occurred during the period of obstruction.[10] The condition may, however, also have a pathologic component secondary to the obliterated concentration gradient within the kidneys and hence a loss of concentration ability. Furthermore, prolonged obstruction can also lead to damage of the tubular cells and the multiple electrolyte transporters. This damage can result in a prolonged deficiency in concentrating ability and thus prolonged diuresis even after the fluid and electrolyte balances are restored. Such a diuresis is usually self-limited. Management is generally supportive with the monitoring of serum electrolytes and maintenance of hydration at a rate slower than that of diuresis to allow the body to gradually arrive at the appropriate fluid balance. Prolonged and nonimproving diuresis may warrant urologic or renal consultation for further workup and management.[11]

The ultimate recovery of renal function may factor into the decision of what type of intervention, if any, is suited for a patient with obstructive uropathy. A prospective study on recovery after treatment of obstruction demonstrated that preoperative renographic GFR and renal perfusion correlated with ultimate recovery. The investigators observed that a preoperative GFR of 10 mL/min/1.73 m^2 for the affected kidney on renographic GFR was the cutoff point below which significant recovery did not occur.[12]

CAUSES OF OBSTRUCTIVE RENAL FAILURE
BPH

BPH can lead to a chronic outlet obstruction, which if left untreated can lead to increasing voiding pressures that ultimately affect the upper tracts.[13] It can also lead to urinary retention that can similarly lead to functional bilateral obstruction and renal damage. In a series of 47 elderly patients with obstructive uropathy leading to renal failure, 38% of the cases were secondary to BPH. Similarly, autopsy-based series show the incidence of hydronephrosis secondary to obstructive uropathy in approximately 3% of women and men younger than 60 years. Men older than 60 years have an incidence of 6%, however, with the 3% increase is largely because of BPH.[10]

The workup of BPH consists of history of signs of lower urinary tract symptoms (LUTS) and obstructive uropathy, including weak stream, postvoid dribbling, hesitancy, and urgency. A physical examination consisting of a digital rectal examination to characterize the prostate size and consistency and lower abdominal percussion and palpation to assess for bladder distention are of particular importance. A bladder scanner can be particularly helpful in determining the volume of postvoid residual urine. In unclear cases, the patient can be referred to a urologist who may perform a urodynamics study to differentiate bladder outlet obstruction from other causes of LUTS.

The primary medical management of BPH consists of a 5α-reductase blocker to reduce the size of the prostate and/or an α-blocker to decrease smooth muscle contraction in the prostate and bladder outlet. Clinical presentations such as renal failure secondary to retention, bladder stones, and failure of maximal medical therapy are all indications for surgical intervention.

Obstructing Stone

Nephrolithiasis is another common cause of ureteral obstruction, which can sometimes lead to renal failure. Most commonly, causes of more-immediate renal failure occur in cases of bilateral simultaneous obstruction, or similarly, unilateral obstruction in a patient with one kidney. However, patients with baseline chronic renal insufficiency sometimes also experience renal failure with the obstruction of one of their kidneys. A more detailed explanation of the management of nephrolithiasis is discussed in the article by Tseng and Stroller elsewhere in this issue. However, the management of kidney stones causing renal failure is discussed further in the article by Margulis and Sagalowsky elsewhere in this issue.

There are few studies describing renal failure secondary to stones causing obstructive uropathy.[14] Most of such studies are in the form of case reports and describe renal failure from bilateral obstructing stones (or unilateral in a uninephric system). Any patient presenting with such a clinical scenario should be referred to the urologist for likely urgent intervention. Patients who are especially at risk for such an event are multiple stone formers (ie, patients with lymphoma and hyperuricosuria undergoing treatment or human immunodeficiency virus–positive patients on indinavir). Treatment of the underlying metabolic derangement is important in such patients.

The case of a patient with a unilateral obstructing stone and increasing creatinine levels is more difficult. Increasing levels of creatinine may be from renal insufficiency, but another common reason for elevated creatinine levels is calyceal rupture with urinary extravasation into the retroperitoneum. The urine is resorbed into the body and causes an artificial elevation of creatinine level. Renal insufficiency is a justified reason for semiurgent intervention, whereas calyceal rupture can often be observed conservatively.

It is the authors' practice to observe patients with a question of borderline, developing renal insufficiency from an obstructing stone without any other reason necessitating intervention. If repeat test demonstrated a persistently worsening creatinine level, intervention is indicated.

The most common methods for decompression include retrograde ureteral stent or percutaneous nephrostomy tube placement. Typically, ureteral stents are favored, except in cases in which cystoscopy or general anesthesia is contraindicated.

Stricture

Ureteral strictures can be an insidious cause of renal deterioration. They can be caused by a multitude of causes including impacted ureteral stones, infection, trauma, periureteral fibrosis, malignancy, or congenital reasons. Workup includes retrograde and/or antegrade ureterography, CT urography, and MAG3 with Lasix renal scan to provide data regarding drainage impairment as well as kidney function. Management options include endoscopic management with ureteral stents, dilation or incision of the stricture, or more involved open surgical procedures. Open surgical options range from simple bladder hitch with reimplantation procedures to reconstructive operations using the ileum as a ureteral substitute. Patients with any ureteral stricture causing hydronephrosis should be referred to a urologist for further workup and management.

UPJ Obstruction

UPJ obstructions are most commonly seen in the pediatric population; however, a significant incidence also occurs in adolescents and adults. The causes of these obstructions are highly variable, ranging from aperistaltic segments of smooth muscle to an aberrantly crossing blood vessel causing compression on the UPJ. The degree of obstruction can be severe enough that over a long period the affected kidney may lose a significant amount of function. The workup of a UPJ obstruction usually includes a MAG3 with Lasix scan, which helps characterize the degree of obstruction and how well the kidney drains as well as the relative function of the kidney. This condition can at times be confused with a large extrarenal pelvis, which is simply an anatomic variant of no consequence to the patient. Typically, treatment is surgical with a laparoscopic or open surgical pyeloplasty because endoscopic management has generally shown low long-term success rates.[15]

Neurogenic Bladder

Neurogenic bladder can lead to lower tract voiding dysfunction and retention that results in high pressures of the upper tract. Patients with a significant history of diabetes especially can develop bladders that have decreased sensation of fullness and may become filled to higher volumes. Changes take place to the bladder wall as it is chronically stretched and, some theorize, made ischemic. There is a decrease in compliance and therefore, an increase in vesical pressures over time. After a resting intravesical pressure of approximately 40 mm Hg is reached, damage can begin to take place to the upper urinary tracts. These patients are often elderly with multiple comorbidities, including chronic renal insufficiency as well as diabetes. If patients are unable to void to sufficiently empty the bladder, they must be maintained on an appropriate drainage regimen for their bladder to avoid a chronic insult on their kidneys.[16]

Tumor Obstruction

Tumors are a common cause of obstructive uropathy, for which intervention can have a significant effect on preserving renal function. Tumors intrinsic to the genitourinary tract are not discussed because their management is discussed elsewhere in detail in this issue. Extrinsic metastatic disease can often obstruct ureters by a compression effect. The most common cancers that cause extrinsic compression are colon, rectal, breast, and ovarian cancer as well as lymphoma. Goals of care are extremely important when faced with a patient who has extrinsic compression from metastatic cancer. The median survival of patients with obstruction caused by metastatic malignancy is about 3 to 7 months.[17] Many of the interventions undertaken to preserve renal function are, in reality, simply palliative. Factors such as pain from the obstruction, potential discomfort from an indwelling stent, or discomfort from a nephrostomy tube are all important. Furthermore, many stents fail, thereby requiring occasional urgent placement of nephrostomy tubes, another event that can be an unnecessary stress on an end-of-life patient.

However, there are many patients who clearly benefit from decompression of the extrinsic ureteral obstruction. Any patient who receives renotoxic chemotherapy stands to benefit greatly from intervention to bypass the obstruction, especially if there is a possibility that the chemotherapy may treat the lesion causing the obstruction. Patients whose disease does not confer a short life expectancy may also benefit from decompression of their kidneys.

The choice of using an internalized indwelling stent or a nephrostomy tube is complex and requires an assessment of risks and benefits for the particular patient, taking into account the disease process. Internalized stents have the benefit of no external appliances to care for and possibly a decreased risk of infection. However, they have a high rate of stent failure (on the order of 40%) in the patient population being studied. Patients with rectal cancer, breast cancer, and lymphoma are particularly prone to stent failure. Stents require visits to the operating room and general anesthesia every 3 to 4 months for stent changes. Stents can also be fairly uncomfortable. It has been observed that baseline creatinine values greater than 1.3, the need for poststent systemic treatment, and the specific type of cancer are predictors of stent failure.[18]

Percutaneous nephrostomy tubes have the benefit of ease of placement when the renal pelvis is dilated and easier to manage. These tubes require changes every 3 months, which can be performed under local anesthesia. The tubes must be managed with a drainage bag and are prone to accidents such as dislodgement.

Miscellaneous Causes of Obstruction

A large list of other causes for obstructive uropathy exist, although the most common causes have been discussed in this article. For example, retroperitoneal fibrosis has a peak incidence in patients aged 40 to 60 years and is predominant in men. The disease is characterized by fibrosis of the retroperitoneal structures, including the vena cava, aorta, and ureters. Pelvic lipomatosis is a condition of pelvic overgrowth of adipose tissue in the retroperitoneum. It has a characteristic radiological appearance of "squeezing" the ureters medially and the bladder into a pear shape. Patients may present with nonspecific symptoms such as constipation and LUTS.

SUMMARY

Obstructive uropathy has a wide spectrum of presentations. Each cause has a different management strategy and variable outcomes. Obstruction can take place anywhere, from the urethra to the kidney with differing outcomes and concerns at each level. Obstruction causing renal failure at essentially any level along the urinary tract should at a minimum lead to a urologic evaluation. Special concern in all of these cases must be paid to concurrent obstruction with fever and infection because they may be an indication for immediate intervention. Ultimately, management decisions should take into account not only expected outcomes but also the morbidity of the intervention and the overall state and goals of care of the patient.

REFERENCES

1. Bell ET. Obstruction of the urinary tract-hydronephrosis. In: Renal diseases. 2nd edition. Philadelphia: Lea & Febiger; 1950. p. 117–45.
2. Back SE, Ljungberg B, Nilsson-Ehle I, et al. Age dependence of renal function: clearance of iohexol and p-amino hippurate in healthy males. Scand J Clin Lab Invest 1989;49(7):641–6.
3. Brown WW, Davis BB, Spry LA, et al. Aging and the kidney. Arch Intern Med 1986;146(9):1790–6.
4. Cockcroft DW, Gault MH. Prediction of creatinine clearance from serum creatinine. Nephron 1976;16(1):31–41.
5. Levey AS, Bosch JP, Lewis JB, et al. A more accurate method to estimate glomerular filtration rate from serum creatinine: a new prediction equation. Modification of Diet in Renal Disease Study Group. Ann Intern Med 1999;130(6):461–70.
6. Levey AS, Stevens LA, Schmid CH, et al. A new equation to estimate glomerular filtration rate. Ann Intern Med 2009;150(9):604–12.
7. Tanrikut C, McDougal WS. Acid-base and electrolyte disorders after urinary diversion. World J Urol 2004;22(3):168–71.
8. Zeidel ML, Pirtskhalaishvili G. Urinary tract obstruction. In: Brenner B, editor. The kidney. Philadelphia: Saunders; 2004. p. 1867.
9. Shoskes DA, McMahon AW. Renal physiology and pathophysiology. In: Wein AJ, Kavoussi LR, Novick AC, et al, editors. Campbells-Walsh urology. Philadelphia: Saunders; 2007. p. 1131.
10. Tseng TY, Stoller ML. Obstructive uropathy. Clin Geriatr Med 2009;25(3):437–43.
11. Klahr S, Morrissey J. Obstructive nephropathy and renal fibrosis. Am J Physiol Renal Physiol 2002;283(5):F861–75.
12. Khalaf IM, Shokeir AA, El-Gyoushi FI, et al. Recoverability of renal function after treatment of adult patients with unilateral obstructive uropathy and normal contralateral kidney: a prospective study. Urology 2004;64(4):664–8.
13. Rule AD, Lieber MM, Jacobsen SJ. Is benign prostatic hyperplasia a risk factor for chronic renal failure? J Urol 2005;173(3):691–6.
14. Gosmanova EO, Baumgarten DA, O'Neill WC. Acute kidney injury in a patient with unilateral ureteral obstruction. Am J Kidney Dis 2009;54(4):775–9.
15. Yong D, Albala DM. Endopyelotomy in the age of laparoscopic and robotic-assisted pyeloplasty. Curr Urol Rep 2010;11(2):74–9.
16. Lawrenson R, Wyndaele JJ, Vlachonikolis I, et al. Renal failure in patients with neurogenic lower urinary tract dysfunction. Neuroepidemiology 2001;20(2):138–43.

17. Kouba E, Wallen EM, Pruthi RS. Management of ureteral obstruction due to advanced malignancy: optimizing therapeutic and palliative outcomes. J Urol 2008;180(2):444–50.
18. Chung SY, Stein RJ, Landsittel D, et al. 15-year experience with the management of extrinsic ureteral obstruction with indwelling ureteral stents. J Urol 2004;172(2): 592–5.

Medical and Medical/ Urologic Approaches in Acute and Chronic Urologic Stone Disease

Timothy Y. Tseng, MD[a], Marshall L. Stoller, MD[b],*

KEYWORDS

- Nephrolithiasis • Urolithiasis • Kidney stones
- Management • Prevention

Urinary stone disease is a condition with far-reaching implications. Patients with their initial presentation of acute renal colic generally enter the health care system through 2 routes. Severe cases are seen in the emergency room, whereas more tolerable cases may be seen by primary care physicians. Patients with urinary stone disease are then managed in the long-term by a urologist. This article reviews the epidemiology, pathogenesis, presentation, and short- and long-term management of acute and chronic urinary stone disease.

EPIDEMIOLOGY

In the United States, the 1988 to 1994 National Health and Nutrition Examination Survey (NHANES III) prospective cohort study found the lifetime prevalence of urinary stone disease to be 5.2%.[1] Stone disease seems to be on the rise, because the 1976 to 1980 NHANES II study recorded a lifetime prevalence of only 3.2%. In NHANES III, lifetime prevalence of stone disease was higher in men at 6.3% compared with 4.1% in women. The risk of stone disease generally seemed to increase as one aged, with the highest prevalence of stone disease in men occurring in the 70- to 74-year-old age group at 13.3%. Women experienced a peak prevalence in their sixth decade of 7.0%. In general, non-Hispanic Caucasian patients had the highest risk of urinary stone disease with a prevalence of 5.9%. Hispanic and African American patients had lower risks of stone disease with prevalences of 2.6% and 1.7%, respectively. Geography

a Department of Urology, University of Texas Health Science Center at San Antonio, San Antonio, TX, USA
b Department of Urology, University of California San Francisco, Box 0738, 400 Parnassus Avenue, UC Clinics A-638, San Francisco, CA 94143-0738, USA
* Corresponding author.
E-mail address: mstoller@urology.ucsf.edu

Med Clin N Am 95 (2011) 169–177
doi:10.1016/j.mcna.2010.08.034
0025-7125/11/$ – see front matter © 2011 Published by Elsevier Inc.

medical.theclinics.com

also seemed to play a role in the risk of stone disease. The US South had the highest age-adjusted lifetime prevalence of stone disease at 6.6%, whereas the West had the lowest prevalence at 3.3%. In the Midwest, the prevalence was 4.6% and in the Northeast, 5.1%.

Regarding costs, as urinary stone disease is increasingly treated on an outpatient basis, the number of inpatient discharges for a diagnosis of urolithiasis has been declining gradually. Nevertheless, in 2007, the Nationwide Inpatient Sample recorded 155,860 urinary stone inpatient discharges. At an estimated true cost of $6128 per inpatient discharge, the total cost of these hospitalizations was $955,192,450.[2] The actual cost for treatment of urinary stone disease would probably be several orders of magnitude greater if outpatient procedures were included. Proper acute and long-term management of such patients is therefore essential.

PATHOGENESIS

The vast majority of patients with urolithiasis have stones composed of calcium oxalate (65%–70%) or calcium phosphate (16%–20%). Approximately 8% of patients have stones composed of uric acid. An additional 2% of patients have cystine stones.[3,4] Stone formation historically has been viewed as a disorder of mineral metabolism. Conditions leading to the supersaturation of urine with various minerals result in their precipitation out of the urine. Predisposing conditions can include low urine volumes, increased urinary mineral excretion, and abnormal urine pH leading to altered solubility.[5,6]

Excluding low urine volumes, the most common abnormality found in patients with urolithiasis is hypercalciuria, defined as a urinary calcium excretion of greater than 200 to 250 mg/d or greater than 4 mg/kg/d. When caused by abnormal intestinal absorption, this condition is termed absorptive hypercalciuria. This form of hypercalciuria is the result of an increased filtered load and a reduced renal tubular reabsorption due to suppression of parathyroid hormone. Absorptive hypercalciuria is further subcategorized as (1) Type I absorptive hypercalciuria, a more severe form in which urinary calcium excretion remains high despite dietary restriction; (2) Type II absorptive hypercalciuria, a milder form in which urinary calcium excretion normalizes with dietary restriction; and (3) Type III absorptive hypercalciuria, a condition caused by a renal phosphate leak in which hypophosphatemia stimulates increased vitamin D synthesis and enhanced intestinal absorption of calcium.

Hypercalciuria may also be due primarily to decreased renal tubular reabsorption of calcium, termed renal leak hypercalciuria. The decreased reabsorption of calcium leads to secondary hyperparathyroidism and increased intestinal absorption of calcium, which further contributes to the increased urinary excretion of calcium. Serum calcium in renal leak hypercalciuria remains normal. In contrast to renal leak hypercalciuria, primary hyperparathyroidism may result in hypercalciuria due to excessive resorption of calcium from bone in addition to increased enteric calcium absorption. In these patients, serum calcium and parathyroid hormone are elevated.

Hyperuricosuria is a disorder defined by excess urinary excretion of uric acid or urate greater than 600 mg/d. This condition may contribute to the formation of uric acid stones. Also, it may be the only abnormality detected in up to 10% of patients with calcium stones and is thought to lead to calcium urolithiasis through a process of heterogeneous nucleation. Another disorder that can lead to uric acid stone formation is gouty diathesis. This is defined by the presence of gouty arthritis and hyperuricosemia or the condition of an abnormally low urine pH less than 5.5 at which the solubility of uric acid is markedly decreased.

Another potential contributor to urinary stone disease is hyperoxaluria, defined as a urinary excretion of oxalate greater than 40 mg/d. This condition may be due primarily to excess enteric absorption or may be secondary to malabsorptive states, such as those seen with inflammatory bowel disease. In the latter case, fat malabsorption results in the sequestering of enteric calcium, thereby reducing the amount of calcium available to bind to and prevent the absorption of oxalate. Citrate is a known inhibitor of stone formation. Thus, hypocitraturia, which is defined as a urinary citrate excretion of less than 450 mg/d and may be due to distal renal tubular acidosis or other metabolic acidoses, may exacerbate stone formation. Inborn errors of cysteine metabolism can also lead to cystinuria, defined as a urinary cystine excretion greater than 250 mg/d and cystine stone formation.

Aside from disorders of mineral metabolism, chronic upper urinary tract infections with urea-splitting bacteria, such as *Proteus*, *Pseudomonas*, *Providencia*, *Klebsiella*, and *Ureaplasma*, can lead to alkalinization of the urine, typically leading to a pH greater than 7.2, potentially resulting in the formation of struvite stones composed of magnesium ammonium phosphate.

MORBIDITY

The consequences of untreated urinary stone disease are significant. In the short term, obstruction of an infected renal unit may lead to severe urosepsis and death. In the long term, stone disease may contribute to recurrent pyelonephritis or permanent ureteral stricture. Persistent urinary obstruction may also cause renal insufficiency and end-stage renal disease. Indeed, in less developed countries, such as Thailand and Indonesia, where access to medical care may be limited, urinary stone disease accounts for 20% of patients on dialysis. In developed countries, only 1% of end-stage renal disease is directly attributable to urinary stone disease.[7] Prompt and appropriate treatment for urinary stone disease is therefore essential to prevent these potential complications.

CLINICAL MANIFESTATIONS AND DIAGNOSIS

Urinary stones are thought to begin as calcifications in renal papillae termed nephrocalcinosis. When these stones erode through the renal papillae and become free within the renal collecting system, nephrolithiasis is the result. Generally, stones that are located peripherally within the collecting system are asymptomatic. Only when one of these stones becomes lodged in the ureter and causes some degree of relative or complete obstruction does a stone typically cause renal colic.

A stone in the proximal ureter tends to cause ipsilateral flank or upper quadrant abdominal pain. As the stone migrates down the ureter, the pain tends to migrate to the ipsilateral lower quadrant and may radiate to the ipsilateral testicle or labium. The pain associated with renal colic is frequently described as sharp, intermittent with acute paroxysms of pain, and similar to or worse than the pains associated with childbirth. The pain is usually not pinpoint or positional. In distinction to patients with appendicitis or peritoneal signs who may appear stiff and immobile, patients with renal colic often find it hard to remain still because of the pain. Stones that reach the junction between the ureter and the bladder (ureterovesical junction) may also cause irritative voiding systems, such as dysuria, urgency, and frequency, that may be confused with a urinary tract infection. Only rarely do patients present without symptoms of colic. These patients may experience only recurrent urinary tract infections or painless hematuria. Such patients may therefore present with longstanding ureteral obstruction resulting in permanent renal damage.

The diagnosis of symptomatic urolithiasis is generally suspected based on the history provided by the patient. On physical examination, the patient may have ipsilateral costovertebral angle tenderness. Tenderness to superficial palpation of the flank or tenderness that crosses the midline is suggestive of a musculoskeletal cause. Examination of the testicles in a man should be performed to exclude testicular torsion as a cause of the patient's symptoms.

When acute urinary stone disease is suspected, the most definitive imaging study is a noncontrast renal stone protocol computed tomographic (CT) scan.[8] A stone protocol CT scan acquires 1- to 2-mm thickness cuts through a patient and is able to identify nearly all stones except those composed of indinavir, an HIV protease inhibitor. Also, a CT scan provides information regarding the potential severity of the obstruction as manifested by the degree of hydronephrosis. A CT scan may also identify other potential causes of a patient's symptoms, such as appendicitis, pyelonephritis, and adnexal disease.[9] A stone protocol CT scan should be performed in the prone position to distinguish between a stone at the ureterovesical junction and one that has passed into the bladder, thus lying in its dependent anterior portion. Stones that pass spontaneously through the ureter almost invariably pass through the urethra without difficulty.

Recently, the fairly high radiation exposure rates from CT scanning in patients with urinary stone disease have been recognized.[10] In an effort to reduce exposure rates, a combination of plain abdominal radiograph (KUB) to detect radiopaque stones and renal ultrasound scan to detect hydronephrosis is considered an acceptable alternative imaging approach in appropriately selected patients. The ultrasound scan should be performed both with the bladder full and drained to properly assess for hydronephrosis and the presence of ureteral jets on Doppler imaging that may suggest an absence of ureteral obstruction. The reduced radiation exposure of this regimen comes at a cost of decreased sensitivity and specificity for detecting urinary calculi compared with CT scan.[11] Alternatively, low-dose renal protocol CT scans with greater "noise" have shown promise with sensitivity and specificity comparable to standard CT scans for identifying stones larger than 2 mm in diameter with radiation dose reductions approaching those of a conventional KUB.[12] Radiation exposure should be avoided, if possible, in patients who may be pregnant. In these patients, a less-than-definitive diagnosis should be made based on clinical suspicion and ultrasound scan alone.

In addition to making an imaging diagnosis, additional laboratory studies should be considered to assess the severity of a patient's condition. In general, a patient with a fever and/or an elevated white blood cell count should be considered infected and obstructed and deserves immediate treatment for relief of the obstruction. Elevated serum blood urea nitrogen and creatinine levels may also suggest significant obstruction. Finally, a urinalysis may be useful, the presence of bacteria suggesting a complicating urinary tract infection. The presence of red blood cells on urinalysis in a less symptomatic patient may suggest the need for further investigation, including an eventual hematuria workup. Finally, a low urine pH in the absence of visible calculi on KUB may suggest the presence of radiolucent uric acid stones.

ACUTE TREATMENT

Once the diagnosis of a urinary stone associated with symptoms of acute renal colic is made, several treatment options may be pursued. If a stone is small, generally less than 5 mm in diameter, there is a high likelihood that the stone may pass spontaneously. In general, when considering distal ureteral stones up to 10 mm in diameter, approximately 50% pass spontaneously with a mean time to passage of up to 2 weeks. Medical expulsive therapy with an α-adrenergic antagonist, such as tamsulosin, with or without a nonsteroidal anti-inflammatory drug (NSAID) increases the spontaneous stone passage rate to 85% and decreases the mean time to stone passage to approximately 1 week.[13,14] In most patients whose pain can be managed with oral analgesics and who do not exhibit signs of infection, renal insufficiency, or massive dilatation of the affected renal collecting system, conservative medical management with an expulsive agent, such as tamsulosin, is warranted for up to 4 weeks. Typically, nonsteroidal anti-inflammatory agents provide the most symptomatic relief, although narcotic analgesics are frequently required. Although most patients are also counseled to increase their fluid hydration during an acute episode of renal colic, based on the theory that increased urine output enhances the expulsion of the stone, a small randomized controlled trial has shown no effect of this intervention on stone passage rates.[15]

Patients who have a fever, elevated white blood cell count, or acute renal insufficiency deserve immediate intervention to relieve the probable obstruction of the urinary tract. Intractable pain is also an indication for such intervention. Generally, this may be accomplished by cystoscopic placement of a ureteral stent by the urologist. However, if a patient has a high fever or is otherwise in extremis, ureteral stent placement may serve as a conduit for ascending infection and urosepsis.[16] In such cases, percutaneous nephrostomy tube placement by an interventional radiologist is recommended.

For any symptomatic stone that does not or cannot be passed spontaneously, an active treatment intervention, such as shock wave lithotripsy, ureteroscopic lithotripsy, percutaneous nephrolithotomy, or laparoscopic/open stone removal, may be undertaken electively by the urologist. Shock wave lithotripsy uses focused high-intensity sound waves to fragment small renal or ureteral calculi. Although less invasive, the disadvantages of this treatment modality include difficulty targeting radiolucent stones; difficulty fragmenting extremely hard stones, such as calcium oxalate monohydrate, brushite, and cystine stones; and a generally lower postprocedure stone-free rate of 73% to 82% compared with other modalities. Ureteroscopy with pneumatic or holmium laser lithotripsy is a common procedure that results in an 81% to 94% postprocedure stone-free rate.[17] For both interventions, patients must still pass the resultant stone fragments themselves.

Larger stones located in the renal collecting system are called staghorn calculi. They are *partial* when they fill only some of the calyces and *complete* when they fill the entire collecting system. Such stones are most appropriately treated with percutaneous nephrolithotomy, in which a rigid nephroscope is passed through one or more 1-cm flank incisions into the renal collecting system. The stones are then fragmented and suctioned out of the collecting system using an ultrasonic and/or pneumatic probe. The stone-free rate after percutaneous nephrolithotomy is approximately 78%.[18] Laparoscopic and open stone-removal procedures result in a stone-free rate similar to that of percutaneous nephrolithotomy and are therefore performed rarely, given the increased risks of such procedures.

LONG-TERM MANAGEMENT

Urinary stone disease can be expected to recur in up to 50% of patients within 5 years.[19–21] For recurrent stone-formers, referral to a urologist for metabolic evaluation to identify predisposing risk factors is warranted. Although frequently uninformative due to the predominance of calcium-based stones, a stone analysis may be useful to identify uric acid, cystine, and other rare stones. Barring such findings, a metabolic evaluation consisting of serum tests and a 24-hour urine panel is more useful. An elevated serum calcium and parathyroid hormone level may suggest a diagnosis of primary hyperparathyroidism and the need for referral to an endocrine surgeon. An elevated uric acid level may suggest gout and the need for treatment with a xanthine oxidase inhibitor, such as allopurinol.

In the absence of any serum abnormalities, a 24-hour urine panel identifies conditions of hypercalciuria, gouty diathesis, hypocitraturia, hyperuricosuria, hyperoxaluria, and cystinuria. Patients with hypercalciuria not due to primary hyperparathyroidism may be treated with a thiazide diuretic. Such agents promote the retention of calcium within the blood, thereby decreasing urinary excretion of calcium. A typical initial regimen is chlorthalidone 25 mg once daily. Patients should have their serum potassium level checked within 1 week of starting a thiazide diuretic to ensure that hypokalemia does not occur. Excess sodium intake, as evidenced by hypernatruria, is also associated with enhanced urinary calcium excretion. Therefore, dietary sodium intake should be limited to maintain urinary sodium excretion at less than 150 to 200 mg/d.

Gouty diathesis and hypocitraturia may be treated by alkalinizing the urine with potassium citrate starting at 60 mEq daily in divided doses. Potassium citrate is available in 10 mEq wax matrix tablets, 30 mEq crystal packets, and liquid preparations. Patients started on potassium citrate should have their serum potassium levels checked within 1 to 2 weeks to identify potential hyperkalemia. In patients who cannot tolerate the added potassium load because of chronic renal insufficiency, sodium bicarbonate 325 mg thrice daily may be used, although it is not ideal because of the increased sodium load. Patients with hyperuricosuria should decrease their intake of purine-rich foods, such as animal meat.[22,23] Hyperuricosuric patients with elevated serum uric acid levels may be treated with allopurinol at a starting dosage of 300 mg/d to decrease uric acid excretion and an alkalinizing agent to increase the urinary solubility of uric acid. Allopurinol is infrequently associated with toxic epidermal necrolysis and should be discontinued for any new-onset dermatologic changes.[24]

For those patients with hyperoxaluria, a reduction in consumption of oxalate-rich foods, such as spinach, nuts, and tea, is recommended. However, dietary changes sometimes make the condition worse because of substitution with other oxalate-rich foods. Therefore, 24-hour urine panels should be repeated to assess the effectiveness of dietary interventions. Because hyperoxaluria may also result from excess intestinal absorption of oxalate under conditions of fat malabsorption, hyperoxaluric patients may be treated further with rapidly dissolving forms of calcium, such as calcium carbonate (TUMS) at meal times. In general, a low dietary calcium intake has been shown to be associated with a higher risk of urinary stone disease.[25–27] For these reasons, calcium restriction is not recommended in patients with urinary stone disease.

Patients with cystinuria may be treated with alkalinization using potassium citrate and a chelating agent, such as α-mercaptopropionylglycine (Thiola). Alkalinization increases the solubility of cystine. Chelating agents bound to cysteine molecules create compounds more soluble than cystine, which is the product of binding between 2 cysteine molecules. Initial α-mercaptopropionylglycine dosing is 100 mg for every 100 mg/d of urinary cystine excretion given in 3 to 4 divided doses daily. α-Mercaptopropionylglycine is frequently associated with side effects, such as asthenia and gastrointestinal problems, resulting in cessation of the medication in approximately 30% of patients. An alternative chelating agent, D-penicillamine, may also be used but is even less well-tolerated. Patients treated with D-penicillamine should also be treated prophylactically with vitamin B6 because of potential drug-induced deficiency.

Regardless of metabolically-directed treatment, increasing urine output remains central to the long-term management of urinary stone disease.[28] As urine output increases, the concentration of the mineral constituents of the urine decreases, resulting in a lower risk of mineral precipitation and stone formation. Stone-forming patients are therefore counseled to increase their fluid intake to produce 1.5 to 2 L of urine per day. Cystine-stone formers are a special group, however. Because there are no known metabolic defect-specific inhibitors of cystine stone formation, such patients are encouraged to increase their fluid intake to produce 3 to 4 L of urine per day. Because relative dehydration occurs during sleep, cystinuric patients are frequently counseled to set alarms to hydrate and void several times during sleep. For chronic stone-formers, periodic metabolic re-evaluation with 24-hour urine panels helps to assess the efficacy of metabolic interventions.

FUTURE DIRECTIONS

Although urinary stone disease has historically been viewed as a disorder of mineral metabolism, a growing body of evidence has demonstrated an association between stone disease and other systemic conditions, most notably, atherogenic risk factors. In particular, obesity, diabetes mellitus, hypertension, and metabolic syndrome itself are associated with increased risks of urinary stone disease.[29–34] General recommendations for urinary stone prevention include decreased sodium and animal protein intake. More specific recommendations based on metabolic evaluations include using antihypertensive thiazide diuretics. Each of these recommendations is used in general medical practice to decrease the risk of cardiovascular disease. It may therefore be appropriate to classify and treat urinary stone disease as one of the many manifestations of cardiovascular disease. Future research into the precise mechanisms through which cardiovascular risk factors increase the risk of stone disease are needed to more fully elucidate the etiology of urinary stone disease.

SUMMARY

Urinary stone disease is a common condition that, when untreated, can result in serious complications, including sepsis and renal failure. Acutely, patients may present with paroxysmal ipsilateral flank, abdominal, or groin pain. A noncontrast CT scan is the most definitive diagnostic imaging test. However, lower radiation dosages may be obtained through a combination of KUB and ultrasound scan. Patients with signs of infection or renal compromise should be referred immediately to a urologist for ureteral stenting or to an interventional radiologist for percutaneous nephrostomy tube placement. In the remaining patients, symptomatic small stones less than 10 mm in diameter may be managed expectantly with medical expulsive therapy using α-adrenergic antagonists and NSAIDs for up to 4 weeks. Patients with larger stones or symptomatic stones that do not pass spontaneously should be referred to a urologist for elective intervention. In the long term, patients with single instances or rare occurrences of spontaneously passed urinary stones may be managed by their primary care physician. Long-term management of chronic urinary stone-formers based on the results of metabolic evaluations should be coordinated by the urologist.

REFERENCES

1. Stamatelou KK, Francis ME, Jones CA, et al. Time trends in reported prevalence of kidney stones in the United States: 1976–1994. Kidney Int 2003;63:1817–23.

2. Healthcare Cost and Utilization Project. Rockville (MA): Agency for Healthcare Research and Quality; 2009. Available at: http://hcupnet.ahrq.gov. Accessed September 24, 2010.

3. Gault MH, Chafe L. Relationship of frequency, age, sex, stone weight and composition in 15,624 stones: comparison of resutls for 1980 to 1983 and 1995 to 1998. J Urol 2000;164:302–7.

4. Saita A, Bonaccorsi A, Motta M. Stone composition: where do we stand? Urol Int 2007;79(Suppl 1):16–9.

5. Delvecchio FC, Preminger GM. Medical management of stone disease. Curr Opin Urol 2003;13:229–33.

6. Pearle M, Lotan Y. Urinary lithiasis: etiology, epidemiology, and pathogenesis. In: Wein AJ, editor. Campbell-walsh urology, vol. 2. Philadelphia: Saunders; 2007. p. 1393–92.

7. Dirks J, Remuzzi G, Horton S, et al. Diseases of the kidney and the urinary system. In: Jamison DT, Breman JG, Measham AR, et al, editors. Disease control priorities in developing countries. 2nd edition. New York: Oxford University Press; 2006. p. 695–706, Chapter 36.

8. Fielding JR, Steele G, Fox LA, et al. Spiral computerized tomography in the evaluation of acute flank pain: a replacement for excretory urography. J Urol 1997; 157:2071–3.

9. Katz DS, Scheer M, Lumerman JH, et al. Alternative or additional diagnoses on unenhanced helical computed tomography for suspected renal colic: experience with 1000 consecutive examinations. Urology 2000;56:53–7.

10. Ferrandino MN, Bagrodia A, Pierre SA, et al. Radiation exposure in the acute and short-term management of urolithiasis at 2 academic centers. J Urol 2009;181: 668–72 [discussion: 673].

11. Catalano O, Nunziata A, Altei F, et al. Suspected ureteral colic: primary helical CT versus selective helical CT after unenhanced radiography and sonography. AJR Am J Roentgenol 2002;178:379–87.

12. Ciaschini MW, Remer EM, Baker ME, et al. Urinary calculi: radiation dose reduction of 50% and 75% at CT–effect on sensitivity. Radiology 2009;251:105–11.

13. Tseng TY, Preminger GM. Medical management of stone disease. In: Dahm P, Dmochowski R, editors. Evidence-based urology. Singapore: Blackwell Publishing; 2010. p. 195–217.

14. Hollingsworth JM, Rogers MA, Kaufman SR, et al. Medical therapy to facilitate urinary stone passage: a meta-analysis. Lancet 2006;368:1171–9.

15. Springhart WP, Marguet CG, Sur RL, et al. Forced versus minimal intravenous hydration in the management of acute renal colic: a randomized trial. J Endourol 2006;20:713–6.

16. Franczyk J, Gray RR. Ureteral stenting in urosepsis: a cautionary note. Cardiovasc Intervent Radiol 1989;12:265–6.

17. Preminger GM, Tiselius HG, Assimos DG, et al. 2007 guideline for the management of ureteral calculi. J Urol 2007;178:2418–34.

18. Preminger GM, Assimos DG, Lingeman JE, et al. Chapter 1: AUA guideline on management of staghorn calculi: diagnosis and treatment recommendations. J Urol 2005;173:1991–2000.

19. Coe FL, Keck J, Norton ER. The natural history of calcium urolithiasis. JAMA 1977;238:1519–23.

20. Johnson CM, Wilson DM, O'Fallon WM, et al. Renal stone epidemiology: a 25-year study in Rochester, Minnesota. Kidney Int 1979;16:624–31.

21. Williams RE. Long-term survey of 538 patients with upper urinary tract stone. Br J Urol 1963;35:416–37.
22. Choi HK, Liu S, Curhan G. Intake of purine-rich foods, protein, and dairy products and relationship to serum levels of uric acid: the Third National Health and Nutrition Examination Survey. Arthritis Rheum 2005;52:283–9.
23. Coe FL, Moran E, Kavalich AG. The contribution of dietary purine over-consumption to hyperpuricosuria in calcium oxalate stone formers. J Chronic Dis 1976;29: 793–800.
24. Halevy S, Ghislain PD, Mockenhaupt M, et al. Allopurinol is the most common cause of Stevens-Johnson syndrome and toxic epidermal necrolysis in Europe and Israel. J Am Acad Dermatol 2008;58:25–32.
25. Taylor EN, Curhan GC. Determinants of 24-hour urinary oxalate excretion. Clin J Am Soc Nephrol 2008;3:1453–60.
26. Curhan GC, Willett WC, Rimm EB, et al. A prospective study of dietary calcium and other nutrients and the risk of symptomatic kidney stones. N Engl J Med 1993;328:833–8.
27. Curhan GC, Willett WC, Speizer FE, et al. Comparison of dietary calcium with supplemental calcium and other nutrients as factors affecting the risk for kidney stones in women. Ann Intern Med 1997;126:497–504.
28. Borghi L, Meschi T, Amato F, et al. Urinary volume, water and recurrences in idiopathic calcium nephrolithiasis: a 5-year randomized prospective study. J Urol 1996;155:839–43.
29. Taylor EN, Stampfer MJ, Curhan GC. Obesity, weight gain, and the risk of kidney stones. JAMA 2005;293:455–62.
30. Obligado SH, Goldfarb DS. The association of nephrolithiasis with hypertension and obesity: a review. Am J Hypertens 2008;21:257–64.
31. Madore F, Stampfer MJ, Rimm EB, et al. Nephrolithiasis and risk of hypertension. Am J Hypertens 1998;11:46–53.
32. Madore F, Stampfer MJ, Willett WC, et al. Nephrolithiasis and risk of hypertension in women. Am J Kidney Dis 1998;32:802–7.
33. Taylor EN, Stampfer MJ, Curhan GC. Diabetes mellitus and the risk of nephrolithiasis. Kidney Int 2005;68:1230–5.
34. West B, Luke A, Durazo-Arvizu RA, et al. Metabolic syndrome and self-reported history of kidney stones: the National Health and Nutrition Examination Survey (NHANES III) 1988–1994. Am J Kidney Dis 2008;51:741–7.

Evaluation and Management of the Renal Mass

David Y.T. Chen, MD*, Robert G. Uzzo, MD

KEYWORDS

- Renal cell carcinoma • Epidemiology • Evaluation • Surgery
- Treatment

The evaluation and management of renal cell carcinoma (RCC) has evolved in recent decades in response to the changing clinical presentation of the disease. Historically, diagnosing RCC has been straightforward, with traditional teaching suggesting that RCC usually presents with signs or symptoms. The textbook patient found to have RCC was described as having a pathognomonic triad of symptoms: gross localizing abdominal or flank pain, and a corresponding palpable mass on physical examination. When discovered this way, however, RCC was usually locally advanced and often metastatic, requiring radical nephrectomy in most cases but often having a poor prognosis.

As contemporary general medical practice began routinely using axial body imaging in the evaluation of many nonspecific abdominal complaints, today more than 70% of RCC cases identified today are "screen-detected" as incidental findings having no attributable symptoms. This change has prompted a significant RCC stage migration over the past 20 years, with most kidney tumors seen in 2010 being smaller, organ-confined, and appropriate for nephron-sparing approaches with the anticipation of a favorable outcome. The approach to addressing patients with these incidentally detected, often localized, small renal masses raises different concerns than for traditional patients presenting with symptomatic RCC. This article reviews the modern epidemiology of RCC, outlines the components of the evaluation of the incidental renal mass, details the current options of management, and discusses the long-term expectations for these patients.

This work was supported in part by Fox Chase Cancer Center via institutional support of the Kidney Cancer Keystone Program.

The authors have nothing to disclose.

Department of Surgery, Fox Chase Cancer Center, Temple University School of Medicine, 333 Cottman Avenue, Philadelphia, PA 19111, USA

* Corresponding author.

E-mail address: david.chen@fccc.edu

INCIDENCE AND PRESENTATION

Although historically associated with symptoms, fewer than 10% of RCC cases today show the classic triad of hematuria, pain, and palpable mass. Most RCCs are currently detected as an incidental renal abnormality found on an imaging study that is requested and performed for unrelated abdominal symptomatology.[1] This change in the manner of RCC diagnosis is suggested to be a major factor in its increasing incidence over the past 3 decades. A steady annual increase of 3% to 4% in the incidence of RCC has occurred since the 1970s (**Fig. 1**).[2] In 2009, an estimated 57,760 new cases of RCC were identified and approximately 12,980 deaths were reported.[3] The largest increase in RCC cases has been in patients having the smallest (<4 cm) tumors, with the mean size of RCC at presentation today approximately 3.6 cm.[4] These small renal masses are now most often found in the elderly, with the peak age at detection approximately 70 years old.[5]

Although improved detection from "screening" imaging is believed to be the main reason for the increasing incidence of RCCs, additional causative factors have also been implicated. A rising RCC incidence is noted worldwide, even in regions where imaging is less frequently used, and well-established risk factors associated with the promotion of RCC include the common diagnoses of hypertension, obesity, and tobacco use.[5]

The nature of RCC presentation, whether incidental or symptomatic, has been recognized to be a prognostic indicator. Survival from RCC is directly correlated with stage at presentation, and symptomatic cases have significantly higher grade and stage than RCC that is detected incidentally.[6] The rise in RCC incidence mostly

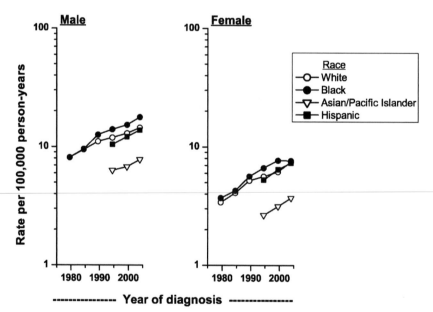

Fig. 1. Trends in age-adjusted (2000 US standard) RCC incidence rates by sex, among whites and blacks in SEER-9 (1977–2005) and among Asian/Pacific Islanders and Hispanics in SEER-12 (1992–2005). SEER, U.S. Surveillance, Epidemiology, and End Results program. (*Reprinted from* Chow WH, Devesa SS. Contemporary epidemiology of renal cell cancer. Cancer J 2008;14(5):288–301; with permission.)

has been in the smallest and earliest-stage cases, and overall a marked downward stage migration of RCC has occurred (**Fig. 2**).[4] Although RCC mortality has risen mostly in parallel with its increasing incidence, a 6.9% fall in the RCC death rate was observed between 1990 and 2006.[7] This most recent drop in RCC mortality suggests that the trend of RCC detection at earlier stages has led to improved overall outcomes.

CLINICAL EVALUATION

Because most RCC cases are now asymptomatic when diagnosed, the value of information obtained from history or physical examination is generally limited. However, a diagnosis of gross hematuria of any amount or frequency must still be considered to be related to a potential undiagnosed malignancy and warrants urologic evaluation. The evaluation of microscopic hematuria is also of potential importance and is the subject of recent American Urological Association guidelines (auanet.org/guidelines). A family history of RCC is of added importance, particularly if the family member was diagnosed at a young age, with multiple tumors, and/or with bilateral disease, because it may suggest the presence of a hereditary RCC syndrome (with von Hippel-Lindau disease the most common). A tobacco history should also be taken because of its association with both RCC and urothelial carcinomas of the upper and lower genitourinary tract.

A negative review of systems is a pertinent parameter to confirm from patient evaluation, because any constitutional symptom, such as fever, weight loss, fatigue, or pulmonary symptoms, can suggest more advanced disease. Physical examination should be attentive to possible supraclavicular, axillary, or groin adenopathy; costovertebral angle tenderness; or a palpable abdominal mass. However, except with larger renal masses, patient history is usually noncontributory and physical

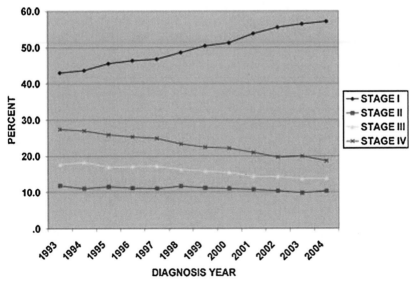

Fig. 2. RCC clinical stage distribution by diagnosis year, from National Cancer Data Base. (*Reprinted from* Kane CJ, Mallin K, Ritchey J, et al. Renal cell cancer stage migration: analysis of the national cancer data base. Cancer 2008;113(1):78–83; with permission.)

examination unremarkable. The most relevant information for evaluation and treatment planning therefore comes from laboratory and imaging test results.

Laboratory testing may be significant in suggesting the presence of disseminated disease. Equally important, it serves to establish the patient's baseline renal function. Anemia or elevated values for liver function tests, lactate dehydrogenase, alkaline phosphatase, or calcium can imply advanced stage, and some of these elements, when abnormal, can predict the estimated survival of patients with metastatic disease.[8] Because the peak incidence of RCC is in individuals of advanced age, a patient's renal function must be determined to appreciate their stage of chronic kidney disease (CKD), because this may impact the choice of management. Glomerular filtration rate (GFR) is the best index of kidney function and can be estimated easily using current Web-based tools.[9] The patient's existing CKD state and risk for progression of renal insufficiency independent of treatment can then be appropriately factored into any treatment decision. Studies have shown that relying on what might be defined as a normal serum creatinine ($\leq$1.4 mg/dL or less) can underestimate the degree of a potentially compromised CKD state, and estimated GFR is a more accurate assessment of renal function than an absolute serum creatinine value. Moreover, 20% to 40% of patients identified with RCC who are older than 70 years present with CKD stage 3 or higher renal dysfunction.[10]

Abdominal/pelvic CT is the optimal imaging modality to evaluate the kidneys and should be performed using multiphase imaging, with and without intravenous contrast. Most urologists will order a dedicated "three-phase CT scan" of the abdomen and pelvis as the primary radiographic study to evaluate hematuria or for a suspected renal mass. A solid renal mass showing an increase greater than 15 to 20 Hounsfield units between precontrast and nephrogram or postcontrast phases indicates RCC and warrants consideration of treatment. CT imaging provides high-resolution anatomic detail that often best defines the tumor and its association to the key structures of the affected kidney, particularly the renal vessels and urinary collecting system, to help in planning for surgical resection. It also informs of the appearance and function of the contralateral kidney and is sensitive for identifying local involvement to regional lymph nodes or the adrenal gland; spread from a small renal tumor to those areas is rarely present if they are normal according to routine CT criteria.[6,11,12] If the initial study detecting the renal abnormality is an ultrasound or single-phase CT, a three-phase CT should be used to confirm the diagnosis, and multiphase CT is nearly 100% sensitive for detecting a renal mass greater than 15 mm in diameter.[13]

An acceptable alternative to multiphase CT is MRI with pre- and post-gadolinium phases, although this is generally not preferred over CT. Multiphase MRI may be required for certain patients with renal insufficiency that prevents the safe receipt of intravenous CT contrast, or may be applied occasionally in cases when the findings of multiphase CT imaging are equivocal, which should be uncommon if interpreted correctly. However, experts have recently recognized that gadolinium nephrotoxicity and acute renal failure can occur in patients with preexisting chronic kidney disease who are at risk for contrast material–induced nephropathy. Therefore, the optimal method of imaging for patients with chronic renal insufficiency remains controversial.[14] The existing options for renal imaging studies and their roles are summarized in **Table 1**.

Although a solid, well-circumscribed enhancing renal mass is the most common appearance suggestive of RCC, other renal abnormalities may be found. These findings are associated with different risks for malignancy and need for intervention. The common renal findings are outlined in **Table 2**.

Besides abdominal imaging, additional studies to assess for metastases or to quantitatively measure renal split function are of benefit only in select patients. In general,

Table 1
Common imaging modalities useful in the renal mass evaluation

Imaging Modality	Advantage	Limitation	Radiation?
Noncontrast CT	Rapid Moderate cost Avoids potential risks of contrast	Limited resolution of intraparenchymal lesions Gives no "enhancement" characteristics Can miss endophytic tumors Considered nondefinitive for evaluation of a renal mass	Yes
Ultrasound	No radiation Low cost Highly sensitive in assessment of simple and complex cystic lesions and solid masses	Limited anatomic detail, especially of normal renal vessels and urinary collecting system Insensitive to isointense renal masses Shows moderate operator dependent variability Considered nondefinitive for the evaluation of a renal mass	No
Three-phase abdominal CT	High sensitivity Excellent anatomic resolution	Requires sufficient renal function for intravenous contrast administration Can generally be performed if eGFR >45 May require hydration or other nephroprotective maneuvers if eGFR 30–45	Yes
Multiphase MRI with gadolinium	No radiation High sensitivity Excellent anatomic resolution Possible with renal insufficiency	Expensive Time-consuming Risk of gadolinium nephrotoxicity and nephrogenic systemic fibrosis if eGFR <30	No
PET/CT	None	Experimental application for renal cell carcinoma Unproven benefit Limited anatomic detail Generally not indicated in the evaluation of renal masses	Yes

Abbreviation: eGFR, estimated glomerular filtration rates.

a chest radiograph is sufficient to evaluate for distant disease, because metastatic disease is unusual for the common small (<4 cm) renal tumor. Chest CT, bone scan, or brain CT imaging are necessary only when the patient has localizing clinical symptoms, or for renal tumors that are large (>7 cm) or have evidence suggesting higher clinical stage, such as adenopathy or adjacent organ or renal vein involvement.[15] Positron emission tomographic imaging currently has no recognized role in the evaluation of RCC. Lastly, in select patients in whom a radical nephrectomy is planned, a renal scan can be considered to confirm sufficient renal function in the uninvolved kidney

Table 2
Common renal mass types and their possible risk for malignancy and diagnosis

Gross Appearance	Additional Details	Likelihood Cancer	Likelihood Benign	Recommend for Treatment	Likely Diagnosis
Solid enhancing renal mass	(a) >15–20 Hounsfield units change on multiphase CT	~80% (more if tumor >4 cm)	~20% (less if tumor >4 cm)	Yes	Renal cell carcinoma (or oncocytoma if benign)
	Same as (a), with macroscopic fat seen on imaging	Very low	High	No (except if tumor >6 cm)	Acute myeloid leukemia
	Same as (a), with irregular border or infiltrative	High	Low	Maybe, consider biopsy	Metastasis Sarcoma Lymphoma Urothelial cancer
Predominant cystic mass	Smooth Symmetric Septa <2 mm (thin) (Bosniak class 1 or 2)	Low	High	No	Simple cyst Atypical cyst
	Irregular wall Calcifications Septa >2 mm (thick) Nodular or enhancing cyst wall (Bosniak class 3 or 4)	High (>70%)	Low	Yes	Cystic renal cell carcinoma

before surgery. However, this can often be determined from prior multiphase abdominal CT or MRI.

Of increasing application is biopsy of a renal mass, which can potentially diagnose the renal tumor before patients are committed to treatment. Historically, a tumor biopsy was not used because of lack of confidence in its accuracy and likely over concerns regarding the possibility of seeding the track, or complications. Assessment of modern biopsy results suggests that it is highly accurate (>90% sensitive) with acceptably low risk.[16] Renal tumor biopsy would be advised for atypical-appearing renal masses that would be treated differently than with upfront surgical excision, such as if a renal abscess or a non-RCC malignancy is suspected (eg, renal pelvis urothelial cancer, renal lymphoma, renal metastasis). It may also have a role in confirming RCC in patients for whom treatment may be of high risk because of medical comorbidity; studies have shown that as many as 20% of renal tumors that are smaller than 4 cm and suspicious for RCC may be benign,[17] and treatment can be deferred in these patients. In one recent retrospective report evaluating 152 patients with renal lesions, biopsy performed before treatment was sensitive for detecting malignancy in 98% of cases, and subjectively impacted subsequent management in more than half of these patients.[18]

MANAGEMENT OPTIONS

Surgical resection is the mainstay of RCC treatment, with patient outcomes excellent if disease is completely excised. For localized RCC, experience over the past decades has shown that contemporary renal tumors are most often solitary and well circumscribed, and are effectively treated when fully resected. For most modern cases, the historic standard surgery of open radical nephrectomy[19] is excessive, and the associated normal kidney loss unnecessary and potentially deleterious. Removal of more than the tumor with a negative margin is considered overtreatment for most of today's incidentally detected renal tumors. Excellent retrospective evidence shows equal long-term cancer-specific survival for small to medium-sized (<7 cm) tumors, whether treated with partial nephrectomy (nephron-sparing surgery), in which only the tumor is removed and the uninvolved aspect of the kidney preserved and maintained, or with radical nephrectomy.[20] The clinical benefit of partial nephrectomy over radical nephrectomy has been shown, with patients with RCC treated with partial nephrectomy having substantially less risk for progression to renal failure. These patients have improved quality of life and better long-term overall survival, with a lower risk of renal morbidity and associated secondary cardiovascular-related events, and non–RCC-related death.[21–23] For these reasons, kidney-sparing treatment of RCC is advised whenever possible. Although radical nephrectomy remains an accepted treatment option, minimizing loss of renal function in the course of RCC treatment should be a critical secondary objective of treatment and strongly emphasized.[24]

Both radical nephrectomy and partial nephrectomy can be performed using traditional open surgery or through minimally invasive surgical (MIS) approaches. In general, the effectiveness of either approach for either surgery is equivalent, with the primary difference being that recovery and convalescence after an MIS approach are often shorter than after an open surgical approach. Although no prospective comparison studies have evaluated these different RCC surgical options, retrospective analyses suggest all surgical options (open radical nephrectomy, MIS radical nephrectomy, open partial nephrectomy, MIS partial nephrectomy) are equally successful RCC treatments. These treatments are all similarly oncologically effective, and only MIS partial nephrectomy has a slightly different but statistically higher rate of perioperative complications compared with the other options (9% vs 1%–6%). This increased risk for complications is attributed to the greater technical demands of this specific approach; MIS surgery is more complex than open surgery, and partial nephrectomy more complex than radical nephrectomy. Despite this higher rate of complications, MIS partial nephrectomy has been suggested by expert opinion to be the optimal treatment for a small renal mass because it results in effective cancer treatment, maintains the integrity of the uninvolved portion of the tumor-bearing kidney, and minimizes the morbidity of surgery.[24] Recently released guidelines on the management of localized renal cancers are available from the American Urological Association (AUA; www.auanet.org/guidelines).

Even though surgical resection is considered to be the gold standard treatment for RCC, ongoing interest has been shown in developing additional interventions. Partial nephrectomy, although effective, is a technically challenging operation that is not readily available in all locales and is recognized to be generally underutilized, mainly because many urologists have insufficient training to perform it safely and effectively. Recent national data suggest that radical nephrectomy is offered far too frequently and accounts for approximately 75% of all surgeries for localized RCC in the United States.[25] The recent guidelines released by the AUA emphasize the long-term peril of overuse of laparoscopic radical nephrectomy in the community instead of MIS or open partial nephrectomy, with surgeons and patients essentially trading the long-term benefit of sustained renal function for the short-term benefit of a potentially quicker postoperative recovery.[24]

Over the past several years, in situ ablation of the renal mass has been introduced as an option that can be performed either laparoscopically or percutaneously. Recognizing that a focused tumor resection seems to be oncologically effective, image-guided ablation has been applied to treat RCC and is hypothesized to be potentially effective as long as the renal mass is adequately targeted. Using either radiofrequency ablation or cryoablation equipment, this approach generates extremes of heat or cold, respectively, that can be lethal to cells and tissues. Thermal ablation is currently approved by the U.S. Food and Drug Administration (FDA) to treat tumors in various organs, including the liver, prostate, lung, and kidney. Initially, patients treated in this manner were ill or elderly and deemed poor risk for routine anesthesia and surgical resection.

With growing experience, in situ ablation is increasingly being applied to treat small renal masses in younger and healthier patients.[26,27] Although it is attractive because of its perceived lower morbidity, it has the disadvantage of having limited long-term efficacy data (mean follow-up in the accumulated literature remains less than 18 to 22 months), and even early results suggest a significantly higher (7–18 times) risk for local recurrence of RCC when treated with either thermal ablation treatment instead of partial nephrectomy.[28] Therefore, in situ ablation should not be recommended over routine surgical resection, preferably with partial nephrectomy, in otherwise healthy individuals who are candidates for surgery.[24]

For patients who are ill or elderly and have incidentally detected RCC, emerging data suggest that many small renal tumors have an indolent behavior and that immediate treatment in these poor-risk patients may not be of benefit. In the setting of advanced age or multiple significant comorbidities, a small RCC might not be clinically meaningful, and active surveillance of the small renal mass can be a viable management strategy. A large meta-analysis at the authors' institution reported on nearly 300 patients with RCC who underwent observation and no immediate treatment.[29] This study showed that development of metastatic RCC during surveillance is a rare event, seen in fewer than 2% of patients, and rarely occurs in tumors smaller than 3 cm. Importantly, in follow-up out to nearly 3 years, no patient died of an untreated RCC. Serial imaging of these patients shows that the interval growth of observed tumors is small, averaging a 3 to 4 mm increase in size per year. Thus, rapid growth above that rate can be used as an indicator to suggest more aggressive behavior and to select for patients who might benefit from delayed treatment. Most tumors do not show rapid growth, although a parameter does not seem to exist that can adequately predict a tumor's growth rate. Active surveillance can be considered an appropriate management for well-selected patients, particularly those who are elderly or infirm, who can be managed by an experienced physician, and may allow avoidance of the recognized risks and morbidity of treatment.[24]

Lastly, for the now-less-common patient who presents with metastatic disease, surgery maintains an important role in management. A cytoreductive radical or partial nephrectomy using either open or MIS techniques before initiating medical treatment is the accepted approach, based on historical level 1 evidence showing that surgery results in improved survival over treatment with systemic (immuno) therapy alone.[30] However, immunotherapy is no longer routinely used because of its very low response rate for metastatic RCC, and its average improvement in survival is only 3 to 4 months.[31] Although no prospective data are available on the benefits of surgery (cytoreduction) in the targeted (antiangiogenic) therapy era, it remains the standard of care in appropriately selected patients.

Major progress has recently occurred in the treatment of metastatic RCC, with the release of six new medications that are FDA-approved for this disease state, all introduced since 2005.[32] Although none of these agents has been able to induce a complete response, they greatly improve the survival of patients with metastatic RCC. Nonetheless, surgery (predominantly nephrectomy because of the typical large size of primary tumors associated with metastases) continues to be recommended as first-line treatment for patients with good performance status who can subsequently receive systemic therapy to treat their remaining disease burden.

RESULTS OF TREATMENT

Because renal mass biopsy remains infrequently performed, confirmation of the presumed RCC diagnosis occurs only after excision in most cases. Surgical resection provides key information, not only in confirming a tumor to be malignant but also in defining pathologic stage and grade, which are the best predictors of disease outcome and a patient's future risk. In the absence of a surgical specimen, such as with RCC treatment with thermal ablation, this information is often not obtained or is inconclusive (40%–60% in contemporary ablative series).[28] This lack of detail is one significant disadvantage of any nonoperative intervention.

Histologically, several different RCC subtypes exist, with clear cell RCC the most common and most aggressive, and constituting approximately 75% of all RCC cases. Less frequently, papillary RCC or chromophobe RCC may be identified, which are generally thought to convey a more favorable prognosis. Regardless of RCC type, in most cases the primary tumor stage, whether it is limited to the kidney (T1 or 2) or not (T3 or 4), and whether evidence of lymph node or distant spread is present are the main parameters that impact outcome. For organ-confined RCC, the recurrence rate is less than 25% and the cancer-specific survival upwards of 95% for the most favorable and smallest tumors (<4 cm) treated with surgical resection. Given the expectation of successful treatment with these cases, follow-up imaging can be considered every 12 to 24 months.[15] In contrast, RCC that shows growth beyond the kidney or local or distant spread has a recurrence risk of 30% to 50%, and more frequent postoperative surveillance is recommended (roughly every 4–6 months).[15] Although these patients are recognized to be at high recurrence risk, no adjuvant therapy currently exists to address this potential. Studies are ongoing examining the benefit of new targeted systemic agents in this role. Results from these trials should be completed within the next 2 to 3 years.

Survival of patients with metastatic RCC traditionally has been poor, averaging less than 12 months.[30] These patients, in particular, benefit from the collaborative management of both medical and urologic oncologists. Patient outcomes with optimal multimodal therapy have shown marked recent improvement, and overall survival for these patients now commonly can extend beyond 2 years.[33] Increasing experience with these new targeted therapies will lead to better disease- and treatment-related symptom management for patients with incurable disease.

SUMMARY

The incidence of RCC has shown a steady increase over recent decades, with the majority of new cases now found when asymptomatic and small. High resolution pre- and post-contrast imaging provides sensitive and accurate clinical staging. Presentation at an early stage has resulted in treatment options that improve on cancer specific outcomes and renal functional preservation. Overutilization of radical nephrectomy for localized disease should be discouraged. Laparoscopic radical nephrectomy may inappropriately trade a more rapid recovery for the future adversities of a lower GFR and CKD. New systemic antiangiogenic agents show great promise in improving the outcome of patients with locally advanced and metastatic kidney cancer.

REFERENCES

1. Parsons JK, Schoenberg MS, Carter HB. Incidental renal tumors: casting doubt on the efficacy of early intervention. Urology 2001;57(6):1013–5.
2. Chow WH, Devesa SS, Warren JL, et al. Rising incidence of renal cell cancer in the United States. JAMA 1999;281(17):1628–31.
3. Jemal A, Siegel R, Ward E, et al. Cancer statistics, 2009. CA Cancer J Clin 2009; 59(4):225–49.
4. Kane CJ, Mallin K, Ritchey J, et al. Renal cell cancer stage migration: analysis of the national cancer data base. Cancer 2008;113(1):78–83.
5. Chow WH, Devesa SS. Contemporary epidemiology of renal cell cancer. Cancer J 2008;14(5):288–301.
6. Tsui KH, Shvarts O, Smith RB, et al. Renal cell carcinoma: prognostic significance of incidentally detected tumors. J Urol 2000;163(2):426–30.
7. Jemal A, Ward E, Thun M. Declining death rates reflect progress against cancer. PLoS One 2010;5(3):e9584.
8. Motzer RJ, Bacik J, Murphy BA, et al. Interferon-alfa as a comparative treatment for clinical trials of new therapies against advanced renal cell carcinoma. J Oncol 2002;20(1):289–96.
9. Available at: http://www.nephron.com/MDRD_GFR.cgi. Accessed September 29, 2010.
10. Lane BR, Demirjian S, Weight CJ, et al. Performance of the chronic kidney disease-epidemiology study equations for estimating glomerular filtration rate before and after nephrectomy. J Urol 2010;183(3):896–901.
11. Zagoria RJ. Imaging of small renal masses: a medical success story. AJR Am J Roentgenol 2000;175(4):945–55.
12. Tsui KH, Shvarts O, Barbaric Z, et al. Is adrenalectomy a necessary component of radical nephrectomy? UCLA experience with 511 radical nephrectomies. J Urol 2000;163(2):437–41.

13. Szolar DH, Kammerhuber F, Altziebler S, et al. Multiphasic helical CT of the kidney: increased conspicuity for detection and characterization of small(< 3-cm) renal masses. Radiology 1997;202(1):211–7.
14. Ledneva E, Karie S, Launay-Vacher V, et al. Renal safety of gadolinium-based contrast media in patients with chronic renal insufficiency. Radiology 2009; 250(3):618–28.
15. Motzer RJ, Agarwal N, Beard C, et al. NCCN clinical practice guidelines in oncology: kidney cancer. J Natl Compr Canc Netw 2009;7(6):618–30.
16. Lane BR, Samplaski MK, Herts BR, et al. Renal mass biopsy—a renaissance? J Urol 2008;179(1):20–7.
17. Frank I, Blute ML, Cheville JC, et al. Solid renal tumors: an analysis of pathological features related to tumor size. J Urol 2003;170(6 Pt 1):2217–20.
18. Maturen KE, Nghiem HV, Caoili EM, et al. Renal mass core biopsy: accuracy and impact on clinical management. AJR Am J Roentgenol 2007;188(2):563–70.
19. Robson CJ. Radical nephrectomy for renal cell carcinoma. J Urol 1963;89:37–42.
20. Uzzo RG, Novick AC. Nephron sparing surgery for renal tumors: indications, techniques and outcomes. J Urol 2001;166(1):6–18.
21. McKiernan J, Simmons R, Katz J, et al. Natural history of chronic renal insufficiency after partial and radical nephrectomy. Urology 2002;59(6):816–20.
22. Huang WC, Elkin EB, Levey AS, et al. Partial nephrectomy versus radical nephrectomy in patients with small renal tumors—is there a difference in mortality and cardiovascular outcomes? J Urol 2009;181(1):55–61 [discussion: 61–2].
23. Thompson RH, Boorjian SA, Lohse CM, et al. Radical nephrectomy for pT1a renal masses may be associated with decreased overall survival compared with partial nephrectomy. J Urol 2008;179(2):468–71 [discussion: 472–3].
24. Campbell SC, Novick AC, Belldegrun A, et al. Guideline for management of the clinical T1 renal mass. J Urol 2009;182(4):1271–9.
25. Hollenbeck BK, Taub DA, Miller DC, et al. National utilization trends of partial nephrectomy for renal cell carcinoma: a case of underutilization? Urology 2006; 67(2):254–9.
26. Uchida M, Imaide Y, Sugimoto K, et al. Percutaneous cryosurgery for renal tumours. Br J Urol 1995;75(2):132–6 [discussion: 136–7].
27. Zlotta AR, Wildschutz T, Raviv G, et al. Radiofrequency interstitial tumor ablation (RITA) is a possible new modality for treatment of renal cancer: ex vivo and in vivo experience. J Endourol 1997;11(4):251–8.
28. Kunkle DA, Egleston BL, Uzzo RG. Excise, ablate or observe: the small renal mass dilemma–a meta-analysis and review. J Urol 2008;179(4):1227–33 [discussion: 1233–4].
29. Chawla SN, Crispen PL, Hanlon AL, et al. The natural history of observed enhancing renal masses: meta-analysis and review of the world literature. J Urol 2006;175(2):425–31.
30. Flanigan RC, Salmon SE, Blumenstein BA, et al. Nephrectomy followed by interferon alfa-2b compared with interferon alfa-2b alone for metastatic renal-cell cancer. N Engl J Med 2001;345(23):1655–9.
31. Coppin C, Porzsolt F, Awa A, et al. Immunotherapy for advanced renal cell cancer. Cochrane Database Syst Rev 2005;1:CD001425.
32. Pal SK, Figlin RA. Renal cell carcinoma therapy in 2010: many options with little comparative data. Clin Adv Hematol Oncol 2010;8(3):191–200.
33. Motzer RJ, Hutson TE, Tomczak P, et al. Overall survival and updated results for sunitinib compared with interferon alfa in patients with metastatic renal cell carcinoma. J Clin Oncol 2009;27(22):3584–90.

Use and Assessment of PSA in Prostate Cancer

Carl K. Gjertson, MD*, Peter C. Albertsen, MD, MS

KEYWORDS

- Prostate-specific antigen • Prostatic neoplasms • Prostate
- Mass screening

Few innovations have had as much impact on men's health and the practice of urology, or been as controversial, as prostate cancer screening with prostate-specific antigen (PSA). PSA is a serine protease that is made almost exclusively by prostate cells and excreted in the ejaculate to liquefy semen.[1] PSA can be detected in blood, normally at a low level. Disruption of normal prostatic architecture by cancer, benign enlargement, inflammation, or trauma can lead to elevated serum levels. When combined with a digital rectal examination (DRE), PSA can be used to screen for prostate cancer (CaP). An abnormal screening test may prompt a prostate biopsy, usually performed in conjunction with transrectal ultrasound, to provide a definitive diagnosis. Unfortunately, serum PSA alone cannot reliably distinguish between benign prostatic hyperplasia (BPH), prostatic infection or inflammation, and prostate cancer, either low or high grade.

Since the introduction of PSA screening in the late 1980s, more prostate cancers have been detected and at an earlier stage. As a consequence, the majority of prostate cancers are now detected years before the emergence of clinically evident disease, which usually represents locally advanced or metastatic cancer. PSA screening has remained controversial, because many of the prostate cancers detected are low grade and slow growing. With this long natural history and a median survival without treatment that often approaches at least 15 to 20 years, many clinicians and researchers have questioned if CaP screening and treatment actually improves survival, as many patients will die *with* prostate cancer rather than *of* prostate cancer.[2] In this review, the authors discuss the rationale for CaP screening and present the current guidelines for the use of PSA.

The authors have nothing to disclose.

Division of Urology, University of Connecticut Health Center, 263 Farmington Avenue, Farmington, CT 06030-3955, USA

* Corresponding author.

E-mail address: gjertson@uchc.edu

Med Clin N Am 95 (2011) 191–200

doi:10.1016/j.mcna.2010.08.024

HISTORY OF PSA

PSA was first described as a marker for prostate cancer in 1987. Higher tumor volumes were shown to correlate with higher PSA levels.[3] PSA as a screening test for CaP was first reported in 1991 and quickly became popular, with a cutoff value of 4.0 ng/mL used to distinguish between a negative or positive screening test.[4] Since then annual testing has become prevalent and many clinicians now use 2.5 ng/mL as the cut point. As a consequence the number of new cases has increased dramatically.[5,6]

The incidence of CaP has been gradually increasing in the United States over the past 30 years, but the use of PSA led to a spike in new cases in the early 1990s. This spike was followed by a decrease and return to a gradual rate of increase, but at a level about twice the previous baseline: a cull effect (**Fig. 1**). During this same period a dramatic stage migration occurred, with far fewer cases of locally advanced or lymph node positive prostate cancer being discovered after surgery.[7,8] Prostate cancer mortality has also been declining since the early 1990s. Though some have suggested that this is evidence of the benefit of PSA screening, others have argued that any benefit from PSA should take many years to be seen.[9] Similar, though less dramatic, declines in CaP mortality have been observed in England where PSA screening is uncommon.[10]

IS PSA A GOOD SCREENING TEST?

Any good screening test should satisfy a few criteria: it should be sensitive, inexpensive, safe, and detect a disease for which early treatment improves survival. It is the

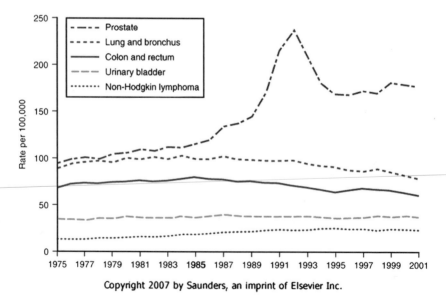

Fig. 1. Cancer incidence rates for men, United States, 1975 to 2001. Source: Surveillance, Epidemiology, and End Results Program, 1975 to 2001, Division of Cancer Control and Population Sciences, National Cancer Institute, 2004. (*From* Klein EA, Platz EA, Thompson IM. Epidemiology, etiology, and prevention of prostate cancer. In: Wein AJ, Kavoussi LR, Novick AC, et al, editors. Campbell-Walsh Urology. 9th edition. Philadelphia: Saunders; 2007. p. 2854–73; with permission.)

final criterion that has been debated extensively since PSA screening became available. At the center of the debate are 2 issues: the natural history of screen detected prostate cancer and the efficacy of treatment.

NATURAL HISTORY OF PROSTATE CANCER

The clinical aggressiveness of prostate cancer is highly variable. Although some men with high-grade disease (Gleason grade 8, 9, or 10) can progress from localized disease to metastasis to death in a short time period, others with low-grade cancer (Gleason grade 6 and lower) may never have any clinical sequelae, even without treatment. Autopsy studies have found high rates of clinically insignificant CaP in up to 75% of male octogenarians.[11] Unfortunately, PSA cannot distinguish between low- and high-grade cancer.

Johansson and colleagues[12–15] published a series of 4 articles between 1989 and 2004 documenting the outcomes of 648 cases of untreated prostate cancer in Sweden. PSA was not yet available when this cohort was assembled. Initial mortality rates at 5 and 10 years were low, suggesting that aggressive treatment (and PSA screening) was unnecessary for many patients with less than a 10-year life expectancy. However, longer follow-up revealed increasing prostate cancer mortality for men surviving 15 to 20 years after diagnosis.

In a cohort of 767 subjects identified from the Connecticut state tumor registry who were similarly followed without definitive treatment, men with Gleason grade 5 and 6 tumors had a 6% to 11% and 18% to 30% cancer-specific mortality at 20 years. Subjects with Gleason scores 7 and 8 to 10 had high rates of death from prostate cancer regardless of age at presentation (42%–70% and 60%–87%, respectively). Few survived more than 15 years.[16,17] These data suggest that men with intermediate- or high-grade CaP (Gleason grade ≥7) have significant risk of cancer-related death within 15 years of diagnosis, and may benefit from PSA screening and definitive treatment. However, many men with low-grade disease (Gleason score ≤6) have a low risk for cancer death, especially older men, and will either not benefit or will suffer harm from PSA screening and cancer treatment.

DOES PROSTATE CANCER TREATMENT IMPROVE SURVIVAL?

Although overall and cancer-specific survival is generally good after treatment, there have been few randomized trials that compared different treatment modalities for prostate cancer. In 2008, Bill-Axelson and colleagues[18] published results of a Scandinavian study of 695 men with clinically localized prostate cancer randomized to radical prostatectomy or watchful waiting between 1989 and 1999. Only 12% had been identified by PSA screening. At 12 years, prostate cancer mortality was 12.5% in the surgery group versus 17.9% in the observation group, for a relative risk reduction of 0.65 (95% confidence interval [CI] = 0.45 to 0.94; $P = .03$). However, subset analysis revealed that only subjects aged younger than 65 years benefitted from treatment. In addition, no significant difference in overall survival was found at a median follow-up of 10.8 years (60.5% in the treatment arm, 55.2% in the control arm, $P = .09$).

Widmark and colleagues[19] recently published findings from a randomized study comparing androgen deprivation therapy (ADT) alone versus ADT plus radiotherapy. Of the 875 subjects, more than 75% had locally advanced (T3) disease and only 2% were identified by PSA screening. The estimated 10-year disease-specific mortality was 23.9% in the ADT alone group compared with 11.9% in the ADT plus radiation group ($P<.001$). Overall mortality was also improved in the combination therapy group, 29.6% versus 39.4% in the controls ($P = .004$).

These 2 studies reveal that treatment with surgery or radiation does indeed reduce prostate cancer mortality, but the effect on overall survival is still unclear. How would these results differ if the subjects had been identified with PSA screening? Because of the lead time and stage migration associated with PSA screening, the relative risk reduction following treatment would likely be similar or greater. The absolute risk reduction, however, would likely be less in a population of screened patients, implying that the number needed to treat to avoid one prostate cancer death would increase.

DOES PSA SCREENING IMPROVE SURVIVAL?

In the spring of 2009, the New England Journal of Medicine published interim results of two highly anticipated randomized trials on PSA screening: the Prostate, Lung, Colorectal, and Ovarian (PLCO) Cancer Screening Trial sponsored by the National Cancer Institute and the European Randomized Study of Screening for Prostate Cancer (ERSPC).[20,21]

The PLCO trial recruited 76,693 men at 10 study centers in the United States between 1993 and 2001. Men were randomized to annual PSA determinations for 6 years and rectal examinations for 4 years, or to usual care. Primary care providers were notified of a PSA of 4.0 ng/mL or greater, and any further intervention was outside of the study protocol. Compliance with PSA screening was 85%. The rate of PSA testing in the control arm was 52% by the sixth year. More prostate cancer was detected in the screening group, 116 cases per 10,000 person-years versus 95 in the control group, (rate ratio, 1.22; 95% CI, 1.16 to 1.29). At 7 and 10 years, prostate cancer mortality was low in both groups and did not differ significantly.

The ERSPC trial is a combination of 7 separate national PSA screening studies conducted between 1991 and 2003. Recruitment, randomization, and screening protocols varied among the countries and by year. Most centers used a serum PSA alone every 4 years as the screening protocol. However, PSA with transrectal ultrasound and DRE were used in the Netherlands and Belgium during the early years of the study, and in Finland and Italy a DRE was added for men with PSA between 2.5 and 3.9 ng/mL. In Sweden the screening interval was every 2 years, and in Belgium every 4 to 7 years because of funding problems. Initially, a PSA of 4.0 ng/mL or greater was considered a positive screening test; later this was lowered to 3.0 ng/mL. Unlike the PLCO trial, an abnormal screening test mandated a transrectal ultrasound and prostate biopsy. A total of 162,387 men aged 55 to 69 years participated.

The incidence of prostate cancer was 8.2% in the screening group compared with 4.8% in the control group at a median follow-up of 9 years. The rate ratio for death from prostate cancer in the screening versus control group was 0.80 ($P = .04$). The absolute risk difference was 0.71 deaths per 1000 men. The investigators concluded that to prevent one prostate cancer death would require 1410 men to be offered PSA screening, 1068 men to actually be screened, and 48 additional cancers to be treated.

Unfortunately, neither trial has resolved the debate over the efficacy of PSA screening. The PLCO trial is primarily limited by its power. Because many subjects in the control arm were screened, it essentially became a study of annual screening versus less frequent screening, and the power to detect a mortality benefit decreased. Because of the wide confidence intervals surrounding the estimate of screening benefit, it will take many additional years of follow-up before a significant difference may be seen. Although the power of the ERSPC trial is much greater, the varying recruitment and screening protocols make it more difficult to interpret. It too will likely require several additional years to see if a more significant mortality benefit is realized.

PSA MANIPULATIONS

Several manipulations and additional tests have been developed in an attempt to make PSA a more sensitive and specific test for prostate cancer. These tests include PSA density, free PSA, age-adjusted PSA, and PSA velocity.

PSA density is calculated by dividing serum PSA by prostate volume. Because benign enlargement of the prostate can elevate PSA, calculating PSA density can adjust for this, increase specificity, and potentially reduce the number of prostate biopsies.[22] However, calculation of prostate volume requires a transrectal ultrasound, which is expensive, uncomfortable, and somewhat cumbersome as a screening test. In practice, transrectal ultrasound is rarely performed unless a prostate biopsy is required, and PSA density is not commonly determined.

PSA circulates in the blood either free or bound to plasma proteins. The amount of free PSA can be determined with a blood test, and is usually expressed as a percentage of the total PSA. For unclear reasons, free PSA is lower in patients with prostate cancer and higher in patients with BPH. Patients with percent-free PSA less than 15% are at a higher risk for prostate cancer; whereas, those with percent-free PSA greater than 25% have significantly lower risk.[23] Using free PSA can provide additional risk stratification and reduce the number of prostate biopsies, especially for men with a PSA between 2.5 and 10. However, it has little role as a screening test and should probably be used only by urologists to help counsel patients considering a prostate biopsy.

Because PSA is known to increase with age, age-specific cut points have been proposed to increase specificity and reduce the number of prostate biopsies in older men while increasing sensitivity in younger men.[24] African American men have higher PSA levels and a higher risk of prostate cancer, so different reference ranges have been proposed based on ethnicity. **Table 1** shows suggested normal PSA levels based on age and ethnicity. Although age-specific ranges for PSA screening are easy to use and understand, their use may increase the risk of missing high-grade prostate cancer in older men and over detecting low-grade disease in younger men.[25]

Changes in PSA over time can also be used in the detection of prostate cancer. PSA velocity (PSAV) can be calculated with 3 PSA values obtained over at least 18 months.[26] For men with a PSA between 4 and 10, a PSAV of 0.75 ng/mL/y or greater can distinguish between men with and without prostate cancer.[27] For those with a PSA less than 4, a PSAV of 0.35 ng/mL/y or greater corresponds to a significantly higher prostate cancer mortality 25 years later.[28] However, when added to total PSA, PSAV was not an independent predictor of positive biopsy in the large randomized Prostate Cancer Prevention Trial, and this has led some to recommend against the routine use of PSAV as a screening test.[29,30]

Table 1 Age-specific PSA reference ranges			
Age	Reference Range African American	Reference Range Caucasian	Median PSA
40–49 years	0–2.0 ng/mL	0–2.5 ng/mL	0.7 ng/mL
50–59 years	0–4.0 ng/mL	0–3.5 ng/mL	0.9 ng/mL
60–69 years	0–4.5 ng/mL	0–4.5 ng/mL	1.2 ng/mL
70–75 years	0–5.5 ng/mL	0–6.5 ng/mL	1.5 ng/mL

Adapted from Greene KL, Albertsen PA, Babaian RJ, et al. Prostate specific antigen best practice statement: 2009 Update. J Urol 2009;182:2232–41.

RACE AND FAMILY HISTORY

Prostate cancer is most prevalent in northern Europe, North America, and Australia, and less common in Asia and Africa. African American men have the highest incidence of prostate cancer: 1.6 times higher than Caucasian men in the United States.[31] African Americans also suffer worse outcomes: 1.8 years shorter survival after prostatectomy, 0.7 years shorter after radiation, and 1.0 year shorter with observation.[32] The risk of death from CaP is 2.4 times greater for African Americans than Caucasians in the United States. This poor prognosis persists after adjustment for other factors, including income and education.

Family history is also an important risk factor for CaP, especially the age at which a relative was diagnosed. Having a first-degree relative (father or brother) with CaP increases the lifetime risk twofold. If the relative was younger than 60 years of age when affected, the risk increases threefold. If 2 first-degree relatives have CaP, the lifetime risk is 4 times greater. Other than age, a family history is the strongest risk factor for prostate cancer.[33]

The increased risk for African Americans and families with CaP has been reflected in previous screening recommendations by the American Urological Association (AUA) and the American Cancer Society, who had urged these men to begin PSA testing 10 years earlier than other men. As the debate over PSA screening as a public health policy continues, we are moving away from the mandatory screening recommendations of the past. However, selective screening for high-risk patients with a positive family history or African American race is still encouraged.

LIMITATIONS OF PSA

Although PSA can be used as a cancer marker and a cancer screening test, its main limitation is that it is not specific for prostate cancer. BPH and large prostate size are known to correlate with higher PSA levels. PSA has been shown to be a marker for prostate growth, acute urinary retention, and progressive urinary symptoms related to BPH.[34] Treatment of BPH with 5-alpha reductase inhibitors (finasteride and dutasteride) reduces the size of the prostate and lowers serum PSA by 50%. Recognition of this correlation between prostate size and PSA has led to the development of PSA density and age-specific PSA reference ranges in an attempt to increase the specificity of PSA screening and reduce the number of biopsies in older men with BPH.

Infection and inflammation, including prostatitis and urinary tract infections, elevate PSA. Trauma to the prostate, such as Foley catheter placement or prostate biopsy, will also increase PSA. PSA should not be checked for at least 4 to 6 weeks after any of these conditions to prevent spurious measurements.

The traditional cut point for determining an abnormal PSA screening test is 4.0 ng/mL. This cut point was used in the PLCO trial. The ERSPC used a cut point of 3.0 ng/mL. A cut point of 2.5 ng/mL has also been proposed to increase the sensitivity of cancer detection. However, PSA is a continuous variable and there is not a PSA threshold below which prostate cancer cannot occur. Selecting an optimal cut point poses many statistical challenges.[35]

Unfortunately, PSA cannot distinguish between low- and high-grade cancers. The majority of cancers detected by PSA testing are low grade (Gleason 6 or less), especially when the cut point is lowered to increase sensitivity.[36] The longer lead time before emergence of clinically detectable disease makes it inevitable that any screening test is more likely to detect slow-growing and low-grade disease versus rapidly progressing high-grade cancer. As more data show little prostate cancer mortality from low-grade disease even without treatment, this becomes a major limitation to PSA screening. PSA is also a poor predictor of progression from low- to high-grade disease for patients on active surveillance protocols.[37] There is certainly a need to develop better markers in the future to distinguish between clinically significant and indolent prostate cancer.

OTHER PROSTATE CANCER MARKERS

Given the limitations of PSA, screening tests using other markers for CaP are in development. The DiaPat urine test (DiaPat GmbH, Hannover, Germany) analyzes urinary polypeptides and is commercially available. A study of 18 subjects having prostate biopsy revealed that the test could correctly predict the biopsy result only 50% of the time.[38]

PCA 3 is an untranslated mRNA overexpressed in 90% to 95% of prostate cancers. It can be detected in urine specimens obtained after prostatic massage. PCA 3 is not influenced by prostate size or PSA level, and has better sensitivity and specificity than PSA to predict CaP on prostate biopsy.[39] However, 1 in 5 patients with a positive prostate biopsy has a negative PCA 3 test, and the cost of PCA 3 is approximately 10 times greater than serum PSA.[40] Although PCA 3 provides additional information and may help guide the decision to biopsy or rebiopsy the prostate, it is not presently recommended for routine prostate cancer screening.

CURRENT RECOMMENDATIONS

Screening for prostate cancer with serum PSA remains controversial. The ERSPC and PLCO trials have thus far shown only a modest or no survival benefit to screening, and its utility as a public health policy is uncertain. The AUA recently revised their recommendations on the use of PSA in a best-practice statement.[26] Because PSA is the only test easily available to detect CaP, selective screening (especially for those at higher risk) is still encouraged. Because PSA is a continuous variable and there is no PSA value at which CaP is definitively ruled out, no specific cutoff value to determine a positive screening test has been accepted. Instead, men are encouraged to discuss with their physician the risks and benefits of prostate cancer screening beginning at 40 years of age and to consider a baseline PSA. At this age, benign prostatic enlargement is uncommon and PSA values are generally low. Men with a PSA greater than the median for their age (see **Table 1**) should be recognized as having a higher risk for being diagnosed with CaP.[41] Patients with an abnormal screening test, either by DRE or age-specific PSA, or an abnormal increase in PSA from a previous result (PSA velocity) should be referred to a urologist. A repeat PSA is appropriate before proceeding to biopsy. The decision for biopsy will be based not simply on a single PSA value but on patients' risk factors, including race and family history; previous PSA values; any previous biopsy results; and an assessment of comorbidities and life expectancy. Because 10-year mortality after clinical diagnosis of CaP is low, men with less than 10 years of life expectancy do not need PSA screening. The average American man reaches 10 years of remaining life expectancy at 75 years of age, and thus the United States Preventive Services Task Force have recommended against PSA screening for men older than 75 years of age.[42]

The appropriate time interval between PSA tests is also unknown. Annual screening was previously encouraged by the AUA and American Cancer Society. However, the ERSPC trial, with a 4-year screening interval, showed a modest cancer-specific survival benefit; whereas, the PLCO trial with annual screening did not. A total of 90% of men in the ERSPC trial with a PSA less than 1.9 ng/mL had a PSA less than 3.0 ng/mL 4 years later.[43] Screening intervals can now be individualized to patients' risk factors.

The American Cancer Society also recently revised their recommendations on prostate cancer screening.[44] Similar to the AUA, they recommend that patients discuss with their physician the risks and benefits of PSA screening starting at 50 years of age for men at average risk. African American men or those with a first-degree relative with CaP should start at 45 years of age, and those with 2 first-degree relatives with CaP should start at 40 years of age.

REFERENCES

1. Balk SP, Ko YJ, Bubley GJ. Biology of prostate-specific antigen. J Clin Oncol 2003;21(2):383–91.
2. Albertsen PC, Hanley JA, Barrows GH, et al. Prostate cancer and the Will Rogers phenomenon. J Natl Cancer Inst 2005;97:1248–53.
3. Stamey TA, Yang N, Hay AR, et al. Prostate-specific antigen as a serum marker for adenocarcinoma of the prostate. N Engl J Med 1987;317:909–16.
4. Catalona WJ, Smith DS, Ratliff TL, et al. Measurement of prostate-specific antigen in serum as a screening test for prostate cancer. N Engl J Med 1991;324(17):1156–61.
5. Smith DS, Catalona WJ, Herschman JD. Longitudinal screening for prostate cancer with prostate-specific antigen. JAMA 1996;276(16):1309–15.
6. Catalona WJ, Smith DS, Ornstein DK. Prostate cancer detection in men with serum PSA concentrations of 2.6 to 4.0 ng/mL and benign prostate examination. Enhancement of specificity with free PSA measurements. JAMA 1997;277(18):1452–5.
7. Jhaveri FM, Klein EA, Kupelian PA, et al. Declining rates of extracapsular extension after radical prostatectomy: evidence for continued stage migration. J Clin Oncol 1999;17:3167–72.
8. Gjertson CK, Asher K, Sclar J, et al. Local control and long term disease free survival for D1 prostate cancer following radical prostatectomy in the PSA era. Urology 2007;70(4):723–7.
9. Etzioni R, Tsodikiv A, Mariotto A, et al. Quantifying the role of PSA screening in the US prostate cancer mortality decline. Cancer Causes Control 2008;19:175–81.
10. Collin SM, Marin RM, Metcalfe C, et al. Prostate cancer mortality in the USA and UK in 1974–2004: an ecological study. Lancet Oncol 2008;9:445–52.
11. Grönberg H. Prostate cancer epidemiology. Lancet 2003;361(9360):859–64.
12. Johansson JE, Adami HO, Andersson SO, et al. Natural history of localized prostatic cancer. A population-based study in 223 untreated patients. Lancet 1989;1(8642):799–803.
13. Johansson JE, Adami HO, Andersson SO, et al. High 10-year survival rate in patients with early, untreated prostatic cancer. JAMA 1992;267:2191–6.
14. Johansson JE, Holmberg JS, Bergrstrom R, et al. Fifteen year survival in prostate cancer. A prospective, population-based study in Sweden. JAMA 1997;277:467–71.
15. Johansson JE, Andren O, Andersson SO, et al. Natural history of early, localized prostate cancer. JAMA 2004;291:2713–9.
16. Albertsen PC, Hanley JA, Gleason DF, et al. Competing risk analysis of men aged 55 to 74 years at diagnosis managed conservatively for clinically localized prostate cancer. JAMA 1998;280:975–80.
17. Albertsen PC, Hanley JA, Fine J. 20 year outcomes following conservative management of clinically localized prostate cancer. JAMA 2005;293:2095–101.

18. Bill-Axelson A, Holmber L, Filen F, et al. Radical prostatectomy versus watchful waiting in localized prostate cancer: the Scandinavian prostate cancer group-4 trial. J Natl Cancer Inst 2008;100:1144–54.
19. Widmark A, Klepp O, Solberg A, et al. Endocrine treatment, with or without radiotherapy, in locally advanced prostate cancer (SPCG-7/SFUO-3): an open randomized phase III trial. Lancet 2009;373:301–8.
20. Andriole GL, Grubb RL, Buys SS, et al. Mortality results from a randomized prostate-cancer screening trial. N Engl J Med 2009;360:1310–9.
21. Schroeder FH, Hugosson J, Roobol MJ, et al. Screening and prostate cancer mortality in a randomized European study. N Engl J Med 2009;360:1320–8.
22. Catalona WJ, Richie JP, de Kernion JB, et al. Comparison of prostate specific antigen concentration versus prostate specific antigen density in the early detection of prostate cancer: receiver operating characteristic curves. J Urol 1994;152:2031.
23. Catalona WJ, Partin AW, Slawin KM, et al. Use of the percentage of free prostate-specific antigen to enhance differentiation of prostate cancer from benign prostatic disease: a prospective multicenter clinical trial. JAMA 1998;279:1542–7.
24. Oesterling JE, Jacobsen SJ, Chute CG, et al. Serum prostate-specific antigen in a community-based population of healthy men: Establishment of age-specific reference ranges. JAMA 1993;270:860.
25. Reed A, Ankerst DP, Pollock BH, et al. Current age and race adjusted prostate specific antigen threshold values delay diagnosis of high grade prostate cancer. J Urol 2007;178:1929–32.
26. Greene KL, Albertsen PA, Babaian RJ, et al. Prostate specific antigen best practice statement: 2009 update. J Urol 2009;182:2232–41.
27. Carter HB, Pearson JD, Metter J, et al. Longitudinal evaluation of prostate-specific antigen levels in men with and without prostate cancer. JAMA 1992;177:2215–20.
28. Carter HB, Ferrucci L, Ketterman A, et al. Detection of life-threatening prostate cancer with prostate-specific antigen velocity during a window of curability. J Natl Cancer Inst 2006;98:1521–7.
29. Thompson IM, Ankerst DP, Chi C, et al. Assessing prostate cancer risk: results from the prostate cancer prevention trial. J Natl Cancer Inst 2006;98:529–34.
30. Vickers AJ, Savage C, O'Brien MF, et al. Systematic review of pretreatment prostate-specific antigen velocity and doubling time as predictors for prostate cancer. J Clin Oncol 2008;27:398–403.
31. American Cancer Society. Cancer facts and figures 2005. Atlanta (GA): American Cancer Society; 2005.
32. Godley PA, Schenck AP, Amamoo A, et al. Racial differences in mortality among Medicare recipients after treatment for localized prostate cancer. J Natl Cancer Inst 2003;95:1702–10.
33. Bratt O. Hereditary prostate cancer: clinical aspects. J Urol 2002;168(3):906–13.
34. McConnell JD, Roehrborn CG, Bautista OM, et al. The long-term effect of doxazosin, finasteride, and combination therapy on the clinical progression of benign prostatic hyperplasia. N Engl J Med 2003;349:2387–98.
35. Altman DG, Lausen B, Sauerbrei W, et al. Dangers of using "optimal" cut points in the evaluation of prognostic factors. J Natl Cancer Inst 1994;86:829–35.
36. Thompson IM, Pauler DK, Goodman PJ, et al. Prevalence of prostate cancer among men with a prostate-specific antigen level < or =4.0 ng per milliliter. N Engl J Med 2004;350:2239–48.

37. Ross AE, Loeb S, Landis P, et al. Prostate-specific antigen kinetics during follow-up are an unreliable trigger for intervention in a prostate cancer surveillance program. J Clin Oncol 2010;28(17):2807–9.
38. Oberpenning F, von Knobloch R, Sprute W, et al. [DiaPat urine test for prostate cancer. Predictive value for results of transrectal ultrasound-guided prostate biopsies]. Urologe A 2008;47:735–9 [in German].
39. Deras IL, Aubin SM, Blase A, et al. PCA3: a molecular urine assay for predicting prostate biopsy outcome. J Urol 2008;179:1587–92.
40. Schilling D, Hennenlotter J, Munz M, et al. Interpretation of the prostate cancer gene 3 in reference to the individual clinical background: implications for daily practice. Urol Int 2010;85(2):159–65.
41. Loeb S, Roehl KA, Antenor JA, et al. Baseline prostate-specific antigen compared with median prostate-specific antigen for age group as a predictor of prostate cancer risk in men younger than 60 years old. Urology 2006;67: 316–20.
42. Screening for prostate cancer. U.S. preventive services task force recommendation statement. Ann Intern Med 2008;149:185–91.
43. Schroeder FH, Raaijmakers R, Postma R, et al. 4-year prostate specific antigen progression and diagnosis of prostate cancer in the European randomized study of screening for prostate cancer, section Rotterdam. J Urol 2005;174:489–94.
44. Wolf AM, Wender RC, Etzioni RB, et al. American Cancer Society guideline for the early detection of prostate cancer: update 2010. CA Cancer J Clin 2010;60(2): 70–98.

Evaluation and Treatment of Erectile Dysfunction

Maarten Albersen, MD[a], Kuwong B. Mwamukonda, MD[b],
Alan W. Shindel, MD[c], Tom F. Lue, MD[d],*

KEYWORDS

- Erectile dysfunction • Phosphodiesterase 5 inhibitors
- Apomorphine SL • Intracavernous injection • Prostaglandin
- Evaluation • Assessment • Treatment

Erectile dysfunction (ED) was defined by the National Institutes of Health Consensus Development Panel on Impotence as the persistent inability to attain and maintain an erection sufficient for sexual intercourse.[1] ED is the most thoroughly studied sexual dysfunction in men and the most common sexual complaint of men presenting to their health care providers.[2] Various large-scale studies (both cross-sectional and longitudinal) have indicated that the worldwide prevalence of ED is between 10% and 20%. ED is strongly correlated with aging, with a steep incline in prevalence rates, from 6.5% in men aged 20 to 39 years to 77.5% in those aged 75 years and older.[3] ED is also associated with various comorbidities, including psychological factors, cardiovascular diseases, diabetes mellitus, and metabolic syndrome, and with smoking.[4] Iatrogenic ED is not uncommon and can be the result of pelvic surgical procedures or the use of various medications.[4]

Although ED is not a direct threat to physical health, it can have dramatic effects on personal sense of well-being and has a significant impact on the quality of life of

Conflicts of interest: Dr Maarten Albersen has received an unrestricted educational grant from Bayer Healthcare Belgium and is a scholar of the European Society for Surgical Oncology, Belgische Vereniging voor Urologie, and the Federico Foundation.
Dr Kuwong B. Mwamukonda has no conflicts of interest to disclose.
Dr Alan W. Shindel has received a research grant from American Medical Systems, and is an informal consultant for Boehringer Ingelheim.
Dr Tom F. Lue is a consultant of Pfizer, Eli Lilly & Co, Bayer, Medtronic, and Auxilium, and is a board member of Genix. He has received a research grant from American Medical Systems.
[a] Laboratory of Experimental Urology, Department of Urology, University Hospitals Leuven, Herestraat 49, Leuven 3000, Belgium
[b] SAUSHEC Urology Program, Brooke Army Medical Center, 3851 Roger Brooke Drive Fort Sam, Houston, TX 78234-6200, USA
[c] UC Davis Department of Urology, Lawrence J. Ellison Ambulatory Care Center, 4860 Y Street, Suite 2200, Sacramento, CA 95817, USA
[d] Department of Urology, University of California at San Francisco, 400 Parnassus Avenue, Campus Box 0738, San Francisco, CA 94143-0738, USA
* Corresponding author.
E-mail address: Tlue@urology.ucsf.edu

Med Clin N Am 95 (2011) 201–212
doi:10.1016/j.mcna.2010.08.016
0025-7125/11/$ – see front matter © 2011 Elsevier Inc. All rights reserved.

patients and their sexual partners. ED is also an independent predictor of cardiovascular morbidity and mortality.[5,6] For these reasons, ED merits consideration from the primary care physician as an important health concern and as a potential sentinel event for serious health problems. This article discusses the physiology and pathophysiology of erectile function in men, how the primary care physician may address the clinical problem of ED in practice, and when specialty referral is indicated.

PHYSIOLOGY AND PATHOPHYSIOLOGY OF ED

Penile erection is often described as a neurovascular process that is controlled by hormones. This article briefly describes the physiologic mechanisms of penile erection. A more elaborate discussion of the mechanisms of penile erection can be found elsewhere.[4,7,8]

Physiology of Penile Erection

During sexual stimulation, the hypothalamus is exposed to input from various neurotransmitters; dopamine seems to be the primary erectogenic central nervous system neurotransmitter. Dopamine-containing nerve endings impinge on oxytocinergic cell bodies contained in pathways descending from the hypothalamus to the brain stem and spinal autonomic centers and produce a "psychogenically mediated" erection.[8] A "tactile-mediated" erectogenic stimulus may result from direct stimulation of the penis. This stimulus occurs via sensory neurons that synapse in the sacral spinal cord.

In either case, the cavernous nerves, which arise from the pelvic plexus, are directly responsible for conducting impulses that generate penile erection. These nerves run alongside the posterolateral side of the prostatic capsule and perforate the urogenital diaphragm to enter the cavernous bodies at the level of the crura. Cavernous nerve activation leads to the release of the gaseous neurotransmitter nitric oxide (NO) from the nonadrenergic, noncholinergic nerve terminals in the corpus cavernosum. Additional NO is released from the endothelium in response to shear stress and the release of acetylcholine from parasympathetic endothelial nerve endings. In both cases, NO is synthesized by the enzyme nitric oxide synthase (NOS), which converts oxygen and l-arginine to NO and citrulline in the cavernous nerve terminals (nNOS) and in the endothelium (eNOS).[4,7,8]

NO passively diffuses into smooth muscle cells in the arterial wall and the trabeculae of the corpus cavernosum, where it binds to and activates soluble guanylate cyclase (GC). GC then catalyzes the breakdown of guanosine triphosphate into 3'5'-cyclic guanosine monophosphate (cGMP). cGMP acts as a downstream messenger and initiates a chain of reactions ultimately resulting in a decrease of intracellular calcium and relaxation of the smooth muscle (**Fig. 1**). Although this pathway is functionally the most important means to produce smooth muscle relaxation, it is supported by the synergistic actions of other pathways using 3'5'-cyclic adenosine monophosphate (cAMP) as a second messenger.

cAMP and cGMP are hydrolyzed by a class of enzymes called *phosphodiesterases*, of which subtype 5 (PDE5), a cGMP-specific phosphodiesterase, seems to be the dominant active isoform in penile tissue. Vasodilation and relaxation of trabecular smooth muscle allow rapid blood flow into the cavernosal sinusoids and the development of an erection, which is maintained by the compression of subtunical venules against the tunica albuginea, and reinforced by contraction of the voluntary ischiocavernosus muscle during the rigid erection phase. These pro-erectogenic parasympathetic pathways are counterbalanced by several sympathetically mediated mechanisms that maintain penile flaccidity. These mechanisms are less relevant for this review and are discussed in detail elsewhere.[4,9]

Pathophysiology of ED

Penile erection requires neural transmission of pro-erectile impulses, an intact arterial blood supply, and functional erectile tissue in the corpus cavernosum. ED can develop from a defect in one of these tissues or, more commonly, from a defect in a combination of tissues. ED is classified as vasculogenic, neurogenic, hormonal, anatomic/structural, drug-induced, or psychogenic.[4,10] **Table 1** summarizes the most prevalent causes of ED.

ED is strongly associated with various comorbidities, including cardiovascular diseases, diabetes mellitus, metabolic syndrome, and late-onset hypogonadism, and with smoking.[8] Aging is another major risk factor for ED.[11] These comorbid conditions and their relationship with ED will be discussed more in detail in the article by Berookhim and Bar-Chama elsewhere in this issue.

ASSESSMENT OF ED
Medical History

ED is often multifactorial in origin and is therefore best managed with a holistic approach that includes lifestyle modification, pharmacologic treatment, and attention to the relationship between partners. It is of particular importance to encourage open and honest communication between the patient and partner. All of these approaches are best facilitated in the context of a trusting patient/provider relationship, and therefore providers must establish rapport with patients when addressing issues of sexuality.[10,11]

The initial evaluation of ED should include a complete medical, psychosocial, and sexual history. A thorough medical assessment is mandatory in evaluating erectile complaints, particularly in older men and patients at intermediate and high risk for cardiovascular disease.[10] These patients should undergo cardiovascular assessment before continuing sexual activity and before beginning therapy for ED (**Fig. 2**).[12] Signs and symptoms of possible underlying conditions should be assessed, such as depression, diabetes, late-onset hypogonadism, metabolic syndrome, and medication/surgically induced causes of ED. Information about the association between ED and tobacco use can be an important tool in helping patients decide to quit use of tobacco products.[10,13] A thorough review of current medications may reveal agents that are known to cause or exacerbate ED (eg, antidepressants, antiandrogens, thiazides, and β-blockers). It is also important to assess for use of nitrate-donors, which are absolute contraindications for therapy with PDE5 inhibitors, and α-blockers that require an interval between use of the two drugs.[10,14] The goal of the history should be to not only understand the specific erectile condition but also identify possible underlying and reversible or treatable disorders.

Sexual History

The use of validated questionnaires, such as the International Index of Erectile Function, can be useful as an "ice-breaker" to initiate the conversation about ED. Numeric scores from instruments such as this may also be helpful in assessing the severity of ED, screening for other sexual dysfunctions, and evaluating treatment outcome.[15,16] These metrics ,however, should not be regarded as a replacement for direct assessment of sexual history.[13] An adequate sexual history should include information about current sexual relationships, the emotional status of the patient and the partner, and the exact nature of the couple's sexual concerns.[10] Issues of sexual orientation and gender identity should also be noted.[13] Descriptive measures such as rigidity

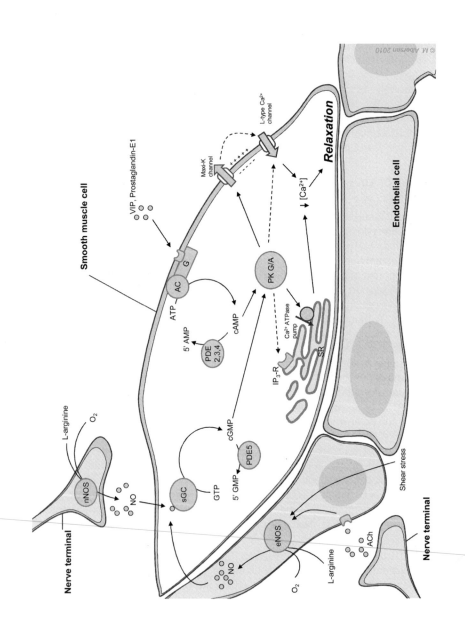

and duration of nocturnal erections, erections during masturbation, and erections after sexual arousal should be discussed, because they can give clues about the cause of ED. The onset of the problem and any situational factors that ameliorate or exacerbate ED should be determined. Problems with arousal, ejaculation, and difficulty reaching orgasm should be discussed because these may be signs of concomitant sexual dysfunctions requiring specialist assessment.[10] The impact of ED and other sexual dysfunctions on general well-being and sexual satisfaction, and issues of partner interest in and satisfaction with sex should be discussed.

Physical Examination

A complete external genital examination should be performed to detect anatomic or structural deformities of the penis, such as Peyronie plaques. Assessment of testicular size is important because small testes and regression of secondary sex characteristics may indicate hypogonadism.[10,11,13] Physical examination should also include a general screening for risk factors and comorbidities that are associated with ED, such as cardiovascular disease, neurologic disease, and obesity. Blood pressure and heart rate should be measured if they were not assessed in the previous 3 to 6 months.[10]

Laboratory Testing

Recommended laboratory tests include a complete blood cell count and measurements of fasting serum glucose, a lipid profile, and free and total testosterone, particularly in patients with signs of hypogonadism.[10,11,13] Additional hormonal testing is only required when low testosterone levels are detected. Baseline prostate-specific antigen screening is advised in patients older than 40 years or when ED is accompanied by lower urinary tract symptoms.[17]

Specific Diagnostic Testing

Radiologic testing, nocturnal penile rigidity testing, vascular and neurologic functional testing, and penile Doppler ultrasound are available for further diagnostic workup of ED. These tests are not routinely indicated in the primary care setting but may be ordered by urologists or sexual medicine specialists in certain cases.[4,10]

◄

Fig. 1. Molecular mechanisms of penile smooth muscle relaxation. Nitric oxide (NO) is released from nerve terminals in the corpus cavernosum in response to a neural stimulus and from the endothelium in response to the release of acetylcholine (Ach) and the shear stress elicited by increased blood flow in the corporeal sinusoids. NO binds to soluble guanylate cyclase (sGC) and thereby activates this enzyme, which catalyzes the breakdown of guanosine triphosphate (GTP) into cyclic guanosine monophosphate (cGMP). Other pathways, which are initiated by vasoactive intestinal polypeptide and prostaglandin E1, activate a G protein (G)–coupled receptor, leading to activation of adenylate cyclase (AC), which catalyzes the breakdown of adenosine triphosphate (ATP) into cyclic adenosine monophosphate (cAMP). cGMP and cAMP exert analogous effects by activating protein kinase G and A (PK G/A), respectively, which modulate potassium and calcium channels in the cell membrane and the inositol triphosphate receptor (IP$_3$-R) and the calcium-ATPase pump in the membrane of the sarcoplasmic reticulum (SR). These events lead to a lowering of the cytosolic calcium concentration, which causes dissociation of calcium from calmodulin. Calmodulin then dissociates from myosin light chain kinase, thus inactivating it, leading to smooth muscle relaxation and ultimately penile tumescence. eNOS, endothelial nitric oxide synthase; NOS, neuronal nitric oxide synthase; PDE, phosphodiesterase; VIP, vasoactive intestinal polypeptide. (*Adapted from* Albersen M, Shindel AW, Mwamukonda KB, et al. The future is today: emerging drugs for the treatment of erectile dysfunction. Expert Opin Emerg Drugs 2010;15:467–80; with permission from Informa Healthcare.)

Table 1
Pathophysiology of ED

Classification	Causes
Vasculogenic	Cardiovascular disease, atherosclerosis Hypertension Diabetes mellitus Hyperlipidemia Smoking Major surgery (retroperitoneum) Radiotherapy (retroperitoneum)
Neurogenic-central causes	Multiple sclerosis Multiple atrophy Parkinson disease Tumors Stroke Disk disease Spinal cord disorders
Neurogenic-peripheral causes	Diabetes mellitus Alcoholism Uremia Polyneuropathy Surgery (pelvis or retroperitoneum, radical prostatectomy)
Anatomic/structural	Peyronie disease Penile fibrosis (after pelvic radiotherapy or pelvic surgery) Penile trauma (penile fracture) Congenital curvature of the penis Micropenis Hypospadias, epispadias
Hormonal	Primary hypogonadism (eg, late-onset hypogonadism) Secondary hypogonadism/hypogonadotropic hypogonadism (eg, hyperprolactinemia) Hyper- and hypothyroidism Cushing disease
Drug- or substance-induced	Antihypertensives (thiazides and ß-blockers are most common) Antidepressants Antipsychotics Antiandrogens Antihistamines Recreational drugs/smoking
Psychogenic	Generalized type (eg, lack of arousability, disorders of sexual intimacy) Situational type (eg, partner-related, performance-related issues, from distress)

Adapted from Wespes E , Amar E, Eardley I, et al. EAU Guidelines on Male Sexual Dysfunction: erectile dysfunction and premature ejaculation. © European Association of Urology 2009; with permission.

When to Refer

The decision of when to refer a patient for management of ED must be made on a case-by-case basis and is determined in large part by the interest and comfort a given primary care provider has in managing ED. Cases that should prompt immediate referral include patients with lifelong ED, a history of pelvic, urethral or perineal

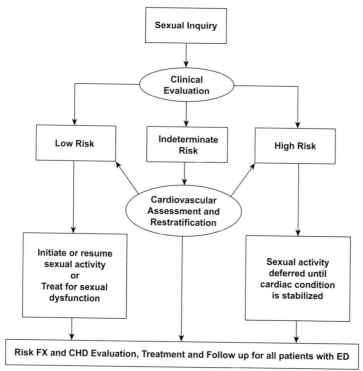

Fig. 2. Sexual dysfunction and cardiac risk (the second Princeton Consensus Conference). CHD, coronary heart disease; Fx, risk factors. (*Reprinted from* Kostis JB, Jackson G, Rosen R, et al. Sexual dysfunction and cardiac risk (the Second Princeton Consensus Conference). Am J Cardiol 2005;96(2):313–21. © 2005; with permission from Elsevier.)

trauma, penile deformities, endocrine disorders detected during standard laboratory testing, and complex or severe psychiatric or psychosexual disorders.[10]

TREATMENT OF ED IN THE PRIMARY CARE SETTING
General Considerations Before Initiating Pharmacologic Treatment

Both the patient's and partner's understanding of ED and results of the diagnostic tests should be reviewed before treatment is initiated, so that a rational selection of treatment options and expectations can be provided. Current pharmacologic treatments for ED do not cure ED but can generally be relied on to greatly improve erectile function. Setting realistic treatment goals and granting permission and legitimacy for engaging in alternative means of sexual intimacy that do not rely on penetrative sexual intercourse should be a goal of therapy. Few older patients with ED will be able to regain full potency, but most should be able to experience restoration of satisfying sexual encounters.

Underlying reversible conditions (obesity, medical comorbidities, relationship issues) should be addressed and treated before or simultaneously with initiating specific ED-directed treatment.[18] Lifestyle changes, such as exercise and smoking cessation, should be suggested where applicable. Referral to exercise physiologists, nutritionists, or personal trainers may be of some benefit in these situations.

Oral Pharmacotherapy

Although many treatment modalities are available for ED, this article mainly focuses on oral pharmacotherapy, which will efficiently treat most patients experiencing ED. When oral therapies fail, referral to a specialist should be considered except when the primary care provider has a particular interest and comfort in dealing with sexuality issues.

PDE5-specific inhibitors

PDE5-specific inhibitors (PDE5Is) are nonhydrolyzable analogs of cGMP and exert their beneficial effects on smooth muscle relaxation through competitively binding to the catalytic site of PDE5. Through slowing the degradation of cGMP, these drugs produce an intracellular accumulation of cGMP in smooth muscle cells in the arteries and trabeculae of the corpus cavernosum (see **Fig. 1**), resulting in relaxation of the smooth muscle, increased arterial blood flow, and penile tumescence.[19]

Treatment of ED with PDE5I

In current treatment guidelines, PDE5Is are recommended as the preferred pharmacotherapy for ED.[10] Numerous trials have established on-demand efficacy rates of 60% to 70% in the general population, and postmarketing data confirms excellent safety profiles of the three compounds currently available in the United States (sildenafil, vardenafil, and tadalafil).[19–22] Although a large crossover study showed an overall equivalence in the subjective perception of treatment benefits among all PDE5Is, the three currently available drugs differ from each other in time to onset of action and duration of action (sildenafil and vardenafil up to 5 hours and tadalafil up to 24–36 hours).[23] The choice of appropriate drug is based on patient and partner preference guided by physician advice.[20]

Before initiation of treatment, patients should be informed that sexual stimulation is essential for the efficacy of the drugs. Although some men may experience limited efficacy after a first trial, these patients should be informed that results generally improve with repeated dosing, and a minimum of six attempts should be made before treatment is considered a failure. The recommended starting doses are 50 mg for sildenafil and 10 mg for vardenafil and tadalafil. The unique pharmacokinetic properties of tadalafil have led to the approval of this drug as a daily treatment for ED at 2.5- and 5-mg doses; this regimen may be best for patients who have frequent intercourse or those who desire to separate the act of taking the drug from sexual interactions. The lowest therapeutic doses (25 mg of sildenafil and 5 mg of vardenafil and tadalafil on-demand) should be used when liver or kidney failure is present or when the patient uses medication that inhibits the CYP34A pathway. Examples of these drugs are ketoconazole, itraconazole, erythromycin, clarithromycin, and HIV protease inhibitors.[10] However, patients taking medications that potentiate the CYP34A pathway, such as rifampin, phenobarbital, phenytoin, and carbamazepine, may need higher doses for efficacy.[10]

Safety profile

Postmarketing surveillance has not shown increased myocardial infarction rates in patients using PDE5Is compared with age-matched controls.[21] However, certain heart-related precautions must be considered in men taking PDE5Is. PDE5Is are relatively contraindicated in patients with unstable angina pectoris, recent myocardial infarction, certain arrhythmias, and poorly controlled hypertension. These patients should undergo cardiovascular examination and treatment for their heart-related condition before initiating ED treatment.[10] Furthermore, patients treated with nitrates or nitrate-donors should not take PDE5Is, and, use of PDE5Is with certain α-blockers may result in postural hypotension.[10] Patients taking α-blockers for prostate symptoms or blood pressure control should take PDE5IS with at least a 4-hour window between dosing because of a theoretical risk of orthostatic hypotension, although some evidence suggests that the risk is low in patients on long-term α-blocker therapy.[14] Patients with prolongation of the QTc interval should not be treated with vardenafil.[22]

Adverse events

The most common adverse events from PDE5Is include headache, facial and ocular hyperemia, nasal congestion, myalgia, dyspepsia, and back pain. These side effects are attributable to specific inhibition of PDE5 and subsequent vasodilatation in tissues other than the penis.[7,21] Congestion and flushing are more common with sildenafil relative to the other PDE5Is, whereas myalgias and dyspepsia are more strongly associated with tadalafil and vardenafil, respectively. Other less-common adverse events involve visual disturbances, most often attributable to the inhibition of PDE6 in the cones of the retina.[7] Adverse events account for approximately 25% of patients who discontinue PDE5I use, whereas the most common reason for discontinuation of PDE5Is is lack of efficacy.[24] More serious adverse events are rare and include seizures, nonarteritic ischemic optic neuritis, and acute hearing loss, although the exact role of PDE5Is in these conditions is debatable and reports are anecdotal.[21,25] Patients can generally be reassured that the risk of serious long-term adverse events is low in appropriately selected candidates for PDE5I therapy.

Nonresponders

Of the patients who do not experience an initial response to PDE5I, between 30% and 50% may be converted to responders through re-education on proper dosing technique and through dose-escalation. Patients who discontinue tadalafil because of side effects may benefit from the daily-dosing option (2.5 or 5 mg/d).[26–28] Furthermore, addition of exogenous testosterone supplementation may enhance PDE5I therapy in individuals in whom hypogonadism is confirmed.[29] Because the efficacy of PDE5I depends on the integrity of the NO pathway in producing cGMP, patients in whom this pathway is disturbed will benefit far less from PDE5I treatment compared with the general population. Disease states that diminish NO availability include denervation of the erectile tissue after radical prostatectomy; severe diabetes; and down-regulation of NOS expression, as may be seen in atherosclerosis, metabolic syndrome, aging, and hypogonadism.[7] These difficult-to-treat patients benefit from referral to a sexual medicine specialist or urologist for second-line treatment.

Alternative Oral Pharmacotherapy

Apomorphine SL

Apomorphine is a centrally acting nonselective dopamine agonist that exhibits D2-like effects. It acts by binding to dopamine receptors in the hypothalamus and enhances naturally occurring pro-erectile signals.[30] It is available in 2- or 3-mg doses but has not been approved in the United States for the treatment of ED.[19] It is rapidly absorbed through the sublingual route of administration and results in the development of an erection within 20 minutes in more than two-thirds of patients.[30] Apomorphine has lower efficacy and satisfaction rates than PDE5Is, and is most effective in patients with mild to moderate ED.[10] It also is a valid alternative to PDE5Is for patients in whom psychogenic ED is suspected and in those who have contraindications to PDE5Is, such as those taking nitrates. The most common adverse events are caused by nonspecific binding to other subtypes of the dopamine receptor and include nausea, headache, and dizziness.[30] These effects occur with relative high frequency, and have limited the usefulness of this drug.

Yohimbine

Yohimbine is a natural peripherally and centrally acting α-blocker. However, little evidence shows its efficacy in treating ED, and therefore it is not currently recommended in most guidelines for management of ED. It may have a role in patients who prefer natural products but should not be considered a recommended mainstream medical therapy.[10]

Vacuum Constriction Devices

The vacuum constriction device (VCD) creates negative pressure around the penis, thereby initiating passive engorgement of the sinusoidal spaces and creating an erection. Maintenance of erection is facilitated by application of a rubber cuff worn around the base of the penis. Although effective in up to 90% of patients, the use of a vacuum device might be perceived as disruptive, especially by younger men.[10] Local side effects are relatively minor and include bruising, some discomfort, and ejaculatory obstruction. It is advised to limit the use of the constriction band to 30 minutes to avoid skin necrosis. Contraindications to VCD use include bleeding disorders and the use of anticoagulants.[10]

Second-Line Treatment

Intracavernous and intraurethral therapy

Before the advent of PDE5I,s intracavernous and intraurethral administration were the only nonsurgical treatment options for ED. The most commonly used substance, and currently the only one approved by the U.S. Food and Drug Administration as a treatment of ED, is prostaglandin E1 (PGE1). PGE1 activates adenylate cyclase and thereby raises intracellular cAMP, with effects analogous to those of cGMP (see **Fig. 1**). These effects are independent of the NO-cGMP pathway, making this treatment an excellent option for patients who do not experience response to PDE5I therapy.[31] Intracavernous PGE1 therapy has an overall satisfaction rate of approximately 80%.[32]

Phentolamine, papaverine, and vasoactive intestinal peptide are also available for intracavernous injection, although their role is limited to combination therapy (commonly referred to as *bimix* or *trimix*).[11] PGE1 is also available for intraurethral administration (medicated urethral system for erection [MUSE]).

Adverse events from these therapies include priapism, variable degrees of pain with injection in approximately half of patients, and penile fibrosis after long-term use.[31] Patients are advised to consult their physician if they experience prolonged penile pain or an erection lasting up to or more than 4 hours, because aspiration of cavernous blood may be necessary for penile decompression.[10] Relative contraindications to injection therapy include a history of priapism or bleeding disorders. Before initiation of therapy, patients follow a short in-office training program. MUSE has many side effects in common with intracavernous PGE1, although it is less likely to cause priapism and may have marginal efficacy in many cases. MUSE has also been associated with hypotension, syncope, urethral burning or pain, and vaginal irritation in the partner.[31]

Third-Line Therapy (Surgery)

Implantation of a penile prosthesis, which can be either inflatable or malleable, is indicated for men in whom pharmacologic therapy is not effective. Implantation of a penile prosthesis has satisfaction rates of 70% to 90%, but patients should be aware of the definitive and irreversible nature of this surgery.[10] Adverse events include mechanical failure after several years of use (50% after a 10-year interval), infection (1%–3%), and, rarely, erosion.[10,11]

Other surgical options available for ED include penile revascularization and venous ligation. Outcomes of these surgeries in the general population of patients with ED are poor. These surgeries should be reserved for a select group of primarily young patients and should be performed in specialized centers only.[10,11]

SUMMARY

ED is a prevalent and important disease that has been associated with various comorbidities. The evaluation of patients with ED should include a general health assessment followed by a discussion of reversible factors and lifestyle changes that might help preserve erectile capacity. Numerous effective treatment options are currently available. A frank discussion about use and side effects of these therapies is required to optimize success. Although oral pharmacologic treatments can be initiated and monitored by the primary care physician, patients who do not experience response to these treatments may be best served by referral to a sexual medicine specialist for further assessment and consideration of other treatment options.

REFERENCES

1. NIH Consensus Conference. Impotence. NIH consensus development panel on impotence. JAMA 1993;270(1):83–90.
2. Uckert S, Mayer ME, Stief CG, et al. The future of the oral pharmacotherapy of male erectile dysfunction: things to come. Expert Opin Emerg Drugs 2007; 12(2):219–28.
3. Saigal CS, Wessells H, Pace J, et al. Predictors and prevalence of erectile dysfunction in a racially diverse population. Arch Intern Med 2006;166(2):207–12.
4. Lue TF. Erectile dysfunction. N Engl J Med 2000;342(24):1802–13.
5. Araujo AB, Travison TG, Ganz P, et al. Erectile dysfunction and mortality. J Sex Med 2009;6(9):2445–54.
6. Guo W, Liao C, Zou Y, et al. Erectile dysfunction and risk of clinical cardiovascular events: a meta-analysis of seven cohort studies. J Sex Med 2010. [Epub ahead of print].
7. Albersen M, Shindel AW, Mwamukonda KB, et al. The future is today: emerging drugs for the treatment of erectile dysfunction. Expert Opin Emerg Drugs 2010; 15(3):467–80.
8. Gratzke C, Angulo J, Chitaley K, et al. Anatomy, physiology, and pathophysiology of erectile dysfunction. J Sex Med 2010;7(1 Pt 2):445–75.
9. Lin CS, Xin ZC, Wang Z, et al. Molecular Yin and Yang of erectile function and dysfunction. Asian J Androl 2008;10(3):433–40.
10. Hatzimouratidis K, Amar E, Eardley I, et al. Guidelines on male sexual dysfunction: erectile dysfunction and premature ejaculation. Eur Urol 2010. [Epub ahead of print].
11. Albersen M, Shindel AW, Lue TF. Sexual dysfunction in the older man. Rev Clin Gerontol 2009;19:b1–8.
12. Kostis JB, Jackson G, Rosen R, et al. Sexual dysfunction and cardiac risk (the second Princeton Consensus Conference). Am J Cardiol 2005;96(2):313–21.
13. Hackett G, Kell P, Ralph D, et al. British Society for Sexual Medicine guidelines on the management of erectile dysfunction. J Sex Med 2008;5(8):1841–65.
14. Kloner RA. Pharmacology and drug interaction effects of the phosphodiesterase 5 inhibitors: focus on alpha-blocker interactions. Am J Cardiol 2005;96(12B): 42M–6M.
15. Rosen RC, Cappelleri JC, Gendrano N III. The international index of erectile function (IIEF): a state-of-the-science review. Int J Impot Res 2002;14(4):226–44.

16. Rosen RC, Cappelleri JC, Smith MD, et al. Development and evaluation of an abridged, 5-item version of the International index of erectile function (IIEF-5) as a diagnostic tool for erectile dysfunction. Int J Impot Res 1999;11(6):319–26.

17. Greene KL, Albertsen PC, Babaian RJ, et al. Prostate specific antigen best practice statement: 2009 update. J Urol 2009;182(5):2232–41.

18. Esposito K, Giugliano F, Di Palo C, et al. Effect of lifestyle changes on erectile dysfunction in obese men: a randomized controlled trial. JAMA 2004;291(24): 2978–84.

19. Eardley I, Donatucci C, Corbin J, et al. Pharmacotherapy for erectile dysfunction. J Sex Med 2010;7(1 Pt 2):524–40.

20. Hatzimouratidis K, Hatzichristou DG. A comparative review of the options for treatment of erectile dysfunction: which treatment for which patient? Drugs 2005;65(12):1621–50.

21. Shindel AW. 2009 update on phosphodiesterase type 5 inhibitor therapy part 2: updates on optimal utilization for sexual concerns and rare toxicities in this class. J Sex Med 2009;6(9):2352–64.

22. Carson CC III. Cardiac safety in clinical trials of phosphodiesterase 5 inhibitors. Am J Cardiol 2005;96(12B):37M–41M.

23. Jannini EA, Isidori AM, Gravina GL, et al. The ENDOTRIAL study: a spontaneous, open-label, randomized, multicenter, crossover study on the efficacy of sildenafil, tadalafil, and vardenafil in the treatment of erectile dysfunction. J Sex Med 2009; 6(9):2547–60.

24. Hatzimouratidis K, Hatzichristou D. Phosphodiesterase type 5 inhibitors: the day after. Eur Urol 2007;51(1):75–88.

25. Bella AJ, Brant WO, Lue TF, et al. Non-arteritic anterior ischemic optic neuropathy (NAION) and phosphodiesterase type-5 inhibitors. Can J Urol 2006;13(5):3233–8.

26. Bella AJ, Deyoung LX, Al-Numi M, et al. Daily administration of phosphodiesterase type 5 inhibitors for urological and nonurological indications. Eur Urol 2007;52(4):990–1005.

27. Shindel AW. 2009 update on phosphodiesterase type 5 inhibitor therapy part 1: recent studies on routine dosing for penile rehabilitation, lower urinary tract symptoms, and other indications (CME). J Sex Med 2009;6(7):1794–808 [quiz: 1793, 1809–10].

28. Rubio-Aurioles E, Kim ED, Rosen RC, et al. Impact on erectile function and sexual quality of life of couples: a double-blind, randomized, placebo-controlled trial of tadalafil taken once daily. J Sex Med 2009;6(5):1314–23.

29. Shabsigh R, Kaufman JM, Steidle C, et al. Randomized study of testosterone gel as adjunctive therapy to sildenafil in hypogonadal men with erectile dysfunction who do not respond to sildenafil alone. J Urol 2004;172(2):658–63.

30. Heaton JP, Altwein JE. The role of apomorphine SL in the treatment of male erectile dysfunction. BJU Int 2001;88(Suppl 3):36–8.

31. Costabile RA, Mammen T, Hwang K. An overview and expert opinion on the use of alprostadil in the treatment of sexual dysfunction. Expert Opin Pharmacother 2008;9(8):1421–9.

32. Alexandre B, Lemaire A, Desvaux P, et al. Intracavernous injections of prostaglandin E1 for erectile dysfunction: patient satisfaction and quality of sex life on long-term treatment. J Sex Med 2007;4(2):426–31.

Medical Implications of Erectile Dysfunction

Boback M. Berookhim, MD, MBA[a], Natan Bar-Chama, MD[a,b],*

KEYWORDS

- Erectile dysfunction • Cardiovascular disease • LUTS
- Endothelial dysfunction

Erectile dysfunction (ED) is defined as the inability to achieve or sustain a penile erection sufficient for sexual performance and is a common condition in aging men. The Massachusetts Male Aging Study (MMAS) has demonstrated a combined prevalence of minimal, moderate, and complete ED in 52% of men, with an increase in the prevalence of complete ED from 5% to 15% and that of moderate dysfunction from 17% to 34% between ages 40 and 70 years.[1] Estimates from a different study evaluating black and Hispanic population groups of a similar age range are 24.4% and 19.9%, respectively.[2] Given the calculated incidence rate of ED, it has been estimated that there are 617,715 new diagnoses of ED among white men annually and there is an estimated prevalence of up to 30 million men in the United States.[3,4]

In the 1970s, ED was thought to have been predominantly a condition of psychogenic origin, leading to likely underreporting of the condition by men. Other causes of ED have been well described over the years, including neurogenic sources (as is often seen in patients after radical pelvic surgery and in those with Parkinson disease, stroke, epilepsy, or Alzheimer disease), endocrinologic sources (hypogonadism), and arteriogenic sources. Evidence exists for the association between ED and several other disorders, including cardiovascular disease (CVD), hypertension, diabetes, obesity, lower urinary tract disorders associated with lower urinary tract symptoms (LUTS), testosterone deficiency/hypogonadism, depression, chronic obstructive pulmonary disease, and a multitude of medications used in the treatment of these conditions. Together, these associations indicate that most cases of ED are secondary to organic causes. Given these associations, there exist data that patients presenting with ED as a primary complaint are at risk for these comorbid conditions and should undergo screening to prevent the sequelae associated with delayed

[a] Department of Urology, Mount Sinai Medical Center, Mount Sinai School of Medicine, One Gustave L. Levy Place, Box 1272, New York, NY 10029, USA
[b] Department of Obstetrics, Gynecology, and Reproductive Science, Mount Sinai Medical Center, Mount Sinai School of Medicine, One Gustave L. Levy Place, Box 1272, New York, NY 10029, USA
* Corresponding author. Department of Urology, Mount Sinai Medical Center, Mount Sinai School of Medicine, One Gustave L. Levy Place, Box 1272, New York, NY 10029.
E-mail address: natan.bar-chama@mountsinai.org

Med Clin N Am 95 (2011) 213–221
doi:10.1016/j.mcna.2010.08.020
0025-7125/11/$ – see front matter © 2011 Elsevier Inc. All rights reserved.

treatment. In this article, the relationships between ED and its most common comorbid diseases are described, so as to better guide practitioners dealing with patients who have a primary complaint of ED.

CVD
ED and Hypertension, Diabetes, Hyperlipidemia, and Obesity

The major comorbidities associated with CVD are also associated with ED. Patients with ED commonly present with some combination of hypertension, diabetes, hyperlipidemia, and obesity. After adjusting for age, the MMAS population had a 15% prevalence of complete ED in patients treated for hypertension, a relationship that was associated with the duration and severity of ED.[1] In a survey of 7689 patients with hypertension and diabetes with a mean age of 59 years, ED was present in a staggering 67% of 3906 patients with hypertension alone, 71% of 2377 patients with diabetes alone, and 78% of patients with both diseases.[5] ED was untreated in 65% of these patients, 69% of whom reported needing treatment, with a strong majority of these saying that they would have welcomed a discussion about ED with their physicians.

Diabetes has long been recognized as a precipitating factor for ED. The prevalence of ED in patients with diabetes is likely a result of a multifactorial relationship because diabetes has both microvascular and neurologic effects. A study of 129 patients with ED has demonstrated the condition to be a presenting symptom of diabetes in 5% of men.[6] A Korean study of more than 1300 men with diabetes has shown a 64% prevalence of ED, nearly 6-fold the rate in the general population, with patients older than 60 years and with a history of diabetes for more than 10 years at a statistically significantly greater risk for ED compared with the reference group.[7] There is also a significantly increased prevalence of hypogonadism in men with type 2 diabetes, which may serve as an additional factor leading to ED.[8,9]

Hyperlipidemia and obesity, the key factors in the metabolic syndrome, have also been associated with ED. Hyperlipidemia is estimated to affect more than 91 million men in the United States alone.[10] Many studies have evaluated the plasma levels of low-density lipoprotein (LDL) in men with ED and found a statistically significant increase in LDL among patients with ED compared with their normal counterparts.[11–13] Treatment of hyperlipidemia with statin has led to mixed results with respect to ED symptoms in several small studies, with some demonstrating improvement of ED and others a worsening in symptoms.[14,15] Obese men are also at an increased risk for ED, particularly those presenting with central obesity. However, there are no multivariate analyses that control for other risk factors.

Prevalence of CVD Among Patients with ED

Given the relationship of ED with cardiovascular risk factors, recent research has shown ED to be a harbinger of CVD and mortality. The placebo arm of the Prostate Cancer Prevention Trial included 9457 men with a mean age of 62 years; of these, 8063 (85%) had no CVD and 3816 (47%) had ED at study entry.[16] In this study population, men with incident ED (n = 2420) during the 5-year study period had a 25% increase in subsequent CVD (hazard ratio [HR], 1.25; 95% confidence interval [CI], 1.02–1.53) compared with their counterparts without ED and men with incident or prevalent ED (n = 6236) had an HR of 1.45 (95% CI, 1.25–1.69). This association was in the range of the risk noted with smoking or a family history of myocardial infarction in this study population. The Olmsted County Study included 1402 men (median age, 55 years) without known coronary artery disease (CAD) and screened for ED for

10 years.[17] Men with ED were approximately 2 times more likely to develop CAD during the study period (univariate analysis: HR, 2.1; 95% CI, 1.5–2.9; multivariate analysis: HR, 1.8; 95% CI, 1.2–2.6). This rate was similar to that seen in patients with diabetes, hypertension, and smoking.

In addition to acting as a marker for future CVD, ED is increasingly associated with cardiovascular mortality. The MMAS, a prospective observational cohort study, evaluated 1709 men during a mean follow-up of 15.2 years.[18] Complete data were available for 1665 men, and 37.7% died of CVD. Men with moderate or complete ED, as evaluated by the International Index of Erectile Function, had an HR of 1.43 (95% CI, 1.00–2.05) for CVD mortality compared with their counterparts with or without minimal ED. Risk of mortality because of CVD increased as ED severity increased (P<.001). In addition, all-cause mortality was considerably higher in patients with moderate or complete ED compared with those with no or mild ED (HR, 1.60; 95% CI, 1.29–1.98). Data from the Erectile Dysfunction Substudy of the ONgoing Telmisartan alone and in combination with Ramipril Global Endpoint Trial/Telmisartan Randomized AssessmeNt Study in ACE iNtolerant subjects with cardiovascular Disease (ONTARGET/TRANSCEND) trial support these results, having been designed to determine whether ED is predictive of death and cardiovascular outcomes in high-risk patients with CVD.[19] In total, 1549 patients with a median age of 64.8 years entered this double-blind randomized trial, which had a median follow-up of 54 months. On multivariate analysis, ED was associated with an HR of 1.93 for cardiovascular death (95% CI, 1.13–3.29), 1.84 for all-cause mortality (95% CI, 1.21–2.81), and 2.02 for myocardial infarction (95% CI, 1.13–3.58).

Proposed Pathophysiology of Comorbid ED and CVD

Montorsi and colleagues[20] have proposed the artery size hypothesis to explain the pathophysiologic association between ED and CVD. The theory relies on the fact that atherosclerosis is a systemic disease, with all vascular beds within the body being affected to the same extent. However, given the varying sizes of arteries throughout the vascular system, symptoms generally present at different time points, with lower extremity claudication often presenting long after a presentation of CAD, given the much larger caliber of the femoral artery compared with the coronary arteries. According to this theory, an occlusion amounting to 50% of the coronary artery would be associated with a near-critical occlusion of the much smaller penile artery despite a nearly equal amount of total atherosclerotic plaque in the 2 arteries. As such, ED often precedes significant CAD despite a common pathophysiologic pathway. Although there is a lack of pathologic evidence verifying this pathway, this mechanism has gained some acceptance because of its plausibility in more advanced diseases.

The role of endothelial dysfunction in both ED and CVD serves as a likely link between pathways in the multifactorial association between these 2 complex disease processes.[21,22] Increased flow and the resultant vasodilation in the penile arteries necessary for erection seem to be mediated largely through nitric oxide (NO) produced by the endothelium. In both ED and CVD, there is a deficiency of NO brought about by either impaired production or increased degradation, leading to a decrease in vasodilation, modulation of smooth muscle cells, and inhibition of cellular adhesion.[23,24] Endothelial dysfunction is, therefore, generally seen as the initiating step in the formation of atherosclerotic plaques. Given the small diameter of the cavernosal arteries and the high content of endothelium and smooth muscle in the penile vascular bed, the inability to achieve an erection may be a sensitive indicator of systemic vascular disease.[25] Endothelial dysfunction in patients with ED but without evidence of other significant CVD was found within the penile vasculature but not within the small arteries of the forearm, suggesting that dysfunction occurs earlier within the penile endothelium than in other vascular beds.[26] The measurement of endothelial function varies across several fairly nonspecific serum markers (eg, endothelin-1, interleukin 6, tumor necrosis factor α, and C-reactive protein), various cellular markers, imaging of carotid artery intima-media thickness, and more specific physiologic measurements, including flow-mediated dilation (FMD) of the brachial artery and reactive hyperemia peripheral arterial tonometry (RH-PAT).

FMD of the brachial artery is the most widely published of these physiologic measurements. The technique is performed by arterial occlusion with a blood pressure cuff for 5 minutes, which leads to reactive hyperemia and local endothelial activation and therefore to endothelium-dependent dilation of the brachial artery. This dilation is measured by ultrasonography and compared with the dilation in the brachial artery by administration of nitroglycerin, which is caused by an endothelium-independent pathway. Several studies using this test have demonstrated significant endothelial dysfunction in men with ED compared with those without ED, without clinical evidence of overt CVD.[27,28] More recently, use of RH-PAT has come into vogue, as it tends to be more reproducible and operator independent (Endo-PAT 2000; Itamar Medical Ltd, Caesarea, Israel). RH-PAT is a Food and Drug Administration (FDA)-approved office-based technique that uses a finger probe to assess the digital volume changes accompanying pulse waves after inducing reactive hyperemia with a blood pressure cuff on the upper arm. Studies using RH-PAT have confirmed the role of endothelial dysfunction in ED, CVD, and diabetes.[29–31] One study evaluating more than 200 patients with ED has demonstrated using RH-PAT that ED is a marker for endothelial dysfunction independent of other cardiovascular comorbidities, including hypertension, diabetes, smoking, and obesity (Berookhim, unpublished data, 2009).

The relationship between ED and endothelial dysfunction is further substantiated by the improvement in endothelial function in patients undergoing phosphodiesterase 5 (PDE5) inhibitor therapy. PDE5 inhibitors decrease the breakdown of cyclic guanosine monophosphate (cGMP) in smooth muscle cells, increasing the effects of NO.[32] Long-term PDE5 inhibitor therapy, as approved by the FDA in the use of tadalafil, leads to persistent improvements in the global endothelial function for up to 2 weeks after cessation of the therapy.[33]

LUTS
ED and LUTS

Recent data have indicated a potential link between LUTS (a symptom complex associated with complaints of urinary frequency, urgency, dysuria, nocturia, hesitancy, and weakness of urinary stream, often indicating benign prostatic hypertrophy [BPH]) and ED, as these 2 conditions tend to occur within the same patient population and are prevalent among aging men. Several studies now indicate that LUTS are an independent predictor of ED after adjusting for known comorbidities for each of the 2 pathologic processes. The National Health and Social Life Survey, which studied sexual dysfunction in 1410 men aged 18 to 59 years, was among the early studies to indicate that LUTS were a significant predictor of ED.[34] Men with LUTS had an adjusted odds ratio of 3.13 of having ED. These results were further elaborated on by the multinational UrEpik study, a population-based study conducted in the United Kingdom, the Netherlands, France, and Korea, evaluating the relationship between LUTS and ED in 4800 men aged 40 to 79 years.[35] ED was present in 21% of patients and was significantly associated with age, diabetes, hypertension, smoking, liver disease, and LUTS after adjusting for age and country of origin. The Cologne Male Survey studied 4489 men with a mean age of 52 years[36] and noted LUTS in 31% of the men. The prevalence of LUTS in patients with ED was 72%, with an odds ratio of 2.11. In addition to diabetes, hypertension, and previous pelvic surgery, LUTS were considered an age-independent risk factor for ED ($P<.001$). A Dutch study of more than 1600 men aged 50 to 78 years[37] also showed a similar relationship between LUTS and ED but differed in that there was a strong dose-response relationship, with the relative risk of ED increasing from 1.8 to 7.5 based on the degree of urinary complaints.

Proposed Pathophysiology of Comorbid ED and LUTS

Recent basic science research has sought to describe a common pathophysiology of ED and LUTS. As described earlier for CVD, endothelial dysfunction is also thought to play a role in the development of LUTS and BPH. Prostatic tissue in patients with BPH has fewer nitrinergic innervations than normal prostate tissue, suggesting a role for NO in BPH/LUTS.[38] Although this relationship needs further study, PDE5 inhibitors seem to improve both BPH/LUTS and ED. A recent prospective randomized controlled trial of 1058 patients who received either placebo or daily tadalafil in varying doses strictly for the treatment of LUTS secondary to BPH indicated significant improvement in the International Prostate Symptom Scores (IPSS) among all patients receiving tadalafil compared with placebo.[39] The IPSS response rates with tadalafil were approximately equal to those described with α-blockers throughout the literature, further suggesting a role for NO in the pathophysiology of ED and BPH/LUTS.

α_1-Adrenergic receptors have been identified throughout the lower urinary tract, with various receptor subtypes in prostatic stromal cells, epithelial cells, urethra, bladder, and detrusor muscle. It has been suggested that these receptors are upregulated in patients with BPH, resulting in increased smooth muscle tone in the prostatic capsule and bladder neck. This upregulation is believed to account for the improvement in symptoms with α_1-adrenergic receptor antagonists in patients with BPH. In addition, detumescence is known to involve norepinephrine in the contraction of penile tissues via activation of α_1-adrenergic receptors in penile vasculature and corpus cavernosum smooth muscle. Murine studies have suggested that androgens may play a role in regulating the responsiveness of these receptors.[40] PDE5 inhibitors increase cGMP levels and decrease prostatic tone in tissues activated by norepinephrine.[41] It is therefore postulated that upregulation of α_1-adrenergic receptors may serve to be a link between LUTS and ED.

ENDOCRINE DISEASE
ED and Testosterone Deficiency

Endocrine diseases and ED have been well linked throughout the literature. The relationship between ED and diabetes mellitus has been discussed earlier. Testosterone deficiency has also been described in patients with ED, with a prospective study estimating a prevalence of testosterone deficiency in up to 27% of men in an ED clinic (mean age, 50 years).[42] Despite the comorbid presentation of these 2 conditions, the role of androgens in ED is controversial because it is not uncommon to find men with very low serum testosterone levels and only mild complaints of ED. No study to date has found an association between the levels of serum total testosterone and the presence and severity of ED.[1,43,44] Testosterone plays a significant role in erectile function in animals, and there is clear evidence linking testosterone deficiency in humans to hypoactive sexual desire and loss of libido.[45–47] Testosterone therapy in patients with ED and testosterone deficiency has yielded mixed results, with some studies showing an increase in the rigidity and duration of erections of patients on testosterone therapy and others simply demonstrating an effect on sexual desire.[48,49] Given this relationship, the Third International Consultation of Sexual Medicine (Paris, 2009) has recommended screening for testosterone deficiency in men presenting with ED and/or hypoactive sexual desire.[50]

Testosterone deficiency has been associated with insulin resistance, type 2 diabetes mellitus, and the metabolic syndrome in several studies.[51,52] Low serum testosterone levels have additionally been associated with CVD and even cardiovascular mortality. Shores and colleagues[53] performed a retrospective review of 858 veterans with a mean age of 68 years. With a median follow-up of 4.3 years and after adjusting for covariates, Kaplan-Meier analysis showed a statistically significant 88% increased risk of mortality in patients with serum testosterone levels less than 250 ng/dL as compared with patients with serum testosterone levels greater than 250 ng/dL. The findings of increased cardiovascular mortality in testosterone deficiency were strengthened by a prospective case-control study from the United Kingdom evaluating more than 2300 patients aged 42 to 78 years with a median follow-up of 7 years.[54] Statistical analysis demonstrated that the age-adjusted odds ratio for all-cause mortality, CVD, CAD, and cancer significantly decreased with increasing quartile group of testosterone. Findings of an increased risk of CVD in testosterone deficiency were furthered in a Surveillance, Epidemiology and End Results Medicare database review of 73,166 men with locoregional prostate cancer, of whom 36% (mean age, 74 years) were treated with gonadotropin-releasing hormone (GnRH) agonists to institute androgen deprivation therapy and followed up for a median of 4.6 years.[55] Patients receiving GnRH agonists had a statistically significant increase in incident diabetes mellitus (HR, 1.44), incident CAD (HR, 1.16), myocardial infarction (HR, 1.11), and sudden cardiac death (HR, 1.16). Testosterone deficiency is therefore increasingly being viewed as an independent risk factor for CVD and diabetes mellitus. The role of testosterone replacement therapy in the treatment and prevention of these sequelae remains nebulous but should alert the practitioner to evaluate these often-comorbid conditions in patients with ED and testosterone deficiency.

SUMMARY

ED is independently associated with CVD, risk of mortality secondary to CVD, and LUTS. It is also associated with testosterone deficiency. Practitioners presented with patients who have a primary complaint of ED must consider these comorbidities, as ED is no longer considered simply a psychogenic condition and a quality-of-life diagnosis. A significant number of patients being evaluated for CVD or LUTS by primary care physicians report ED that was unaddressed by their doctor, despite wanting to discuss treatment options and causes of the condition. The relationship between ED and risk factors for CVD has been well established, and ED may be the presenting symptom of diabetes. Significant research demonstrates the presence of endothelial dysfunction in patients with ED, giving the physician an opportunity for earlier intervention against CVD, the primary cause of death among American men. In addition, men with ED are often at risk for bothersome LUTS often secondary to BPH. The presence of ED in patients with testosterone deficiency and its potential role in the pathogenesis of the metabolic syndrome and CVD needs further elucidation. These conditions may have significant quality-of-life consequences if not adequately assessed and treated.

REFERENCES

1. Feldman HA, Goldstein I, Hatzichristou DG, et al. Impotence and its medical and psychosocial correlates: results of the Massachusetts Male Aging Study. J Urol 1994;151:54.
2. Laumann EO, West S, Glasser D, et al. Prevalence and correlates of erectile dysfunction by race and ethnicity among men aged 40 or older in the United States: from the male attitudes regarding sexual health survey. J Sex Med 2007;4:57.
3. Johannes CB, Araujo AB, Feldman HA, et al. Incidence of erectile dysfunction in men 40 to 69 years old: longitudinal results from the Massachusetts Male Aging Study. J Urol 2000;163:460.
4. Lue TF. Erectile dysfunction. N Engl J Med 2000;342:1802.
5. Giuliano FA, Leriche A, Jaudinot EO, et al. Prevalence of erectile dysfunction among 7689 patients with diabetes or hypertension, or both. Urology 2004;64: 1196.
6. Sairam K, Kulinskaya E, Boustead GB, et al. Prevalence of undiagnosed diabetes mellitus in male erectile dysfunction. BJU Int 2001;88:68.
7. Cho NH, Ahn CW, Park JY, et al. Prevalence of erectile dysfunction in Korean men with Type 2 diabetes mellitus. Diabet Med 2006;23:198.
8. Shabsigh R. Testosterone therapy in erectile dysfunction and hypogonadism. J Sex Med 2005;2:785.
9. Kapoor D, Aldred H, Clark S, et al. Clinical and biochemical assessment of hypogonadism in men with type 2 diabetes: correlations with bioavailable testosterone and visceral adiposity. Diabetes Care 2007;30:911.
10. Executive Summary of the Third Report of the National Cholesterol Education Program (NCEP) Expert Panel on Detection, Evaluation, and Treatment of High Blood Cholesterol in Adults (Adult Treatment Panel III). JAMA 2001;285:2486.
11. Nikoobakht M, Nasseh H, Pourkasmaee M. The relationship between lipid profile and erectile dysfunction. Int J Impot Res 2005;17:523.
12. Roumeguere T, Wespes E, Carpentier Y, et al. Erectile dysfunction is associated with a high prevalence of hyperlipidemia and coronary heart disease risk. Eur Urol 2003;44:355.
13. Sullivan ME, Miller MA, Bell CR, et al. Fibrinogen, lipoprotein (a) and lipids in patients with erectile dysfunction. A preliminary study. Int Angiol 2001;20:195.
14. Bank AJ, Kelly AS, Kaiser DR, et al. The effects of quinapril and atorvastatin on the responsiveness to sildenafil in men with erectile dysfunction. Vasc Med 2006;11:251.
15. Solomon H, Samarasinghe YP, Feher MD, et al. Erectile dysfunction and statin treatment in high cardiovascular risk patients. Int J Clin Pract 2006;60:141.
16. Thompson IM, Tangen CM, Goodman PJ, et al. Erectile dysfunction and subsequent cardiovascular disease. JAMA 2005;294:2996.
17. Inman BA, Sauver JL, Jacobson DJ, et al. A population-based, longitudinal study of erectile dysfunction and future coronary artery disease. Mayo Clin Proc 2009; 84:108.
18. Araujo AB, Travison TG, Ganz P, et al. Erectile dysfunction and mortality. J Sex Med 2009;6:2445.
19. Bohm M, Baumhakel M, Teo K, et al. Erectile dysfunction predicts cardiovascular events in high-risk patients receiving telmisartan, ramipril, or both: the ONgoing Telmisartan alone and in combination with Ramipril Global Endpoint Trial/Telmisartan Randomized AssessmeNt Study in ACE iNtolerant subjects with cardiovascular Disease (ONTARGET/TRANSCEND) Trials. Circulation 2010;121:1439.

20. Montorsi P, Ravagnani PM, Galli S, et al. The artery size hypothesis: a macrovascular link between erectile dysfunction and coronary artery disease. Am J Cardiol 2005;96:19M.
21. Guay AT. ED2: erectile dysfunction = endothelial dysfunction. Endocrinol Metab Clin N Am 2007;36:453.
22. Billups KL, Bank AJ, Padma-Nathan H, et al. Erectile dysfunction is a marker for cardiovascular disease: results of the Minority Health Institute Expert Advisory Panel. J Sex Med 2005;2:40.
23. Tamler R, Bar-Chama N. Assessment of endothelial function in the patient with erectile dysfunction: an opportunity for the urologist. Int J Impot Res 2008;20:370.
24. Ross R. Atherosclerosis—an inflammatory disease. N Engl J Med 1999;340:115.
25. Jackson G, Montorsi P, Adams MA, et al. Cardiovascular aspects of sexual medicine. J Sex Med 2010;7:1608.
26. Kaiser DR, Billups K, Mason C, et al. Impaired brachial artery endothelium-dependent and -independent vasodilation in men with erectile dysfunction and no other clinical cardiovascular disease. J Am Coll Cardiol 2004;43:179.
27. Chiurlia E, D'Amico R, Ratti C, et al. Subclinical coronary artery atherosclerosis in patients with erectile dysfunction. J Am Coll Cardiol 2005;46:1503.
28. Kaya C, Uslu Z, Karaman I. Is endothelial function impaired in erectile dysfunction patients? Int J Impot Res 2006;18:55.
29. Bonetti PO, Pumper GM, Higano ST, et al. Noninvasive identification of patients with early coronary atherosclerosis by assessment of digital reactive hyperemia. J Am Coll Cardiol 2004;44:2137.
30. Rozanski A, Qureshi E, Bauman M, et al. Peripheral arterial responses to treadmill exercise among healthy subjects and atherosclerotic patients. Circulation 2001;103:2084.
31. Kuvin JT, Patel AR, Sliney KA, et al. Assessment of peripheral vascular endothelial function with finger arterial pulse wave amplitude. Am Heart J 2003;146:168.
32. Goldstein I, Lue TF, Padma-Nathan H, et al. Oral sildenafil in the treatment of erectile dysfunction. Sildenafil Study Group. N Engl J Med 1998;338:1397.
33. Rosano GM, Aversa A, Vitale C, et al. Chronic treatment with tadalafil improves endothelial function in men with increased cardiovascular risk. Eur Urol 2005;47:214.
34. Laumann EO, Paik A, Rosen RC. Sexual dysfunction in the United States: prevalence and predictors. JAMA 1999;281:537.
35. Boyle P, Robertson C, Mazzetta C, et al. The association between lower urinary tract symptoms and erectile dysfunction in four centres: the UrEpik study. BJU Int 2003;92:719.
36. Braun MH, Sommer F, Haupt G, et al. Lower urinary tract symptoms and erectile dysfunction: co-morbidity or typical "aging male" symptoms? Results of the "Cologne Male Survey". Eur Urol 2003;44:588.
37. Blanker MH, Bohnen AM, Groeneveld FP, et al. Correlates for erectile and ejaculatory dysfunction in older Dutch men: a community-based study. J Am Geriatr Soc 2001;49:436.
38. Bloch W, Klotz T, Loch C, et al. Distribution of nitric oxide synthase implies a regulation of circulation, smooth muscle tone, and secretory function in the human prostate by nitric oxide. Prostate 1997;33:1.
39. Roehrborn C, McVary KT, Elbion-Mboussa A, et al. Tadalafil administered once daily for lower urinary tract symptoms secondary to benign prostatic hyperplasia: a dose finding study. J Urol 2008;180:1228.

40. Reilly CM, Stopper VS, Mills TM. Androgens modulate the alpha-adrenergic responsiveness of vascular smooth muscle in the corpus cavernosum. J Androl 1997;18:26.
41. Uckert S, Sormes M, Kedia G, et al. Effects of phosphodiesterase inhibitors on tension induced by norepinephrine and accumulation of cyclic nucleotides in isolated human prostatic tissue. Urology 2008;71:526.
42. Somani B, Khan S, Donat R. Screening for metabolic syndrome and testosterone deficiency in patients with erectile dysfunction: results from the first UK prospective study. BJU Int 2010;106:688.
43. Rhoden EL, Teloken C, Mafessoni R, et al. Is there any relation between serum levels of total testosterone and the severity of erectile dysfunction? Int J Impot Res 2002;14:167.
44. Corona G, Mannucci E, Mansani R, et al. Aging and pathogenesis of erectile dysfunction. Int J Impot Res 2004;16:395.
45. Steidle C, Schwartz S, Jacoby K, et al. AA2500 testosterone gel normalizes androgen levels in aging males with improvements in body composition and sexual function. J Clin Endocrinol Metab 2003;88:2673.
46. O'Carroll R, Shapiro C, Bancroft J. Androgens, behaviour and nocturnal erection in hypogonadal men: the effects of varying the replacement dose. Clin Endocrinol (Oxf) 1985;23:527.
47. Wang C, Swerdloff RS, Iranmanesh A, et al. Transdermal testosterone gel improves sexual function, mood, muscle strength, and body composition parameters in hypogonadal men. J Clin Endocrinol Metab 2000;85:2839.
48. Carani C, Granata AR, Bancroft J, et al. The effects of testosterone replacement on nocturnal penile tumescence and rigidity and erectile response to visual erotic stimuli in hypogonadal men. Psychoneuroendocrinology 1995;20:743.
49. O'Connor DB, Archer J, Wu FC. Effects of testosterone on mood, aggression, and sexual behavior in young men: a double-blind, placebo-controlled, cross-over study. J Clin Endocrinol Metab 2004;89:2837.
50. Buvat J, Maggi M, Gooren L, et al. Endocrine aspects of male sexual dysfunctions. J Sex Med 2010;7:1627.
51. Corona G, Mannucci E, Petrone L, et al. NCEP-ATPIII-defined metabolic syndrome, type 2 diabetes mellitus, and prevalence of hypogonadism in male patients with sexual dysfunction. J Sex Med 2007;4:1038.
52. Corona G, Mannucci E, Petrone L, et al. Association of hypogonadism and type II diabetes in men attending an outpatient erectile dysfunction clinic. Int J Impot Res 2006;18:190.
53. Shores MM, Matsumoto AM, Sloan KL, et al. Low serum testosterone and mortality in male veterans. Arch Intern Med 2006;166:1660.
54. Khaw KT, Dowsett M, Folkerd E, et al. Endogenous testosterone and mortality due to all causes, cardiovascular disease, and cancer in men: European Prospective Investigation into Cancer in Norfolk (EPIC-Norfolk) Prospective Population Study. Circulation 2007;116:2694.
55. Keating NL, O'Malley AJ, Smith MR. Diabetes and cardiovascular disease during androgen deprivation therapy for prostate cancer. J Clin Oncol 2006;24:4448.

Male Factor Assessment in Infertility

Zamip P. Patel, MD[a],*, Craig S. Niederberger, MD[a,b]

KEYWORDS
- Male • Infertility • Assessment • Review

Often in the course of a couple's infertility work-up, the man is considered only in terms of a semen analysis. Because the management of infertility is often initiated by the female partner's gynecologist, and the couple sent directly to a fertility clinic staffed by physicians who had their basic training in obstetrics/gynecology, the male factor is often distilled into two questions: (1) Is the semen analysis within World Health Organization (WHO) normal boundaries? and, if not, (2) Does the man have any usable sperm for either intrauterine insemination, in vitro fertilization, or intracytoplasmic sperm injection? If the answer to these both is no, the couple is often told to use donor sperm.

This article reviews the current modalities for the evaluation of male factor infertility from both urologist and primary care physician points of view and discusses the implications male factor infertility have on overall male health. The authors hope to dispel the notion that the male factor infertility work-up is simply a semen analysis. With a properly done assessment, many men who otherwise would not be able to sire children, even through artificial means, will be able to father healthy progeny.

EPIDEMIOLOGY, PATHOPHYSIOLOGY, AND DEFINITIONS

Male factor infertility is the sole cause of infertility in approximately 20% of infertile couples, and in 30% to 40% of couples both male and female factors contribute.[1,2] Thus half of all infertility can be attributed in part or completely to the male factor. Current American Society for Reproductive Medicine (ASRM) guidelines consequently recommend that both the man and woman be evaluated in an infertility work-up and that both evaluations start concurrently at the first year of being unable to conceive and earlier if known pre-existing conditions are present.[3]

The authors have nothing to disclose.

[a] Department of Urology, University of Illinois College of Medicine, Clinical Science North, Suite 515, 840 South Wood Street, Chicago, IL 60612, USA

[b] Department of Bioengineering, College of Engineering, University of Illinois at Chicago, Suite 515, 840 South Wood Street, Chicago, IL 60612, USA

* Corresponding author.

E-mail address: zamip.patel@gmail.com

To diagnose a man as infertile, it is necessary to define the condition. Although routine history and physical examination are necessary for the complete assessment of an infertile man, most times a work-up is prompted by a semen analysis, because it is the most obvious way to evaluate the man. To understand some of the clues that may appear during the course of a history and physical examination, it becomes necessary to discuss what a semen analysis represents and where its parameters may lead in diagnosis. Early investigation into ejaculated semen parameters set the foundation for the semen analysis that is used today. These early studies examining the nature of sperm were done using a microscope, pipette, and basic chemical analysis.[4] By examining characteristics that varied between ejaculates of male partners in infertile versus fertile couples, scientists determined a set of parameters validated by further efforts.[5,6] Those gave rise to the first set of WHO[7] standards, published in 1987. These currently exist in their fifth edition and are used as a standard for laboratories worldwide.

These measures were determined by analyzing a large heterogenous population of fertile men. Fertility was determined by a given man having a currently pregnant partner or a partner who had been pregnant within the previous 12 months. Using one-sided lower reference limits, the fifth centiles (with 95% CIs) were generated.[8] These reference values are listed in **Table 1**. The importance of each of these reference values is discussed.

Semen Volume

Semen volume is often used as a surrogate marker for assessing the anatomy of semen delivery. Secretions from the testis, epididymis, bulbourethral gland, periurethral glands, prostate, and seminal vesicles comprise normal seminal fluid.[9] Periurethral glands account for 0.1 to 0.2 mL, prostatic secretions account for 0.5 mL, and secretions from the seminal vesicles account for 1.5 to 2.0 mL of total semen volume. Little of the total volume of seminal fluid comes from the testis. The contribution of sperm (primarily from the distal epididymis) accounts for only 1% to 5% of total semen volume.[9] Thus, low semen volumes are more likely to be indicators of abnormalities with semen delivery. These include but are not limited to retrograde ejaculation, obstruction of the ejaculatory duct (either acquired or secondary to congenital conditions, such as a prostatic cyst), previous urologic surgery, anatomic absence of the seminal vesicles and complete absence of the vas deferens, and other congenital malformations of wolffian duct structures.

Table 1 2010 WHO parameters	
	Percentile (95% CI)
Semen volume	1.5 mL (1.4–1.7)
Total sperm number	39 Million (33–46)
Sperm concentration	15 Million/mL (12–16)
Vitality	58% Live (55–63)
Progressive motility	32% (31–34)
Total (progressive + nonprogressive) motility	40% (38–42)
Morphologically normal forms	4.0% (3.0–4.0)

Data from Cooper TG, Noonan E, von Eckardstein S, et al. World Health Organization reference values for human semen characteristics. Hum Reprod Update 2010;16(3):231–45.

Total Sperm Number and Sperm Concentration

Total sperm numbers are calculated by pouring specimens on a grid, examining them under the microscope, and extrapolating the number of sperm to the total sample. The total sperm number is simply the sperm concentration multiplied by volume. Although it may seem intuitive that the higher the total number of sperm, the increased likelihood of achieving a pregnancy, in practice this is only partially true. Although total numbers of sperm do correlate with higher pregnancy rates, the correlation is loose when taken as a sole indicator. In conjunction with the rest of the semen parameters, the total sperm number gains greater relevance.[10]

Decreased total sperm numbers can be due to several causes, both physiologic and pathologic. Total sperm numbers have a normal variation that occurs cyclically. There is a diurnal variation in semen quality, including total count.[11] There is also a seasonal variation in the quality and count of sperm.[12] Finally, although most evidence suggests that increased male age is associated with a mild decline in semen volume, sperm motility, and sperm morphology, there is some debate as to whether or not a decline in sperm concentration concurrently decreases.[13] Still, a large body of evidence suggests that total sperm numbers decline to a small degree with advancing age.[14,15]

Pathologic reasons for a decrease in total sperm number are many. Contributing causes range from exogenous factors, such as heat (regular hot water baths, sauna, and so forth), drugs, infection (systemic), and gonadotoxins, to endogenous factors, such as varicocele, endocrinopathy, febrile or systemic illness, and childhood conditions, such as cryptorchidism. DNA-targeted cancer chemotherapeutic agents can alter semen parameters.[16] Spironolactone may affect semen parameters through its antiandrogenic activity.[9] Long-term use of nitrofurantion, sulfasalazine, and colchicine may decrease semen parameters, although short-term use likely does not.[9] There is a large body of evidence demonstrating a causal effect of chronic opioid use and hypogonadotropic hypogonadism, causing a decrease in sperm parameters.[17] One of the most effective ways to decrease sperm counts, in occasional cases permanently, is exogenous testosterone.[9,16] All of these factors that decrease sperm counts decrease motility as well. Although these conditions usually do not result in a complete loss of sperm in a specimen, many can result in azoospermia. Thus it is necessary to distinguish obstructive azoospermia (OA) from nonobstructive azoospermia (NOA). The diagnosis of OA from NOA is discussed later.

Vitality

Vitality refers to a laboratory technique in which sperm are exposed to a dye (commonly eosin-based stains) and the percentage of sperm that do not stain, representing the sperm that are able to exclude the stain from their intracytoplasmic environment, are reported. This is commonly used as an adjunct test to a low motility score (commonly <5%–10%) to differentiate necrospermia from nonmotile but viable sperm.[9]

Motility

Motility refers to the degree and percentage of sperm movement. Although there is a clear distinction under a microscope between "moving" and "nonmoving" sperm, not all the moving sperm in a given specimen act uniformly. To account for these differences, the WHO classifies sperm in four categories. Category A refers to rapid progressive motility, B to slow but progressive motility, C to nonprogressive motility, and D to no motility.[18] Category A plus B is reported as progressive motility and A plus B plus C is total motility.[8]

A useful measure often used by andrologists is the total motile count (TMC) or total motile sperm. This is calculated by the total sperm count multiplied by motility. This is a useful measure because it incorporates the three most important validated measures into a single number that represents the total number of motile, viable sperm in a given specimen. When gauging the probabilities of a natural conception, and by extension of assisted reproductive technologies, the TMC becomes a standard measure to assess the male factor infertility.[19]

Morphology

Of all the identified semen parameters, morphology (the external shape of the sperm) is the most subjective. More than one classification system is used to determine normal versus abnormal morphology, and even within andrology centers there is variability between technicians using the same classification system.[20] Kruger proposed a rigid classification system using exact numbers to determine sizes of particular anatomic areas of sperm, referred to interchangeably as strict, Kruger, or Tygerberg morphology.[21] Strict criteria identify normal sperm as having a single ellipse-shaped head with specific measurements for the head, the acrosome percentage of the head, midpiece width and length, tail length and appearance, and the amount and location of cytoplasmic droplets.[21] Using this classification in its past three semen analysis specifications, the WHO reported a 4% normal morphology (95% CI, 3–4) as the fifth centile in its most recent update.[8] This low number reflects the high degree of variability of morphology within even a fertile population. Once a diagnosis of teratozoospermia is made, there is significant debate as to its clinical significance. For patients with isolated teratozoospermia, there is no consensus as to the appropriate artificial reproductive technology to use.[22,23]

Genetics is expected to play a role in the etiology of many cases of teratozoospermia. Many investigators have suggested subdividing abnormal morphology based on appearance and genetic information to identify those men who are most likely to succeed with assisted technologies. Karyotype testing in teratozoospermia for aneuploidy is the most recognized in this quest, but other assays, including chromatin structural analysis, Y-microdeletion, and fluorescence in situ hybridization–based assays, have been suggested as important in the decision-making process.[24,25]

Additional Semen Analysis Tests

Other tests are often included in a semen analysis but are of limited use. According to the latest WHO guidelines, there are currently few reference values for the pH of semen from fertile men; thus, the consensus pH of 7.2 is accepted as a threshold for normal.[26] Because the seminal vesicles secrete a fluid rich in fructose and alkaline fluid, and because a large proportion of normal ejaculate is from the seminal vesicles, a decrease in pH and a decrease in fructose are both considered indicators of possible obstruction, especially when combined with a low volume.

As useful as a semen analysis can be in guiding care, it is only a surrogate marker for fertility. A full understanding of male infertility remains elusive, as evidenced by the fact that approximately 15% of patients with male factor infertility have a normal semen analysis.[27] Furthermore, a semen analysis can theoretically only indicate that the azoospermic patient is infertile, because even severely oligoasthenoteratospermic patients have a small but finite chance of conceiving naturally. As knowledge of the genetic basis of male infertility broadens, so does the ability to link those changes with pathologic states observed. This proliferation has led to a battery of candidate genes and tests, outlined in the following sections.

Karyotype

One of the first tests developed to evaluate the genetic makeup of an infertile man was karyotyping. The most common diagnosis from karyotype analysis is the mosaic or nonmosaic XXY (Klinefelter syndrome) but, besides numerical anomalies in chromosome count, structural, translocation, and inversion defects can also be identified.[28] Approximately 6% of all infertile men have abnormalities in their karyotype, with proportionately more men having an abnormality as sperm counts decline.[29]

Y chromosome microdeletions

Loci collectively known as the azoospermia factor (AZF) are on the long arm of the Y chromosome. This region is the most common identified genetic cause of male infertility, accounting for approximately 7% of infertile men.[30] It consists of at least three subregions (AZFa, AZFb, and AZFc), which seem to encode for proteins involved in germ cycle regulation and meiosis.[29] Deletions in any portion of AZFa and AZFb are consistent with male sterility, whereas some men with isolated deletions in AZFc are able to father children with assisted reproduction.[31]

Cystic fibrosis

Most male patients with cystic fibrosis have azoospermia secondary to congenital bilateral absence of the vas deferens (CBAVD). In otherwise phenotypically normal men, however, a mild form of the cystic fibrosis transmembrane regulator (CFTR) mutation responsible for cystic fibrosis can lead to the isolated condition of CBAVD. The diagnosis is made simply by physical examination. Because the carrier rate is 1 in 25, and because men with CBAVD are frequently heterozygotes for many mutations within the large encoding region for CFTR,[28] it is important to perform genetic testing of both male and female partners to determine the probability of transmitting the condition to progeny. The most common screening tests identify a few dozen of the most prevalent cystic fibrosis–associated mutation,[28] but a more detailed (and consequently more expensive) assay can be performed to include the rarer mutations. Even more detailed screening does not rule out the possibility of an unidentified mutation within the CFTR region, and couples should be counseled accordingly.

Sperm DNA integrity testing

One of the unique characteristics of spermiogenesis is that it results in DNA that is more tightly wound and packed and, therefore, less susceptible to injury, than somatic DNA.[28] Infertile men may have dysfunction in this structure and, therefore, sperm is more likely to become damaged in an environment unable to repair it. The theoretic consequence of this is twofold: DNA with more damage leads to less viable sperm, and a substantial increase in DNA injury may supercede the oocyte's ability for repair, resulting in a higher rate of miscarriage and a lower rate of fertilization.[28] To assess this, many different assays have been developed. The sperm chromatic structure assay exposes sperm to acid, incorporates a dye, and then uses flow cytometry to measure the proportion of damaged DNA. Comet and terminal deoxynucleotidyl transferase-mediated deoxyuridine triphosphate nick end labeling (TUNEL) assays directly measure DNA breaks.[28] Although highly positive assays imply a higher risk of pregnancy failure,[32] an ASRM practice committee did not find that testing for sperm integrity led to clinically improved outcomes.[33]

INITIAL EVALUATION

A physician's history taking and physical examination play a large role in the initial evaluation of a patient with suspected or known male infertility. A thorough sexual history, including history of intercourse timing, possible lubricants, previous and current birth control methods, and previous history of children, are questions for a couple on initial evaluation. Assuming normal female ovulation, optimal timing of intercourse should be performed every 2 days near the time of ovulation.[34]

Pertinent questions specific to the man should center on developmental, surgical, medical, and family history. Developmental questions include a history of cryptorchidism as a child and, if the condition was present, the age of orchidopexy. Lee and colleagues[35] reported a 38% infertility rate in men with a positive bilateral cryptorchidism history versus 10.5% in unilateral and 6% in age-matched controls. Although there is some debate as to the optimal time to perform an orchidopexy, data suggest that spermatogenesis may be at least partially preserved if orchidopexy is performed before puberty.[36] Other developmental abnormalities may be uncovered by inquiring about age of puberty. Precocious puberty may be secondary to a pathologic excess of androgen, including such causes as Leydig cell tumor, whereas delayed or incomplete puberty may be secondary to hypogonadotropic hypogonadism (Kallmann syndrome). History of gynecomastia can suggest either androgen or estrogen excess (eg, tumor or androgen insensitivity) or, conversely, androgen deficiency states, such as Klinefelter syndrome. History of multiple epididymal cysts or absence or malformation of renal structures may suggest ureteric bud and genital ridge anomalies that may manifest as unilateral absence of the vas, seminal vesicle cysts, or genital tract obstruction.

Surgical influences on fertility may be secondary to orchidopexy (discussed previously). Other causes can be secondary to neurologic damage to the ejaculation reflex (eg, retroperitoneal or spinal surgery), vasectomy, trauma, or inguinal hernia surgery. Although congenital unilateral absence of a testis (either secondary to malformation or in utero torsion) does not seem to affect fertility potential, there is some evidence to suggest that torsion later in life may adversely affect semen and testosterone parameters.[37,38]

Orchiectomy for testicular cancer does not itself predispose to infertility; however, testis cancer is associated with spermatogenic dysfunction, chemotherapy may have an effect on semen parameters, and retroperitoneal surgery may result in retrograde ejaculation or anejaculation. An increased probability of cancer in the contralateral testis has been reported.[39] Thus, sperm banking soon after orchiectomy is strongly urged to counter the consequences of a possible future bilateral orchiectomy.

The complete list of medical conditions that can affect fertility is long. Any effect on vascular function can adversely affect testosterone levels and thus reflect the decreasing quality of the intratesticular environment, leading to a decrease in semen parameters. Vascular effects often also coincide with changes in endocrine function and can have a direct effect on semen parameters. The list of medical conditions affecting fertility includes hypertension, diabetes, obesity, any systemic or chronic disease or illness (including infections), and endocrinopathies.[9] Many routine medications have a direct gonadotoxic effect as well as endocrine effects (eg, spironolactone and chronic opiod use as described previously).[16] Besides systemic conditions, infections localized to the genitourinary tract, such as sexually transmitted diseases, can lead to pyospermia and decreases in semen parameters. Even with treatment, scarring from the initial insult can lead to genital tract obstruction.[40] Environmental exposures should be assessed as well. Smoking is a common lifestyle exposure linked to male infertility. A history of pesticide or heavy metal exposure is also an example of a possible gonadotoxic insult.[41]

Because a genetic link has been implicated in if not fully responsible for, cryptor-chidism, cystic fibrosis, hypogonadism, and idiopathic infertility, family history for any of these conditions is relevant.[42]

Part of the medical history should include an assessment of a patient's testosterone status. Testosterone has many functions in men, not limited to differentiation of primary and secondary sexual characteristics. Testosterone is involved, in bone, cardiovascular, sexual, and cognitive functions. Although the link between testos-terone and erectile dysfunction is not as simple as cause and effect, low levels of testosterone can contribute to erectile dysfunction. Conversely, erectile dysfunction may be one of the first signs of testosterone deficiency.[43] Erectile function is important in the reproductive process and thus should be a part of the medical history. Testos-terone is also vital to the growth and maturation of sperm, however. High testicular concentrations of testosterone are required to maintain spermatogenesis,[44] and intra-testicular testosterone levels are approximately 40 times higher than serum levels.[45] Thus, small variations in serum testosterone levels represent large fluctuations in the intratesticular environment. Therefore, evidence of hypoandrogenism, such as erectile dysfunction as well as decreased energy, decreased libido, sudden onset of cognitive difficulties, sudden decrease in muscle mass, early onset of osteoporosis, and evidence of endothelial dysfunction in an otherwise healthy men, should be noted. Many disease states can give any one or a constellation of these symptoms.

The physical examination can also be revealing. Global abnormalities in secondary sexual characteristics may be indicative of androgen insensitivity or of Klinefelter syndrome. Gynecomastia can accompany these findings in these two disease states or may be secondary to high prolactin levels from a prolactinoma. The genital exam-ination can be particularly helpful. Hypospadias or chordee can lead to improper semen placement and can contribute to infertility.[9] Particular attention should be paid to the testes. The testes should be palpated for masses and consistency. A decrease in the turgor of the testes may be indicative of infertility. The testes should be measured using sonography or an orchidometer during an infertility assessment. Testes size directly reflects spermatogenesis.[9] Next, the epididymis and vas should be examined. Dilation of the epididymis is suggestive of obstruction. Although epidid-ymal cysts are common and not a sign of obstruction, multiple cysts within the epidid-ymis may be a sign of abnormalities with development and should indicate ultrasound examination of the kidneys. A prostate examination is recommended to evaluate for seminal vesicle cysts.[9]

The spermatic cord should be palpated first for the vas deferens. The vas should be followed to determine areas of atrophy or, in the case of a previous vasectomy, the presence of granulomata. The cord should also be inspected for varicocele. Varico-celes are more likely to occur on the left due to the anatomy of the left testicular vein drainage at a right angle into the left renal vein rather than directly into the inferior vena cava. An isolated right varicocele raises the question of situs inversus or retroper-itoneal or renal tumor. Varicoceles have been implicated in male infertility related to the increase in testicular temperature that accompanies the venous pooling of blood.[9] Clinical varicoceles are divided into three categories. Grade I is a varicocele identified by radiographic assessment, such as ultrasound, but is not palpable. A grade II vari-cocele is palpable but not visible. A grade III varicocele is visible. Many studies eval-uating the repair of grade I varicoceles report that reproductive potential is not improved, and consideration of varicocelectomy should be reserved for grade II and III varicoceles.[46,47]

Thirty five percent to 40% of infertile men have a palpable varicocele, whereas the prevalence of a palpable varicocele in the general male population is approximately

15%.[48] Most investigators agree that grade II and III varicoceles should be considered for treatment, because studies questioning varicocele outcomes generally include treating grade I varicoceles, which is not recommended.[49] In the case of azoospermia, although a small percentage of patients with NOA and concurrent varicoceles have regained sperm in the ejaculate, there is as yet no study elucidating the most appropriate way to select patients who would benefit most from repair.[50] Should varicocelectomy be performed, the preferred method for repair is using the surgical microscope. A recent meta-analysis confirmed that microscopic varicocelectomy results in higher spontaneous pregnancy rates and lower postoperative recurrence and hydrocele formation.[51]

LABORATORY AND RADIOLOGIC EVALUATION

The extent of laboratory examination in the assessment of infertile men is predicated on the history and physical examination. Semen analysis is necessary in the evaluation of infertile men to determine diagnosis, because only the diagnosis of CBAVD or known history of vasectomy precludes this test. In the case of vasectomy, a semen analysis demonstrating azoospermia should have been performed shortly after the procedure. Although almost always necessary, however, a single semen analysis alone is not sufficient to diagnose male infertility. There is significant physiologic variation in semen parameters, and therefore at least two and sometimes three semen analyses are necessary to suggest a pattern of infertility.[9]

Key to the evaluation of any infertile man is a hormone evaluation. As discussed previously, testosterone is essential to spermatogenesis, mediated through the hypothalamic-pituitary-gonadal (HPG) axis. There is no consensus, however, as to what should constitute the initial endocrine evaluation in infertile men.[9] Based on clinical experience and an exhaustive review of the literature, the authors believe that all infertile men should have a morning serum testosterone and luteinizing hormone (LH) as an initial evaluation. The caveat with a simple testosterone test, however, is that it may not be a true reflection of the intratesticular environment. Declining semen parameters, as well as clinical symptoms of hypoandrogenism, correlate more strongly with bioavailable testosterone,[52,53] which accounts for sex hormone–binding globulin (SHBG) and albumin effects on the HPG axis. The authors, consequently, perform testosterone, SHBG, and albumin levels for all men presenting for a fertility evaluation, because bioavailable testosterone may be easily calculated from these stable laboratory assays. (For a calculator, see http://www.issam.ch/freetesto.htm.)

Evidence also suggests that high estradiol levels in some infertile men can play a significant role in suppression of testosterone via the HPG axis. When the testosterone/estradiol ratio was returned to normal values, semen parameters improved.[54] Prolactin levels may be performed to screen for the possibility of a prolactinoma causing a suppression of the HPG axis. Clinically significant prolactin-secreting tumors in men are rare, however, with macroadenomas (>1 cm) resulting in prolactin levels typically greater than 50 ng/mL.[9] The much more common mild elevation in prolactin is of questionable significance, because it may be due to medications as well as to a host of medical conditions. Thus, the authors recommend prolactin assessment when symptoms of headache, visual disturbances, or gynecomastia are present.

Assessment of follicle-stimulating hormone (FSH) is a useful test to diagnose many pathologic processes. One of its uses is in differentiating OA from NOA. Approximately 89% of azoospermic men with testicular length less than 4.6 cm and an FSH above 7.6 have NOA, whereas 96% of azoospermic men with FSH below 7.6 and testicular length greater than 4.6 cm have OA.[55] This finding not only is helpful in providing clinical guidelines as to diagnosis but also underscores the role FSH plays as a surrogate marker for testicular dysfunction. Only approximately 12.4% of Klinefelter syndrome patients demonstrate gynecomastia versus more than 50% who demonstrate elevated FSH levels.[56] Decreased levels of FSH and LH in conjunction with decreased testosterone identify hypogonadotropic hypogonadism.

Other serum tests that may be pertinent include thyroid function tests if there is suspicion of thyroid disease. Antisperm antibodies can be useful in the event of a previous vasectomy and reversal to explain oligoasthenospermia. In an ideal world, all patients with moderate to severe oligoasthenospermia (<5 million TMC) would also obtain a karyotype and Y-microdeletion assay, according to AUA and ASRM guidelines. Unfortunately, the expense of these tests often precludes a universal approach. Because of the high geographic disparity in rates of genetic disorders detected by these tests and their high cost, it is necessary to carefully choose patients for screening. In patients with a clinical picture suggestive of a disease state consistent with a positive test (eg, gynecomastia and a female escutcheon pattern suggestive of Klinefelter syndrome or strong family history of infertility suggestive of a genetic basis for disease), the authors advise a karyotype and/or a Y-microdeletion assay for diagnosis.

Should physical examination reveal unilateral or bilateral vasal absence, renal ultrasound should be performed to investigate renal abnormality or aplasia. For low seminal volumes in the absence of CBAVD, transrectal ultrasound is recommended to evaluate for dilation of the ejaculatory ducts and/or seminal vesicles, to investigate if ejaculatory ductal obstruction is present.

FOLLOW-UP

Short-term follow-up depends on diagnosis. In the reproductive years, mild to moderate hypogonadotropic hypoandrogenism is treated with stimulation of HPG axis output either with a weak estrogen agonist, such as clomiphene citrate, or, failing therapy, direct stimulation with human chorionic gonadotropin (hCG). hCG shares homology with LH to spur intratesticular testosterone, thus promoting spermatogenesis and increasing androgen levels. Severe hypogonadotropic hypogonadism (Kallmann syndrome) is treated with hCG and recombinant FSH. Because testosterone has prostatic effects as well as effects on hemoglobin levels, prostate-specific antigen and hemoglobin levels are recommended every 3 months for the first year and then biannually after pending normal values.[57] NOA patients or severely oligoasthenospermic patients may undergo surgical intervention to obtain sperm directly from seminiferous tubules suitable for assisted reproduction.

Long-term follow-up is essential for any man identified with male infertility. Men with infertility are at increased cancer risk and have a 2.6-fold increase in high-grade prostate cancer.[58] Hypoandrogenic men are at increased risk of cardiovascular disease, obesity, and osteoporosis.[59,60] As a result of the disease processes that lead to infertility, men with diagnosed primary or secondary infertility represent a high-risk population that requires surveillance and early prevention.

SUMMARY

Male infertility is more than a semen analysis. Diagnosis and subsequent treatment depend on the recognition of a semen analysis as a surrogate marker for fertility. Future efforts will help bridge the gap between basic understanding of the genetics of infertility and comprehension of the pathophysiology of disease states. Work-up consists of a thorough history and physical as well two to three semen analyses and an endocrine profile, preferably with determination of LH, FSH, estradiol, testosterone, albumin, and SHBG (to calculate bioavailable testosterone). Genetic, other endocrine, and radiologic tests should be ordered when indicated. Short-term and long-term efforts should focus not only on restoring fertility when possible but also on aiding and educating an at-risk population to avoid sequelae of disease.

REFERENCES

1. Mosher WD, Pratt WF. Fecundity and infertility in the United States: incidence and trends. Fertil Steril 1991;56:192–3.
2. Thonneau P, Marchand S, Tallec A, et al. Incidence and main causes of infertility in a resident population (1,850,000) of three French regions (1988–1989). Hum Reprod 1991;6:811–6.
3. Sharlip ID, Jarow JP, Belker AM, et al. Best practice policies for male infertility. Fertil Steril 2002;77:873–82.
4. MacLeod J, Gold RZ. The male factor in fertility and infertility, IV. Sperm morphology in fertile and infertile marriage. Fertil Steril 1951;2:394–414.
5. Freund M. Standards for rating of human sperm morphology. Int J Fertil 1966;11: 97–118.
6. Eliasson R. Analysis of semen. In: Behrman SJ, Kistner RW, editors. Progress in infertility. Boston (MA): Little Brown and Co; 1975. p. 691–702.
7. World Health Organization. WHO laboratory manual for the examination of human semen and sperm-cervical mucus interaction. 2nd edition. Cambridge: Cambridge University Press; 1987. p. 67.
8. Cooper TG, Noonan E, von Eckardstein S, et al. World Health Organization reference values for human semen characteristics. Hum Reprod Update 2010;16(3):231–45.
9. Sigman M, Jarrow JP. Male infertility. In: Wein AJ, Kavoussi LR, Novick AC, et al, editors. Campbell-walsh urology. 9th edition. Philadelphia (PA): Saunders Elsevier Press; 2007. p.577–653.
10. Bartov B, Eltes F, Pansky M, et al. Estimating fertility potential via semen analysis data. Hum Reprod 1993;8(l):65–70.
11. Cagnacci A, Maxia N, Volpe A. Diurnal variation of semen quality in human males. Hum Reprod 1999;14(1):106–9.
12. Baker HW, Burger HG, de Kretser DM, et al. Factors affecting the variability of semen analysis results in infertile men. Int J Androl 1981;4(6):609–22.
13. Kidd SA, Eskenazi B, Wyrobek AJ. Effects of male age on semen quality and fertility: a review of the literature. Fertil Steril 2001;75(2):237–48.
14. Eskenazi B, Wyrobek AJ, Sloter E, et al. The association of age and semen quality in healthy men. Hum Reprod 2003;18(2):447–54.
15. Cardona MW, Berdugo J, Cadavid JA. The effects of male age on semen parameters: analysis of 1364 men attending an andrology center. Aging Male 2009; 12(4):100–3.
16. Delbès G, Hales BF, Robaire B. Toxicants and human sperm chromatin integrity. Mol Hum Reprod 2010;16(1):14–22.
17. Vuong C, Van Uum SH, O'Dell LE, et al. The effects of opioids and opioid analogs on animal and human endocrine systems. Endocr Rev 2010;31(1):98–132.
18. World Health Organization. World Health Organization: WHO laboratory manual for the examination of human semen and sperm-cal mucus interaction. New York: Cambridge University Press; 1999.

19. Merviel P, Heraud MH, Grenier N, et al. Predictive factors for pregnancy after intrauterine insemination (IUI): an analysis of 1038 cycles and a review of the literature. Fertil Steril 2010;93(1):79–88.
20. Menkveld R, Kruger TF. Advantages of strict (Tygerberg) criteria for evaluation of sperm morphology. Int J Androl 1995;18(Suppl 2):36–42.
21. Menkveld R, Stander FS, Kotze TJ, et al. The evaluation of morphological characteristics of human spermatozoa according to stricter criteria. Hum Reprod 1990; 5(5):586–92.
22. Keegan BR, Barton S, Sanchez X, et al. Isolated teratozoospermia does not affect in vitro fertilization outcome and is not an indication for intracytoplasmic sperm injection. Fertil Steril 2007;88(6):1583–8.
23. Spiessens C, Vanderschueren D, Meuleman C, et al. Isolated teratozoospermia and intrauterine insemination. Fertil Steril 2003;80(5):1185–9.
24. Machev N, Gosset P, Viville S. Chromosome abnormalities in sperm from infertile men with normal somatic karyotypes: teratozoospermia. Cytogenet Genome Res 2005;111(3–4):352–7.
25. Sun F, Ko E, Martin RH. Is there a relationship between sperm chromosome abnormalities and sperm morphology? Reprod Biol Endocrinol 2006;4:1.
26. World Health Organization. WHO laboratory manual for the examination of human semen and sperm-cervical mucus interaction. 5th edition. Cambridge: Cambridge University Press; 2010. p. 16.
27. Agarwal A, Allamaneni SS. Sperm DNA damage assessment: a test whose time has come. Fertil Steril 2005;84:850–3.
28. McLachlan RI, O'Bryan MK. Clinical review: state of the art for genetic testing of infertile men. J Clin Endocrinol Metab 2010;95(3):1013–24.
29. Bourrouillou G, Bujan L, Calvas P, et al. Role and contribution of karyotyping in male infertility. Prog Urol 1992;2:189–95.
30. Simoni M, Bakker E, Krausz C. 2004 EAA/EMQN best practice guidelines for molecular diagnosis of Y-chromosomal microdeletions. Int J Androl 2004;27:240–9.
31. Hopps CV, Mielnik A, Goldstein M, et al. Detection of sperm in men with Y chromosome microdeletions of the AZFa, AZFb and AZFc regions. Hum Reprod 2003; 18:1660–5.
32. Collins JA, Barnhart KT, Schlegel PN. Do sperm DNA integrity tests predict pregnancy with in vitro fertilization? Fertil Steril 2008;89:823–31.
33. Practice Committee of the American Society for Reproductive Medicine. The clinical utility of sperm DNA integrity testing. Fertil Steril 2006;86:S35–7.
34. Wilcox AJ, Weinberg CR, Baird DD. Timing of sexual intercourse in relation to ovulation: effects on the probability of conception, survival of the pregnancy, and sex of the baby. N Engl J Med 1995;333:1517–21.
35. Lee PA, O'Leary LA, Songer NJ, et al. Paternity after bilateral cryptorchidism. A controlled study. Arch Pediatr Adolesc Med 1997;151(3):260–3.
36. Lipshultz LI, Caminos-Torres R, Greenspan CS, et al. Testicular function after orchiopexy for unilaterally undescended testis. N Engl J Med 1976;295: 15–8.
37. Ozkan KU, Küçükaydin M, Muhtaroğlu S, et al. Evaluation of contralateral testicular damage after unilateral testicular torsion by serum inhibin B levels. J Pediatr Surg 2001;36(7):1050–3.
38. Romeo C, Impellizzeri P, Arrigo T, et al. Late hormonal function after testicular torsion. J Pediatr Surg 2010;45(2):411–3.
39. Fosså SD, Oldenburg J, Dahl AA. Short- and long-term morbidity after treatment for testicular cancer. BJU Int 2009;104(9 Pt B):1418–22.

40. Nudell DM, Monoski MM, Lipshultz LI. Common medications and drugs: how they affect male fertility. Urol Clin North Am 2002;29(4):965–73.

41. Ochsendorf FR. Sexually transmitted infections: impact on male fertility. Andrologia 2008;40(2):72–5.

42. O'Flynn O'Brien KL, Varghese AC, Agarwal A. The genetic causes of male factor infertility: a review. Fertil Steril 2010;93(1):1–12.

43. Yassin AA, Saad F. Testosterone and erectile dysfunction. J Androl 2008;29(6): 593–604.

44. O'Shaughnessy PJ, Verhoeven G, De Gendt K, et al. Direct action through the sertoli cells is essential for androgen stimulation of spermatogenesis. Endocrinology 2010;151(5):2343–8.

45. Coviello AD, Bremner WJ, Matsumoto AM, et al. Intratesticular testosterone concentrations comparable with serum levels are not sufficient to maintain normal sperm production in men receiving a hormonal contraceptive regimen. J Androl 2004;25(6):931–8.

46. McClure RD, Khoo D, Jarvi K, et al. Subclinical varicocele: the effectiveness of varicocelectomy. J Urol 1991;145:789–91.

47. Yarborough MA, Burns JR, Keller FS. Incidence and clinical significance of subclinical scrotal varicoceles. J Urol 1989;141:1372–4.

48. Zini A, Boman JM. Varicocele: red flag or red herring? Semin Reprod Med 2009; 27(2):171–8.

49. Evers JL, Collins JA. Assessment of efficacy of varicocele repair for male subfertility: a systematic review. Lancet 2003;361:1849–52.

50. Schlegel PN, Kaufmann J. The role of varicocelectomy in men with non-obstructive azoospermia. Fertil Steril 2004;81:1585–8.

51. Cayan S, Shavakhabov S, Kadioğlu A. Treatment of palpable varicocele in infertile men: a meta-analysis to define the best technique. J Androl 2009;30(1): 33–40.

52. Itoh N, Kumamoto Y, Akagashi K. The assessment of bioavailable androgen levels from the serum free testosterone level. Nippon Naibunpi Gakkai Zasshi 1991;67(1):23–22.

53. Ashok S, Sigman M. Bioavailable testosterone should be used for the determination of androgen levels in infertile men. J Urol 2007;177(4):1443–6.

54. Pavlovich CP, King P, Goldstein M, et al. Evidence of a treatable endocrinopathy in infertile men. J Urol 2001;165(3):837–41.

55. Schoor RA, Elhanby S, Niederberger CS, et al. The role of testicular biopsy in the modern management of male infertility. J Urol 2002;167:197–200.

56. Okada H, Fujioka H, Tatsumi N. Klinefelter's syndrome in the male infertility clinic. Hum Reprod 1999;14(4):946–52.

57. Wang C, Nieschlag E, Swerdloff R, et al. ISA, ISSAM, EAU, EAA and ASA recommendations: investigation, treatment and monitoring of late-onset hypogonadism in males. Int J Impot Res 2009;21(1):1–8.

58. Walsh TJ, Schembri M, Turek PJ, et al. Increased risk of high-grade prostate cancer among infertile men. Cancer 2010;116(9):2140–7.

59. Tajar A, Forti G, O'Neill TW, et al. Characteristics of secondary, primary, and compensated hypogonadism in aging men: evidence from the European Male Ageing Study. J Clin Endocrinol Metab 2010;95(4):1810–8.

60. Lunenfeld B, Saad F, Hoesl CE. ISA, ISSAM and EAU recommendations for the investigation, treatment and monitoring of late-onset hypogonadism in males: scientific background and rationale. Aging Male 2005;8(2):59–74.

The Diagnosis and Management of Scrotal Masses

Jeffrey S. Montgomery, MD, MHSA*, David A. Bloom, MD

KEYWORDS

• Scrotum • Testicular neoplasms • Epididymis • Spermatic cord

Scrotal and inguinal masses are common patient concerns that require some level of diagnostic competency in primary care practices. Diagnosis of scrotal pathology is challenging because of the multiple anatomic structures found within the confined space of the scrotum. When evaluating a scrotal mass, it is important to be systematic in collecting the history, performing the scrotal examination, and evaluating diagnostic studies. Each component can add important clues. This article reviews the diagnosis and treatment of benign and malignant scrotal masses of children and adults according to anatomic location (scrotal wall, paratesticular, testicular, and spermatic cord).

HISTORY

Scrotal or inguinal masses may be the chief complaint, a secondary concern, or identified incidentally during physical examination. The history is the cornerstone in diagnosing scrotal pathology (**Box 1**). Establishing when the patient first noticed the mass, the rate of growth, documentation of trauma, infectious conditions, and other relevant symptoms, such as fever, dysuria, urethral discharge, or nausea, may each be important in diagnosing the problem. If pain is a symptom, ascertaining if it is constant or intermittent, dull or sharp, and what precipitates or relieves it may provide valuable information. The acute onset of severe pain generally indicates a urologic emergency, such as testicular torsion. As scrotal pathology may be associated with other conditions, obtaining a general medical history, surgical history, documenting any previous scrotal or inguinal procedures, and medication use will also be important. Previous evaluations and scrotal imaging should be reviewed.

SCROTAL EXAMINATION

The scrotal contents include the testicles, epididymides, and spermatic cords (**Fig. 1**). The testicles should be nearly equal in size, uniform in texture, firm but not hard, and

The authors have nothing to disclose.
Department of Urology, University of Michigan Health System, 1500 East Medical Center Drive, Taubman Center 3875, Ann Arbor, MI 48109, USA
* Corresponding author.
E-mail address: montrose@umich.edu

smooth. The normal testicular length by age group ranges from 1.5 to 2 cm for prepubertal boys and 4 to 5 cm postpuberty. The epididymides are located posterolaterally from the testicle and are normally separated from the testicle by a palpable sulcus. The head of the epididymis is superior and the tail inferior. The vas deferens emanates from the tail of the epididymis and coalesces with the vascular pedicle of the testicle to form the spermatic cord. The spermatic cord travels superiorly and enters the inguinal canal at the external ring.

An inguinal-scrotal examination should be part of a thorough general physical examination (**Box 2**). Note the general appearance of the scrotum, assessing for scars, lesions or masses on the skin. Evaluate for any swelling or obvious bulges of the scrotum or inguinal canal. Then palpate the scrotal contents. Assure that the testicles are descended, symmetric, nontender, and without masses. The epididymides should be without tenderness or mass. The vasa and vascular components of the spermatic cord should be palpated, noting any fullness that may indicate a varicocele or hernia, and the external inguinal ring should be intact without laxity or obvious hernia with Valsalva (increased abdominal pressure). Any palpable masses or abnormalities should be noted, and the location, size, texture (eg, firm, cystic), and associated tenderness characterized. Keep in mind that a mass in the epididymis is usually benign, whereas one in the testis is likely malignant.

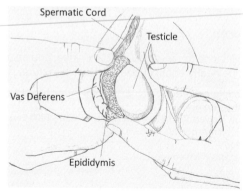

Fig. 1. Scrotal structures.

Box 2
Aspects of the scrotal exam
Inspect
Appropriate pubic hair distribution
Identify scrotal skin lesions
Look for bulging masses
Evaluate symmetry of left & right hemi-scrotum
Palpate
Testes should be firm but not hard
Epididymides
Identify vasa bilaterally
Vascular cord structures
Intact external ring upon Valsalva
Characterize masses
Location
Size
Texture (eg, hard, cystic)
Tenderness

DIAGNOSTIC TESTS

If the diagnosis of a scrotal mass is not obvious based on history or examination alone, further diagnostic tests may be warranted. **Table 1** lists different types of scrotal masses. If fluid surrounds the testicle, use a penlight or otoscope to transilluminate the scrotum to discern a hydrocele from a hernia. Ultrasonography is the principal radiologic study used to evaluate scrotal masses. This test is relatively inexpensive, often readily available, and can usually be performed with little delay. The ultrasound extends physical examination findings, confirming mass location and cystic or solid nature. The Doppler feature can evaluate testicular and epididymal blood flow. Ultrasonography is also useful for evaluating the inguinal canal for hernia.

On ultrasonography, inflammatory conditions, such as epididymitis and orchitis, will result in increased blood flow to the structure, swelling, and often a reactive hydrocele. With trauma, ultrasonography can document the integrity of the testicular capsule, or tunica albuginea, assuring that no testicular fracture has occurred. Ultrasonography can also be used as an adjunct to the history and physical examination in diagnosing testicular torsion, showing the lack of blood flow to the testicle, or characterizing a firm mass as potentially neoplastic. In adults, additional scrotal imaging with CT scan or MRI is rarely indicated. In children, most urologists move to scrotal exploration if ultrasonography is inconclusive.

SCROTAL WALL MASSES

Scrotal skin has many normal variations, and most conditions of the scrotal wall are benign. Fibroepithelial polyps (ie, skin tags) on the scrotum can easily be excised if bothersome to the patient. Other cutaneous variations, such as nevi, hemangiomas, and

Table 1
Scrotal mass types

Location	Adult	Pediatric
Scrotal skin/wall	Fibroepithelial polyp Nevi Sexually transmitted disease Wall cyst Lipoma Carcinoma	Henoch-Schönlein purpura
Paratesticular	Adenomatoid tumor Cystadenoma Leiomyoma Epididymal cyst Spermatocele Carcinomas Epididymitis	Rhabdomyosarcoma Leiomyosarcoma Fibrosarcoma Liposarcoma Epididymitis
Testicular	Seminoma Nonseminoma Leydig cell tumor Sertoli cell tumor Fibroma Neurofibroma Leiomyoma Angioma Torsion	Yolk sac tumor Teratoma Stromal tumor Leydig cell tumor Sertoli cell tumor Torsion
Spermatic cord	Hydrocele Hernia Varicocele Lipoma Liposarcoma Leiomyosarcoma	Hydrocele Hernia Varicocele Rhabdomyosarcoma

telangiectasia, also can be seen on the scrotum. Scrotal melanoma is fortunately rare. The same criteria for identifying a concerning nevus on other areas of the body apply to the scrotum: asymmetry, irregular borders, color variation, and changing size or character. It is important to question the patient as to the stability of these lesions.

Sexually transmitted diseases (STDs) can manifest on the scrotum, especially condyloma and herpetic ulcers. Other STDs, such as syphilis, chancroid, lymphogranuloma venereum, and molluscum contagiosum, can manifest on the scrotal skin. Ulcers associated with herpes and chancroid are painful, whereas those of primary syphilis and lymphogranuloma venereum are painless. Syphilis is associated with nontender inguinal lymphadenopathy, whereas it is frequently tender in association with herpes, chancroid, and lymphogranuloma venereum. If these conditions are suspected, a complete sexual history should be obtained.

Scrotal wall cysts (epidermoid or sebaceous) are common and pose no threat to the patient. These cysts are often isolated findings but can be multiple. Benign lipomas of the scrotal wall present as rubbery subcutaneous masses. If the patient finds these masses unsightly or they are painful, become infected, or intermittently or persistently drain, then they can be easily excised under local anesthesia. Frequently, patient reassurance is all that is required.

Malignant carcinomas of the scrotal skin are very rare, and most information concerning these entities is provided by individual case reports. Primary squamous cell carcinoma of the scrotum is generally related to occupational exposures, especially direct contact with industrial oils. Cutaneous scrotal malignancy also was once common in chimney sweepers. It can also be associated with poor hygiene, human papilloma virus infection, surgical scar or sites of trauma, or immune-related conditions, such as psoriasis.[1] Extramammary Paget disease and basal cell carcinoma of the scrotum have also been reported.[2,3] These primary malignancies of the scrotal skin often appear erythematous, raised, shiny, and scaly, and do not improve with conservative treatment measures.

Direct extension of cancer from neighboring structures to the scrotal skin can occur; spread of colorectal, bladder, prostate, ureteral, and urethral cancers to the scrotal skin has been reported. More distant metastases from sites such as the lung and kidney also have been reported.[4,5] When uncertainty exists as to the diagnosis of a scrotal skin lesion, the patient should be referred to a urologist for biopsy.

Masses of the scrotal wall or skin are rare in pediatric patients. Henoch-Schönlein purpura (HSP) is a systemic vasculitis of unknown origin. It is usually characterized by a palpable skin rash, abdominal pain, and polyarthralgia. It has been reported that up to 38% of cases of HSP have scrotal manifestations.[6] Patients can present with scrotal wall swelling and ecchymosis and, in extreme cases, with an acute scrotum, mimicking testicular torsion.

PARATESTICULAR MASSES

Paratesticular structures include the epididymis, gubernaculum, and supporting tissues. Most paratesticular masses are benign, and only require intervention if they become massive or cause pain to the patient. Adenomatoid tumors are the most common solid paratesticular masses, representing 30% of these lesions and up to 77% of the benign tumors arising from the epididymis.[7,8] These are most commonly identified in men in their 20s to 40s but may be found in any age group. They rarely arise in the testicular tunicae or spermatic cord. They are round, firm, smooth, discrete masses measuring 0.5 to 5 cm in diameter that are usually asymptomatic and slow growing. Ultrasonography can confirm the extratesticular nature of these masses, but is not essential. Papillary cystadenomas and leiomyomas account for most of the other benign epididymal solid tumors. Two-thirds of papillary cystadenomas occur in patients with von Hippel-Lindau syndrome and are frequently bilateral.[9] Leiomyomas can also be bilateral and may accompany a hydrocele or hernia.[10] These masses are smooth and firm and can grow to be large.

Cysts of the epididymis occur in up to 40% of men.[11] True epididymal cysts account for 75% of these masses and contain lymphatic fluid. Spermatoceles form as a result of efferent duct obstruction and contain spermatozoa, lymphocytes, and debris.[12] Ultrasonography cannot differentiate between these cyst types, but can distinguish epididymal cysts from hydroceles. Epididymal cysts can displace the testicle, whereas hydroceles envelop it.

Primary malignancies of the epididymis or paratesticular structures are extremely rare in adults. Adenocarcinomas or sarcomas can develop but are so uncommon that most information available on these cancers comes from single case reports. These tumors tend to extensively invade local structures and increase in size at a rapid rate.

Rhabdomyosarcoma, however, accounts for a large proportion of the paratesticular tumors in the pediatric population. Paratesticular rhabdomyosarcoma has a better prognosis than rhabdomyosarcoma of other sites because of its more favorable histology and earlier detection.[13] Other rarer pediatric paratesticular sarcomas include leiomyosarcomas, fibrosarcomas, and liposarcomas. A child with a paratesticular mass requires prompt referral to a urologist for management.

Epididymitis is one of the most common urologic diagnoses. It can be caused by bacterial, viral, or fungal infections or idiopathic inflammation.[14] Acute epididymitis presents with pain and swelling, usually unilateral and developing over several days. Fever, scrotal skin erythema, urethritis, dysuria, and testicular pain can also be present. Epididymitis can mimic testicular torsion, requiring emergent evaluation. When a scrotal ultrasound is obtained in this setting, the epididymis is often hyperemic on Doppler evaluation, and an associated hydrocele may be present. If any scrotal fluctuance is identified, or a patient's symptoms do not improve as expected with treatment, an ultrasound should be obtained to assure that a scrotal abscess has not developed. Generally, though, ultrasound is not required to diagnose epididymitis.

If epididymitis is suspected, a mid-stream urinalysis and microscopy should be performed. If concern exists for a urinary tract infection, a sterile urine sample should be sent for culture. In patients with suspected sexually transmitted infection or urethritis, submit not only a urine culture, but also perform a urethral swab for gonorrhea and chlamydia. Once cultures are sent, epididymitis can be treated empirically with antibiotics, adjusting the antibiotics as needed based on urine culture results. Other measures that can alleviate symptoms include bed rest, scrotal elevation, and nonsteroidal anti-inflammatory medications.

TESTICULAR MASSES

The testicles descend into the scrotum by week 38 of gestation. Three percent of fullterm and 30% of premature infant boys are born with at least one undescended testicle.[15] On examination, most undescended testicles can be identified with careful palpation of the inguinal canal, but can be located anywhere along the path of testicular descent. Most will descend into their anatomic scrotal location within the first 6 months of life. After this, spontaneous descent is unlikely, and most pediatric urologists recommend surgical exploration and orchiopexy to preserve fertility. In addition, the risk of malignancy in males with an undescended testis is 10 times greater than that in the general population. Early orchiopexy may not alter this rate of malignancy, but the scrotal location aids in surveillance.

In adults, upwards of 95% of all testicular tumors are derived from the germ cells.[16] These lesions are categorized as either seminomatous or nonseminomatous germ cell tumors. They are the most common cancers diagnosed in men aged 15 to 34 years and are five times more common in Caucasians than in African Americans. Patients often describe a painless mass that was incidentally identified. On examination, these masses are generally firm, nodular, and discrete from the normal testicle. Of patients with testicular cancer, 30% present with metastatic disease at diagnosis, usually to the retroperitoneal lymph nodes. Risk factors include family and personal history of germ-cell tumor, cryptorchidism, testicular atrophy, previous orchitis, and history of Klinefelter syndrome. Prompt inguinal orchiectomy is required, not only as treatment but also to establish a pathologic diagnosis that will dictate further therapy.

Evaluation of a testicular mass includes history, inguinoscrotal examination, and evaluation of the testis cancer tumor markers alpha fetoprotein (AFP), ß-human chorionic gonadotropin (ß-hCG) and lactate dehydrogenase. A testicular ultrasound is helpful to confirm the diagnosis but is not obligatory if the mass is obvious. At some point in the workup, either before or after orchiectomy, the patient requires staging imaging, including a CT scan of the abdomen and pelvis and chest radiograph. If abdominal or pelvic metastases are seen, a chest CT also should be obtained.

Seminoma is the most common form of germ cell tumor, diagnosed in approximately 50% of cases. It occurs most frequently in men aged 35 to 45 years. These tumors can produce ß-hCG, but usually the tumor markers are normal. Nonseminomatous tumors include embryonal carcinoma, yolk sac tumor, choriocarcinoma, and teratoma. These tumor types occasionally present in their pure form but most commonly present as a component of a mixed germ cell tumor.

Seminoma is also often a component of mixed tumors; in these situations, the tumor is treated as a nonseminomatous germ cell tumor. Additional treatments for germ cell tumors are determined by tumor type and stage, and can range from observation after orchiectomy, retroperitoneal radiation for lower-staged seminoma, and systemic chemotherapy for nonseminomatous, mixed germ cell tumors, and more advanced seminomas.

Non–germ cell tumors are rare, but most commonly arise from Leydig or Sertoli cells. Leydig cells are the principle source of male testosterone. Leydig cell tumors represent fewer than 3% of all testis tumors and have two peak incidences: 5 to 10 years of age and 30 to 35 years of age.[16] Patients often present with a palpable testicular mass and either precocious virilization (ie, genital maturation, pubic hair, voice changes) in pediatric cases or gynecomastia and infertility in adults.

Sertoli cell tumors represent approximately 1% of testicular tumors and can occur in children and adults. In addition to a testicular mass, gynecomastia frequently develops.[17] Few Leydig or Sertoli cell tumors are malignant. If diagnosed before or at surgery, testis-sparing resection can be considered.

Several benign tumors can arise in the tunica albuginea surrounding the testis. These include fibromas, angiomas, neurofibromas, and leiomyomas, which are concerning because of their location and confusion with malignant germ cell tumors. These tumors are localized to the surface of the testicle and can range from small, shotty, nontender nodules to tumors several centimeters in size. Ultrasonography is essential in defining the location and nature of these masses.

Testicular tumors in infants and children are rare, representing only 1% of all pediatric solid tumors, and metastasize less frequently than those in adults.[18] Age distribution is bimodal, with one peak incidence within the first 5 years of life and a gradual increase in frequency during adolescence.[19] They are classified as either germ cell (81%) or non–germ cell tumors (19%), and most commonly present as a painless testicular mass (88%) and are identified after scrotal trauma (5%), during evaluation for hydrocele (1%), or with a wide range of other symptoms (6%).[18] In these patients, tumor markers should be obtained and testicular ultrasound considered. Evidence of precocity may hint at tumors that have hormonal activity.

Based on tumor registries, yolk sac tumor is by far the most common type of tumor diagnosed in the pediatric population (62%), followed by unknown pathology (17%), teratoma (14%), stromal (6%), Leydig cell (1%), and Sertoli cell tumors (1%).[18] Most (85%) of patients with yolk sac tumors present with disease confined to the testicle, but staging with CT scan, chest radiograph, and tumor markers is still necessary.[20] AFP, which is produced by yolk sac tumors, remains elevated for up to 6 weeks after birth, and therefore is not useful for diagnosis in this age group. It still should be obtained to establish a baseline level and assure proper marker decay after tumor removal. ß-hCG levels are not needed before puberty, because choriocarcinoma, which produces ß-hCG, is not found in this age group.[21] Teratoma does not have the same malignant potential as in adults. Epidermoid cyst is a monolayer expression of teratoma also found in children. If identified at surgery, these tumors can be enucleated, sparing the remainder of the testicle.

Testicular torsion usually presents with acute, severe, constant, unilateral testicular pain. Patients may have a previous history of similar pain, indicating a torsion/detorsion event. Torsion can be associated with other symptoms, such as nausea, vomiting, and anorexia. Examination is often difficult because of patient discomfort. The torsed testicle may be noticeably high-riding in the scrotum and the cremasteric reflex absent. The overlying scrotal skin may be erythematous. If torsion is the obvious diagnosis, prompt surgical exploration is the only chance to preserve testicular viability. If the diagnosis is questionable, a Doppler scrotal ultrasound will show lack of blood flow to the affected testicle.

SPERMATIC CORD MASSES

The spermatic cord contains the vas deferens and the testicular vascular pedicle. The vasa should be palpable bilaterally; absence of the vas deferens may be associated with cystic fibrosis. The vascular pedicle contains the testicular venous plexus, testicular artery, and lymphatics. It should be palpable distinctly from the vas deferens. The external ring of the inguinal canal should be free of bulging peritoneal contents.

Congenital hernia and hydrocele are a result of failure of the processus vaginalis to obliterate, resulting in peritoneal fluid (hydrocele) or viscus (hernia) entering inguinal canal. The incidence of congenital hernia is 4%, with a risk of incarceration up to 60% in the first 6 months of life.[22,23] It is generally accepted that, once diagnosed, pediatric hernias should be surgically repaired. In children, hydroceles can be communicating, allowing fluid to pass between the peritoneum and inguinal canal, or noncommunicating. Noncommunicating hydroceles are either reactive (from inflammation or trauma) or nonreactive (idiopathic). A penlight or otoscope will transilluminate the fluid contained within a hydrocele. When in doubt, a scrotal ultrasound is useful to differentiate hydroceles from hernias. Hydroceles frequently resolve spontaneously, but if they persist beyond 1 year, elective exploration and repair is advised.

A varicocele is a dilation of the venous pampiniform plexus of the spermatic cord, which coalesces into a single testicular vein. Varicocele usually first appears in midpuberty and occurs in up to 15% of the male population.[24] A varicocele can present as a mass and is often described as a "bag of worms" on examination, at times with pain or discomfort. Most varicoceles are diagnosed in adult men, discovered in evaluation for infertility. Varicoceles are graded from 1 to 3: grade 1 is detected with the patient standing and performing a Valsalva maneuver; grade 2 is palpable on standing, but is not evident when the patient is supine; and grade 3 persists even in the supine position. Varicoceles are most commonly left-sided but occasionally bilateral. Isolated right-sided varicoceles or any acute onset of varicocele in an adult deserves investigation with abdominal imaging to rule out the presence of an obstructing mass in or along the vena cava. Adolescents with pain, grade 3 varicoceles, or growth failure of the testis should undergo varicocelectomy.

Lipomas of the spermatic cord are very common, can be unilateral or bilateral, and often present as asymptomatic fullness of the spermatic cord. It is important to confirm that these masses do not represent inguinal hernias by noting the intact external inguinal ring on examination. If any doubt exists, a scrotal ultrasound can be useful to rule out the presence of a hernia. Rhabdomyosarcomas may occur in the spermatic cord in children, and liposarcoma is the most common malignant tumor arising in the spermatic cord in adults, although fortunately both are rare. Leiomyosarcomas also have been reported.

SUMMARY

When evaluating a patient with a scrotal mass, a careful history and inguinoscrotal examination are necessary. Malignant scrotal wall, paratesticular, or spermatic cord tumors are rare. Scrotal ultrasound can confirm the precise location of a mass or rule out the presence of an inguinal hernia. Testicular masses deserve a formal workup, with serum tumor markers, a scrotal ultrasound as needed, and prompt consultation with a urologist for further staging and intervention. Scrotal masses in children are much rarer than in adults and should be evaluated by a urologist.

REFERENCES

1. Lowe FC. Squamous-cell carcinoma of the scrotum. Urol Clin North Am 1992; 19(2):397–405.
2. Chave TA, Finch TM. The scrotum: an unusual site for basal cell carcinoma. Clin Exp Dermatol 2002;27(1):68.
3. Quinn AM, Sienko A, Basrawala Z, et al. Extramammary Paget disease of the scrotum with features of Bowen disease. Arch Pathol Lab Med 2004;128(1): 84–6.
4. Aridogan IA, Satar N, Doran F, et al. Scrotal skin metastases of renal cell carcinoma a case report. Acta Chir Belg 2004;104:599–600.
5. Mori K, Kitazawa R, Kondo T, et al. Lung adenocarcinoma with micropapillary component presenting with metastatic scrotum tumor and cancer-to-cancer metastasis: a case report. Cases J 2008;1:162.
6. Hara Y, Tajiri T, Matsuura K, et al. Acute scrotum caused by Henoch-Schönlein purpura. Int J Urol 2004;11:578–80.
7. Broth G, Bullock WK, Morrow J. Epididymal tumor: 1. report of 15 new cases including review of literature. 2. Histochemical study of the so-called adenomatoid tumor. J Urol 1968;100:530–6.
8. Woodward PJ, Schwab CM, Sesterhenn IA. From the archives of AFIP: extratesticular scrotal masses. Radiographics 2003;23:215.
9. Billesbolle P, Nielsen K. Papillary cystadenoma of the epididymis. J Urol 1988; 139:1062.
10. Kuhn MT, MacLennan GT. Benign neoplasms of the epididymis. J Urol 2005;174: 723.
11. Leung ML, Gooding GA, Williams RD. High-resolution sonography of scrotal contents in asymptomatic subjects. Am J Roentgenol 1984;143(1):161–4.
12. Tracy C, Steers W. Anatomy, physiology and diseases of the epididymis. AUA Update Series 2007;26(12):114–23.
13. Rypens F, Garel L, Franc-Guimond J, et al. Paratesticular rhabdomyosarcoma presenting as thickening of the tunica vaginalis. Pediatr Radiol 2009;39:1010–2.
14. Tracy CR, Steers WD, Costabile R. Diagnosis and management of epididymitis. Urol Clin North Am 2008;35:101–8.
15. Hutson JM, Clarke MC. Current management of the undescended testicle. Semin Pediatr Surg 2007;16(1):64–70.
16. Dilworth JP, Farrow GM, Oesterling JE. Testicular tumors of non-germ cell origin. AUA Update Series 1992;11(3):399–417.
17. Gabrilove JL, Freiberg EK, Leiter E. Feminizing and non-feminizing Sertoli cell tumors. J Urol 1980;124:757.
18. Kaplan GW. Prepubertal testicular tumors. World J Urol 1984;2:238.
19. Green DM. Testicular tumors in infants and children. Semin Surg Oncol 1986;2(3): 156–62.
20. Grady RW, Ross JH, Kay R. Patterns of metastatic spread in prepubertal yolk sac tumor of the testis. J Urol 1995;153:1259.
21. Kay R. Prepubertal testicular tumor registry. J Urol 1993;150:671.

22. Bronsther B. Inguinal hernia in children—a study of 1000 cases and review of the literature. J Am Womens Med Assoc 1972;27:524.
23. Rowe M. Incarcerated and strangulated hernias in children. A study of high risk factors. Arch Surg 1970;101(2):136–9.
24. Paduch DA, Niedzielski J. Repair versus observation in adolescent varicocele: a prospective study. J Urol 1992;158:1128–32.

Assessment and Initial Management of Urologic Trauma

Jeremy B. Tonkin, MD*, Britton E. Tisdale, MD,
Gerald H. Jordan, MD

KEYWORDS

- Urogenital injury • Bladder trauma • Abdominal trauma
- Renal injury

Acute injury to the urogenital organs may be the result of blunt trauma, penetrating trauma, burns, and avulsion injuries. Both self-inflicted and iatrogenic injuries are part of these problems. These types of injuries may be commonly encountered by physicians and surgeons whose primary focus is not urology and are working in the emergency room, urgent care, or office setting.

Appropriate assessment, initial management, and timely referral to a urologist are critical in minimizing morbidity from these injuries. It is trite but true to say that urogenital trauma can be occult in its initial presentation and to be found it must be considered. Likewise, in many cases, aggressive diagnosis is far more important than aggressive treatment. This article focuses on the signs and symptoms, assessment, and initial care in the broad categories of blunt and penetrating trauma, as each may affect the structures of the genitourinary tract.

BLUNT ABDOMINAL TRAUMA

Blunt trauma to the abdomen is a leading cause of morbidity in all age groups and may result in injury to the kidneys, bladder, urethra, and, more rarely, the ureter.[1] Injuries may result from crushing or decelerating forces. Automobile-related trauma accounts for a majority of these injuries.[2]

Initial assessment includes a history of the injury, mechanism of injury, history of the emergency medical course, and physical examination. Particular attention should be given to the location of pain, patterns of bruising, and any apparent lacerations. Vaginal, penile, and rectal examinations should be performed. The patient should be hemodynamically stabilized and any concomitant injuries to the airway or breathing apparatus should be addressed. Initial laboratory examinations include: complete blood cell count, complete metabolic profile, coagulation studies, serum human chorionic gonadotropin

Department of Urology, Eastern Virginia Medical School, Norfolk, VA, USA
* Corresponding author.
E-mail address: quiksand25@yahoo.com

Med Clin N Am 95 (2011) 245–251
doi:10.1016/j.mcna.2010.08.033
0025-7125/11/$ – see front matter © 2011 Published by Elsevier Inc.

for female patients where pregnancy status is pertinent, and urine analysis. Gross or microscopic hematuria is a significant predictor of intra-abdominal injury.[3]

At most centers, initial imaging should include abdominal ultrasonography (focused abdominal sonography for trauma) or CT scan of the abdomen and pelvis with and without administration of intravenous contrast. Delayed images must \be obtained if considering the possibility of urologic injury and specifically ureteral injury. Other imaging studies may include intravenous pyelogram (IVP) or MRI. Cystogram may be performed if suspicion exists for bladder injury. The cystogram portion of an IVP or CT scan is not sufficient. If a bladder injury is to be ruled out, it needs to be done with a pressure cystogram. Retrograde urethrography (RUG) should be performed to evaluate for urethral injury, if suspected.

PENETRATING ABDOMINAL TRAUMA

Penetrating trauma is usually the result of stab or gunshot wounds. Such trauma is assessed in a manner similar to that for blunt trauma, except that penetrating trauma is likely to lead to a higher rate of surgical exploration. Entrance and exit wounds may give clues regarding potentially involved organs. Unlike blunt trauma, penetrating trauma more often causes ureteric injury.

With ballistic trauma, often the course of the bullet is deceptively unpredictable. Initial laboratory and imaging studies are the same as they are for blunt trauma.

RENAL INJURY

The kidney is the most commonly injured urogenital organ; and renal injury can result from either blunt or penetrating abdominal trauma. Seventy to eighty percent of renal injuries are a consequence of blunt trauma,[4] but can also present after surgical intervention for stones, or other intra-abdominal procedures. Common signs and symptoms include flank pain or bruising, abdominal pain, and/or hematuria. Fracture of ribs or spinal transverse processes, often apparent on plain radiograph should prompt suspicion. Clinical suspicion of such injuries should always prompt further evaluation for renal injury. Gross or microscopic hematuria with hemodynamic instability is a symptom of clinically significant renal injury.[5–8] Falls from significant heights or other suspicious mechanisms of injury should also be evaluated for renal injury and not uncommonly present with hematuria or flank hematoma.[9]

Injuries may be classified as renal lacerations, renal contusions, or renovascular injuries. These are usually identified on radiologic imaging, with CT scan performed with the use of intravenous contrast being the most sensitive.[10] On CT scan, renal injury, in the case of a contusion, may be quite subtle; occasionally the subcapsular hematoma is noted as a fluid or mass effect, immediately beneath the renal capsule. In more severe injuries, the disruption of the parenchyma is noted, and the depth of the laceration relates to the severity of the injury. In the case of vascular injury, a number of findings are listed, all or some of which may be noted. In the case of renal artery injury, nonuptake of contrast is noted. In the case of some renovascular injuries, all that may be noted is a medial paranephric hematoma. The classic findings are of disruption of the renal contour, with attendant fluid mass effect in the space of Gerota. In the case of disruption of the collecting system associated with parenchymal injury, contrast is seen within the mass of the paranephric hematoma on delayed images.

Initial management of most renal injuries includes fluid resuscitation, bed rest, and serial monitoring of vital signs and hemoglobin levels. Urologic consultation should be promptly obtained, especially in cases of hemodynamic instability, evidence of or suspicion for renovascular injury, urine extravasation noted on imaging studies, or expanding perirenal hematoma, where operative management may be warranted. It is imperative that the history of "hemodynamic stability or instability" begin with the first assessment at the scene, if available. The emergency medical technicians answering the trauma call must be questioned regarding this information. In the setting of clinical instability, anytime in the posttrauma course, radiologic evaluation must be promptly accomplished—with emergent surgical intervention sometimes required and sometimes taking precedence over all further evaluation. These interventions include partial nephrectomy, nephrectomy, ureteral stent placement, and endovascular embolization. Remarkably, significant injuries to the renal parenchyma can be observed and will heal with observation only. However, there are situations when a patient can rapidly deteriorate; thus, all management needs to be closely monitored by the surgical specialist.

Hypertension is a potential long-term sequela of renal injury, and can occur in the immediate posttrauma course, or can be a delayed presentation. Rarely, vascular malformations can result from renal trauma. These can be associated with the development of hypertension or, more likely, with unexplained presence or persistence, or development of hematuria. In the patient who has a history of renal trauma, the discovery of these symptoms or findings must be presumed to be a result of the trauma until evaluation proves otherwise.

URETERAL INJURY

Ureteral injuries represent less than 1% of urogenital injuries; 95% are a result of gunshot wounds.[11] The ureter is highly mobile within the retroperitoneal fat and is protected by the psoas muscle. These factors have been proposed to prevent injury during blunt trauma. As many as 80% of ureteral injuries may be missed on initial imaging and subsequently discovered on follow-up imaging studies.[12]

Suspicion for ureteral injury should be especially raised with gunshot wounds to the flank, as previously noted; the course of a bullet in soft tissue is quite unpredictable. Iatrogenic ureteral injuries should be suspected after abdominal or endoscopic stone procedures, and pelvic procedures (especially laparoscopic procedures), when serum blood urea nitrogen and creatinine levels (due to reabsorption of urine) are noted to be "inexplicably" increased. Such injuries may also present as nonspecific abdominal pain, malaise, and fever. In some cases, fluid will leak from a surgical wound and can be diagnosed as urine by its elevated serum creatinine level (not consistent with serum). Ultrasonography or CT scan may demonstrate evidence of urinoma in these cases. Urinoma appears as a mass that is clearly fluid, unlike hematoma, which, depending on its age, can appear as almost identical to urinoma or, with organization, can become more dense on CT scan.

In cases of suspected ureteral injury, it has been recommended to obtain delayed CT scan images at 5 to 8 minutes after administration of contrast to increase sensitivity of diagnosis.[13] To properly "clear the ureters," both distal ureters need to be visualized on delay. If they are not, then the possibility of ureteral injury always remains. If a ureteral injury is identified, whether by contrast extravasation or luminal abnormality, urologic consultation should be initiated. Retrograde Ureteropyelogram (RUPG) must be done to localize and confirm the extent of the injury. On RUPG, the ureteral defect is usually accurately defined by extravasation. Open repair, placement of a ureteral stent, or percutaneous nephrostomy tube may be required.

Ureteral stricture may develop after ureteral injury and may be asymptomatic in some cases.[14] Thus, follow-up with imaging is important, even with lack of symptoms, to diagnose and address this occurrence. The development of "silent hydronephrosis" can result in significant deterioration of kidney function.

BLADDER INJURY

Blunt trauma accounts for a majority of bladder injuries, often because the trauma occurs with the bladder distended with urine. Presenting symptoms include lower abdominal pain, hematuria, palpable fullness, azotemia from urine reabsorption, concomitant pelvic fracture, or inability to void. Bladder injuries occur in approximately 10% of all pelvic fractures.[15] In most series, 85% to 95% of patients who sustain pelvic fractures resulting in bladder injuries presented with gross hematuria.[16–18] The remainder had significant microscopic hematuria (>30 red blood cells per high-power field) from rupture or contusion of the detrusor muscle.[19]

A majority of patients with a bladder injury demonstrate pelvic fluid on CT scan.[20] Without cystography, the findings suggesting bladder injury are often quite subtle, and when noted appear as stranding in the paravesical tissues. In cases of suspected bladder injury, cystography should be obtained using trauma protocols, as already discussed. CT cystography should be performed only if the patient is undergoing CT scan for other injuries, and that also should be a pressure cystogram. CT must be regarded as the modality for imaging, not the procedure. It has a similar sensitivity and specificity to conventional cystography, but otherwise confers no additional benefit in detection of injury.[21] On cystography, the pattern of contrast extravasation is of paramount importance. In the case of extraperitoneal injuries, the classic "flame" configuration of extravasation is noted as the contrast infiltrates the paravesical tissues. If the point of extravasation is near the base of the bladder, then injury to the bladder neck must be considered and further evaluated by the urologist. With intraperitoneal bladder injuries, contrast can be seen outlining the bowel loops.

Extraperitoneal injuries are usually managed with placement of an indwelling catheter only after evaluation for a urethral injury has been performed. In these cases, the involvement of a urologist is an absolute necessity. Any attempts at blind indwelling catheter placement can result in extension of a urethral injury. Special procedures, such as catheter placement associated with endoscopy and guide wire, or the use of a coude tip catheter may be useful. Injuries to the bladder neck, concomitant rectal injuries, or bony fragments within the bladder may require open surgical management. Intraperitoneal injuries virtually always require surgical intervention.

Typically, injuries to the bladder heal well and do not cause long-term issues. Rarely, stones, fistulae, diverticula, or voiding dysfunction may present subsequent to the injury. In the setting of poor healing of the bladder wall, protrusion of the bladder epithelium without the backing of the detrusor muscle leads to these sequela. If the bladder epithelium does not heal, then, rarely, fistula can occur—particularly if there is coincident injury of an adjacent viscous, or a large urinoma develops and decompresses through the skin. Stones can occur when any of these conditions leads to stasis of urine, or poor bladder emptying.

URETHRAL INJURY

Urethral injuries are most commonly the result of displaced anterior arch pelvic fractures[22] or iatrogenic manipulation. Common symptoms and findings include gross hematuria, blood at the urethral meatus, inability to void, dysuria, perineal hematoma prostatic displacement, and inability to pass an indwelling catheter. Absence of these findings does not exclude urethral injury.[23] Patients examined within 1 hour of injury may not exhibit any of these physical findings and, in fact, the ability to place a catheter does not exclude a small but possibly important urethral tear or perforation.[24]

Urethral injury is diagnosed with RUG. Contrast extravasation is pathognomonic for urethral injury. It is imperative that RUG be carefully performed, so that contrast extravasation is limited. The goal of a trauma RUG, is to determine if the urethra "is water-tight." Exact definition of the extent of trauma rarely influences the subsequent management and, if necessary, further evaluation will be done by the consulting urologist.

A catheter may sometimes be placed with the aid of fluoroscopy or flexible endoscopy. In most cases of significant disruption, a suprapubic cystostomy catheter is placed.

In the case of suspected urethral injury, evaluation by a urologist must be done. Subsequent development of a urethral stricture or stenosis may present as lower urinary tract symptoms at any time after the urethral injury. Weakened force of stream, urinary tract infection, dysuria, hematuria, or urinary retention are signs or symptoms of disruption of the voiding pattern resulting from obstruction to urine passage. In the case of the patient who has sustained known urethral trauma in the past, stricture or stenosis of the urethra must be ruled out. Referral back to the urologist is appropriate.

PENILE TRAUMA

The penis is less commonly injured as compared with the kidneys or bladder. In addition to iatrogenic injuries and blunt and penetrating trauma, burns, avulsions, and sexual trauma can occur.[25] When compared with internal organs, which usually require radiographic studies to evaluate, the penis can often be evaluated with a thorough physical examination. In some cases, ultrasound or MRI have been used. On ultrasound, occasionally the defect of the tunica albuginea can be seen. Ultrasound is very technician dependent, and thus not accurate in many instances. MRI is very accurate; however, it often is difficult to obtain in timely fashion and, in many instances, only delays the surgical exploration that ultimately is required. Injuries to the penis may also require evaluation of the urethra with RUG; again, looking for extravasation of contrast that is indicative of disruption of the urethral epithelium. There are no definitive algorithms for treating penile trauma[26] and classification of injuries is currently insufficient.

Sexual trauma, causing penile fracture, may present with penile ecchymosis, a recognized "pop" during intercourse, sudden detumescence, or delayed onset of penile curvature. These are caused by trauma to or the tearing of the tunica albuginea. Delayed presentation occurs because of embarrassment about the location or mechanism of the injury. Immediate management includes pain control, urinalysis, and consideration of urethrography. Urologic consultation is warranted as prompt correction may decrease subsequent erectile dysfunction and penile curvature.[27,28] Although MRI can be helpful in very select cases, surgical exploration generally leads to accurate diagnosis in cases where penile fracture is suspected.

Burns or avulsion injuries to the penis are treated as they would be on any other part of the body. Prophylactic antibiotics and tetanus prophylaxis should be administered. Appropriate debridement of devitalized tissues, irrigation of the wound, and placement of surgical dressings should be performed. Patients should be monitored for progression of infection after injury. Tissue reconstruction depends on extent of injury, but is usually performed in a delayed fashion. Pain, poor cosmesis, erectile dysfunction, and penile curvature may be long-term sequelae.

SCROTAL AND TESTICULAR TRAUMA

Like the penis, the scrotum and testicles are located externally and are thus subject to burns and avulsion injuries as well as to the other injuries discussed. They are also readily amenable to physical examination.

Scrotal trauma occurs most frequently in males aged 15 to 40 years.[29] Like the penis, embarrassment may delay presentation. Pain, hematoma, and obvious skin disruptions should be noted during examination. Blunt injury presentations should also be considered for testicular mass or torsion.

Scrotal ultrasonography, aided by Doppler, is a useful adjunct to physical examination and is greater than 95% sensitive and specific for testicular rupture/fracture.[30,31] On ultrasound, in the case of testicular fracture, the classic findings are of hematocele (fluid in the space surrounding the testes), with the seminiferous tubules seen in the fluid, protruding through the disruption of the tunica albuginea. However, there are circumstances where the classic findings are not seen. To rule out fracture of the testicle with ultrasound, it is necessary that there be no distortion of the intraparenchymal appearance of the testis. CT scan is rarely used, but pelvic CT scan done for other injuries may image the upper scrotum and testicles as well. Surgical exploration often is necessary for correct diagnosis.

Burns and avulsion injuries are handled in a fashion similar to those of the penis. Injuries that do not cause testicular fracture, expanding hematoma, large hematocele, or loss of blood flow may be managed conservatively. Scrotal support, ice, and pain management, including antiinflammatories may be prescribed. Penetrating injuries and those injuries listed above warrant prompt surgical exploration. Salvage rates after testicular fracture decrease from 90% to 45% if there is a delay greater than 72 hours.[32] Testicular pain and atrophy may be long term-sequelae after traumatic injury. Thus, prompt urologic consultation is necessary.

SUMMARY

Urologic trauma may result from a wide range of events and is often seen in combination with injuries to other systems. A high level of suspicion is required for prompt evaluation of the urinary tract. As with all trauma patients, care should be taken to address cardiopulmonary and neurologic injuries first and to achieve hemodynamic stability. Appropriate laboratory and physical examinations, as well as radiologic imaging, are paramount to obtaining accurate diagnosis and to providing appropriate initial treatment. Most significant injuries require immediate or early care of the specialist.

REFERENCES

1. American College of Surgeons Committee on Trauma. Abdominal trauma. In: ATLS student course manual. 8th edition. Chicago (IL): American College of Surgeons; 2008.
2. Cooper A, Barlow B, DiScala C, et al. Mortality and truncal injury: the pediatric perspective. J Pediatr Surg 1994;29(1):33–8.
3. Knudson MM, McAninch JW, Gomez R, et al. Hematuria as a predictor of abdominal injury after blunt trauma. Am J Surg. 1992;164(5):482–5 [discussion: 485–6].
4. Holevar M, DiGiacomo JC, Ebert J, et al. Practice management guideline for the evaluation of genitourinary trauma. The EAST Practice Management Guideline Work Group 2003.
5. Guice K, Oldham K, Eide B, et al. Hematuria after blunt trauma: when is pyelography useful? J Trauma 1983;23:305–11.
6. Eastham JA, Wilson TG, Ahlering TE. Radiographic evaluation of adult patients with blunt renal trauma. J Urol 1992;148:266–7.
7. Herschorn S, Radomski SB, Shoskes DA, et al. Evaluation and treatment of blunt renal trauma. J Urol 1991;146:274–6.
8. Wilson RF, Ziegler DW. Diagnostic and treatment problems in renal injuries. Am Surg 1987;53:399–402.

9. Brandes S, McAninch JW. Urban free falls and patterns of renal injury: a 20-year experience with 396 cases. J Trauma 1999;47:643–9.

10. Shanmuganathan K. Multi-detector row CT imaging of blunt abdominal trauma. Semin Ultrasound CT MR 2004;25(2):180–204.

11. Brandes SB, Chelsky MJ, Buckman RF, et al. Ureteral injuries from penetrating trauma. J Trauma 1994;36:766–9.

12. Mulligan JM, Cagiannos I, Collins JP, et al. Ureteropelvic junction disruption secondary to blunt trauma: excretory phase imaging (delayed films) should help prevent a missed diagnosis. J Urol 1998;159(1):67–70.

13. Brown SL, Hoffman DM, Spirnak JP. Limitations of routine spiral computerized tomography in the evaluation of blunt renal trauma. J Urol 1998;160:1979–81.

14. Weizer AZ, Auge BK, Silverstein AD, et al. Routine postoperative imaging is important after ureteroscopic stone manipulation. J Urol 2002;168(1):46–50.

15. Brandes S, Borrelli J Jr. Pelvic fracture and associated urologic injuries. World J Surg 2001;25:1578.

16. Morey AF, Iverson AJ, Swan A, et al. Bladder rupture after blunt trauma: guidelines for diagnostic imaging. J Trauma 2001;51:683–6.

17. Carroll PR, McAninch JW. Major bladder trauma: mechanisms of injury and a unified method of diagnosis and repair. J Urol 1984;132:254.

18. Corriere JN Jr, Sandler CM. Management of the ruptured bladder: seven years of experience with 111 cases. J Trauma 1986;26:830.

19. Avey G, Blackmore CC, Wessells H, et al. Radiographic and clinical predictors of bladder rupture in blunt trauma patients with pelvic fracture. Acad Radiol 2006; 13:573.

20. Morgan DE, Nallamala LK, Kenney PJ, et al. CT cystography: radiographic and clinical predictors of bladder rupture. AJR Am J Roentgenol 2007;174:89–95.

21. Peng MY, Parisky YR, Cornwell EE 3rd, et al. CT cystography versus conventional cystography in evaluation of bladder injury. AJR Am J Roentgenol 1999;173: 1269–72.

22. Koraitim MM, Marzouk ME, Atta MA, et al. Risk factors and mechanism of urethral injury in pelvic fractures. Br J Urol 1996;77:876–80.

23. Lowe MA, Mason JT, Luna GK, et al. Risk factors for urethral injuries in men with traumatic pelvic fractures. J Urol 1988;140:506–7.

24. Rohner TJ Jr, Blanchard TW. Management of urethral injuries in war casualties. Mil Med 1970;135:748–51.

25. Mydio JH, Harris CF, Brown JG. Blunt, penetrating and ischemic injuries to the penis. J Urol 2002;168:1433–5.

26. Morey AF, Metro MJ, Carney KJ, et al. Consensus on genitourinary trauma: external genitalia. BJU Int 2004;94:507–15.

27. Nicolaisen GS, Melamud A, Williams RD, et al. Rupture of the corpus cavernosum: surgical management. J Urol 1983;130:917–9.

28. Orvis BR, McAninch JW. Penile rupture. Urol Clin North Am 1989;16:369–75.

29. Buckley JC, McAninch JW. Diagnosis and management of testicular ruptures. Urol Clin North Am 2006;33:111–6.

30. Anderson KA, McAninch JW, Jeffrey RB, et al. Ultrasonography for the diagnosis and staging of blunt scrotal trauma. J Urol 1983;130:933.

31. Cass AS, Luxenberg M. Testicular injuries. Urology 1991;37:528.

32. Gross M. Rupture of the testicle, the importance of early surgical treatment. J Urol 1969;101:196–7.

Major Urologic Problems in Geriatrics: Assessment and Management

Thomas J. Guzzo, MD, MPH*, George W. Drach, MD

KEYWORDS

- Geriatric urology • Urologic cancer • Urinary incontinence
- Urinary infection • Erectile dysfunction

The percentage of the US population over age 65 is now 17% and will be greater than 20% by 2030. This represents approximately 72 million people.[1] Currently, 1 in every 10 individuals in the world is more than 60 years old; by 2050 this number will double to 1 in 5.[2] To illustrate, in 2004, the median life expectancy after age 65 was 17.1 years and at age 75, 10.7 years.[3] Although many health care specialists will feel the impact of this growing elderly population, few will be more affected than those in the field of urology. Although urologic diseases affect a broad spectrum of age groups (from prenatal to advanced age), many urologic disorders have increased prevalence among the elderly. As the elderly population expands and there is a lack of urologists, primary care physicians will likely take a more active role in the diagnosis and management of urologic diseases in the elderly.

Thus, the elderly urology patients merit special assessment on several fronts. Many nonoperative urologic conditions are now treated with medications that can affect cognition and/or interact with other daily medications. Hence, careful drug integration remains necessary. Urinary issues, such as incontinence or frequency, can lead to significant morbidity in the functionally impaired, often leading to falls. Surgical intervention is common for urologic disease, both oncologic and benign, and must be carefully considered before initiation in geriatric patients.

Aside from a general history and physical examination, elderly urologic patients require additional assessment in several key areas. Careful review of medications is important because 40% of individuals ages 65 and older take 5 or more medications.[4] An overall assessment of the geriatric patient's functional ability is also paramount. Within this context, the concept of frailty has been introduced. The Cardiovascular Health Study identified five variables that make up the phenotype of frailty, including

---

Division of Urology, Department of Surgery, The Hospital of the University of Pennsylvania, 3400 Spruce Street, 9 Penn Tower, Philadelphia, PA 19104, USA
* Corresponding author.
E-mail address: Thomas.guzzo@uphs.upenn.edu

Med Clin N Am 95 (2011) 253–264
doi:10.1016/j.mcna.2010.08.026
0025-7125/11/$ – see front matter © 2011 Elsevier Inc. All rights reserved.

recent weight loss, weakness, poor endurance, slowness of gait, and low physical activity.[5] Cardiovascular Health Study described an association between frailty and adverse outcomes, including increased hospitalization, falls, worsening activities of daily living, worsening disability, and death.[5]

Within the context of balance of risk and benefit, common urologic conditions of the elderly are reviewed in this article, with particular emphasis on their management in the geriatric population. Voiding dysfunction, urologic malignancies, and certain other urologic conditions are reviewed.

VOIDING DYSFUNCTION
Benign Prostatic Hyperplasia

Incidence of benign prostatic hyperplasia (BPH) increases with each decade of life.[6] Increasing age also seems to be a risk factor for greater lower urinary tract symptoms associated with BPH.[7] BPH can lead to bladder outlet obstruction from a combination of static obstruction (prostatic enlargement) and dynamic obstruction (increased smooth muscle tone). Medical therapy in the form of alpha-blockade and 5α-reductase inhibition is now considered first-line treatment for BPH.[8] Although both drugs are used to treat BPH, they have different mechanisms of action. α-Blockers cause relaxation of prostatic smooth muscle, thus treating the dynamic component of bladder outlet obstruction. By inhibiting conversion of testosterone to the more potent dihydrotestosterone, 5α-reductase inhibitors reduce overall prostatic glandular volume. Uroselective α-blockers, such as tamsulosin, offer the advantage of rapid onset of action and require no dose titration.[9] Attention must be paid to an elderly patient's medication regimen, especially antihypertensives, to minimize the potential for drug-drug interactions leading to hypotension, increasing the risk of falls in this age group. Adding a 5α-reductase inhibitor, such as finasteride, to reduce prostatic size (especially for those with prostatic volume of over 30 g) is considered maximum medical therapy and has been shown to decrease the incidence of acute urinary retention and surgical intervention for BPH.[10] For elderly men who cannot tolerate or fail medical therapy, surgery remains a viable option. Transurethral resection of the prostate is reasonably tolerated in the elderly population with perioperative morbidity and mortality rates of less than 20% and 1%, respectively.[11] For men who are at significant surgical risk, less-invasive options include transurethral prostatic laser vaporization or enucleation, microwave therapy, or needle ablation. Laser procedures may offer the advantage of minimizing or alleviating the need to discontinue oral anticoagulants in the perioperative period. Several retrospective studies have shown that both KTP laser vaporization of the prostate and holmium laser enucleation of the prostate can be safely performed on patients maintained on oral anticoagulation regimens with acceptable morbidity and transfusion rates.[12] Prostatic stenting may be used where any ablative intervention is contraindicated; however, complications related to prostatic stenting can be significant, including worsening of lower urinary tract symptoms, stent migration, obstruction, sexual dysfunction, and recurrent urinary tract infection.[13,14]

Nocturia

The incidence of nocturia is similar for men and women and increases significantly with age.[15] Nocturia can result in sleep deprivation, leading to exacerbation of medical illness and worsening of cognitive function in the elderly. Additionally, nocturia places elderly individuals at an increased fall risk. Stewart and colleagues[16] have demonstrated that individuals with nocturia greater than or equal to 2 times per night were at high fall risk.

Nocturia has three basic etiologies: diurnal polyuria (increased urine production over 24 hours), nocturnal polyuria (increased urine production at night), and reduced nocturnal bladder capacity.[15] A variety of causes exist for nocturia within these three broad etiologies, including diabetes mellitus and insipidus for diurnal polyuria; overactive bladder and bladder cancer for reduced nocturnal bladder capacity; and altered ADH secretion, congestive heart failure, and excessive fluid intake for nocturnal polyuria. A voiding diary, including voiding times and volume, is a useful tool for nocturia assessment. Other causes of sleep disturbances, such as sleep apnea, anxiety, depression and dementia, should be excluded.[17]

After medical conditions have been searched for and addressed and behavior modification has been attempted (eg, limiting fluid intake in the evening), therapy in the form of desmopressin or anticholinergic medications may be considered. Anticholinergic medications relax the bladder detrusor muscle, thereby treating nocturia caused by overactive bladder. Desmopressin directly increases water reabsorption in the collecting duct of the nephron acting to directly decrease nighttime urine output. Estimating the potential for drug-drug interactions and adverse side effects is essential before starting such medications. For example, desmopressin-induced hyponatremia is more common in the elderly population, and regular serum sodium monitoring is recommended.[18] Anticholinergic medications can also have significant side effects, including dry mouth, constipation, dizziness, constipation, urinary retention, and exacerbation of cognitive deficits.[19] Although multiple anticholinergic medications have been marketed with theoretic benefits from efficacy and side-effect profile standpoints, little evidence exists to substantiate such claims.

Incontinence

Urinary incontinence (UI) is estimated to affect between 15% and 30% of independent adults ages 65 and older.[20] In addition to significant alterations in quality of life (QOL), the economic burden of UI is not small. In 2000, total incontinence-related costs in the United States were estimated at $20 billion.[21] Two basic presentations of incontinence exist: acute and chronic. Acute UI, as its name implies, refers to a sudden onset of UI and generally is secondary to a treatable condition.[22] Potential causes include urinary tract infection, surgery, constipation, medications, worsening cognition, and metabolic disturbances. Also, causes of acute UI can exacerbate chronic UI and, therefore, a change in a patient's chronic UI symptoms warrants further investigation. Chronic UI can be stratified into four basic categories: urge (bladder overactivity), stress (sphincteric deficiency), functional (inability to get to bathroom on time), and overflow incontinence (in the setting of urinary retention).

UI often goes untreated in the elderly population. Elderly patients are hesitant to discuss UI and often accept it as a fact of normal aging. Hence, physicians should discuss UI with all elderly patients openly. A complete and quick work-up for UI can be done in the office and often leads to the cause and type of UI. A detailed history is the first step in any patient, elderly or not, with UI. Important information that can be elucidated from the history includes onset and frequency, symptom type, medication changes, and severity. A physical examination focusing on total volume status, neurologic deficits, suprapubic palpation (for bladder fullness), and rectal and pelvic examinations can cue a physician to potential causes of UI. Tests that can routinely be done in the office setting and are inexpensive to perform include urinalysis and culture, postvoid residual measurement, and voided volume measurement.[22] Often a simple office work-up can cue a physician to the cause of a patient's UI. For example, a history of UI with sneezing or laughing and demonstration of UI with Valsalva maneuver are diagnostic of stress UI. UI in the setting of a large postvoid residual and low voided volume is suggestive of overflow UI. UI in the setting of urgency and frequency with small voided volumes and minimal postvoid residual is consistent with urge incontinence.

The first step in UI intervention is assessing the degree of bother for individual patients. This simple assessment often guides aggressiveness of the treatment intervention. Behavioral interventions for patients with stress incontinence, such as pelvic floor exercises, are noninvasive but require a motivated patient. Anticholinergic medications are most commonly used to treat UI caused by bladder overactivity, but these drugs can have significant side effects (discussed previously).[19] Anticholinergic therapy is contraindicated in patients with overflow UI or in patients at high risk for urinary retention. Reduction in cognitive function in the elderly population can have devastating consequences, including loss of functional independence and independent living. Antimuscarinic properties can also potentiate side effects of other medications, including over-the-counter antihistamines, eye drops, and antidepressants.[17] Comorbid conditions must also be taken into account before starting anticholinergic therapy because many medical conditions can be exacerbated by these medications.[19] Common medical conditions in the elderly that can be exacerbated by anticholinergic therapy include glaucoma, bronchitis, chronic airway disease, constipation, congestive heart failure, diabetes mellitus, and dementia.[19]

When considering surgical intervention for incontinence, age alone should not be considered a contraindication. Overall patient comorbidity, desire to pursue aggressive management, and a willingness to accept the potential morbidity of surgical intervention are important factors to consider. Reduced perioperative morbidity due to recent adoption of less-invasive surgical procedures in the form of urethral slings may make surgical intervention for stress UI a viable option for larger numbers of geriatric patients than in the past. Recently, Carr and colleagues[23] reported that pubovaginal sling procedures can be performed safely with outcomes equivalent to those seen in younger women. Similarly, minimally invasive surgical approaches exist for refractory urge UI, including sacral nerve modulation and botulinum toxin injection; however, these have not been extensively studied in the elderly population.[24,25] External appliances and indwelling Foley catheters should be avoided because they can lead to significant skin breakdown, urethral erosion, and urinary tract infections. If catheterization is needed to reduce incontinence episodes, clean intermittent catheterization is superior to appliances and indwelling catheters in reducing complications.[26]

UROLOGIC MALIGNANCIES IN THE ELDERLY
Surgical Considerations in Elderly Cancer Patients

Currently, approximately half of all surgical procedures performed in the United States are in patients ages 65 and older.[27] Furthermore, 50% of new cancer diagnoses are made in patients 70 and older.[28] Many elderly patients have complex physiologic and functional issues that merit consideration from a surgical perspective. The aging process is associated with changes in many organ systems that can have an impact on an elderly patient's ability to withstand and tolerate a major surgical procedure. The cardiac, pulmonary, hepatobiliary, immune, and renal systems all undergo deterioration and loss of physiologic reserve with aging. Knowledge of such changes with regard to perioperative management is essential in the evaluation of the elderly surgical candidate. Renal function decreases with age and serum creatinine is not a good surrogate for glomerular filtration rate in elderly patients.[29] Renal drug dose adjustment in the elderly and proper fluid balance in the perioperative period are important points to minimize morbidity. Cardiac changes that accompany aging include a lower sensitivity to β-adrenergic modulation, altered calcium regulation, and an overall reduction in ejection fraction.[28] Occult coronary artery disease is not uncommon and a high index of suspicion for underlying cardiac pathology and prompt preoperative cardiology referral is essential. A decline in immunologic function in the elderly has two important implications. First, immunologic decline may predispose individuals to the development and progression of cancer.[29] Altered immunologic function may also lead to an increased susceptibility to infection during cancer therapy.[29] A significant reduction in liver volume with aging is also accompanied by an overall decrease in hepatic function, which can have implications on dosage of chemotherapeutic drugs. Finally, decreased respiratory function from intrinsic lung disease, weakened respiratory musculature, pulmonary vascular disease, or a combination of the three can predispose elderly patients to postoperative complications, such as pneumonia.[28]

Multiple comorbidities may have an impact on clinical decision making with regard to the pursuit of aggressive therapy. Comorbidity status is also a valuable predictor of perioperative outcomes. Comorbidity scores are useful tools to quantify an elderly patient's surgical risk. Several useful scores to assess overall comorbidity include the Cumulative Illness Rating Scale for geriatrics, the Charlson Comorbidity Index (CCI), and the American Society of Anesthesiologists classification. The Cumulative Illness Rating Scale for geriatrics and CCI have been validated in elderly populations and found associated with increased perioperative morbidity and mortality.[30,31] Overall comorbidity is a more useful predictor of perioperative outcome than chronologic age alone. Sanchez-Sales and colleagues[32] recently evaluated their laparoscopic radical prostatectomy outcomes in men 70 and older. In this cohort of 297 men, a CCI greater than or equal to 2 was associated with a higher risk of short-term postoperative complications compared those with lower CCI. Similarly, with regard to laparoscopic renal surgery, Guzzo and colleagues[33] found a CCI greater than or equal to 2 a significant predictor of perioperative complication in patients ages 75 and older.

Although comorbidity is an important indicator of outcome, it generally does not take into account overall global functioning. Careful preoperative attention to functional status in the elderly surgical candidate can help predict the need for social support and physical rehabilitation services.[28] Functional assessment tools that have been validated in the elderly include the activities of daily living dependency score and the instrumental activities of daily living dependency score (IADL).[28] More recently a comprehensive multidisciplinary approach, the Comprehensive Geriatric Assessment, has proved effective in risk stratifying patients before intervention and in minimizing postoperative morbidity.[28] The Comprehensive Geriatric Assessment before surgical intervention improves functional status postoperatively and reduces hospital and nursing home stays, thus decreasing overall costs.[34]

Recent data show that 56% of newly diagnosed cancers and 71% of cancer deaths occur in individuals older than 65.[35] Many factors often need to be addressed when considering cancer treatment in the geriatric population. The impact of treatment on QOL must be minimized and long-term functioning and independence maximized. Physiologic and cognitive changes associated with aging can have an impact on an elderly patient's ability to receive standard oncologic therapies and also may make them more at risk for potential treatment-related side effects and complications. Functional status, cognition, comorbidity, life expectancy, and risk of functional decline all must be considered in elderly cancer patients.[36] Unfortunately, few oncology clinical trials include significant numbers of elderly patients, making it difficult to extrapolate standard cancer therapy to this age group. Thus, pretreatment assessment of the elderly cancer patient's overall health status is imperative.

Prostate Cancer Screening and Treatment

The incidence of prostate cancer increases with increasing age, both clinically and in autopsy studies.[37] Despite little evidence to support the benefit of prostate-specific antigen (PSA) screening in elderly populations, the prevalence of screening in the United States population is high.[38] Two recent, large, randomized trials looked for a beneficial impact of PSA screening on prostate cancer mortality with contradictory results.[39,40] Despite these trials, PSA screening remains controversial. (For a more detailed review of prostate cancer screening, readers are referred to article by Gjertson and Albertsen elsewhere in this issue.) The appropriate use of PSA screening in older men remains even less clear. Generally, the authors' practice is that prostate cancer screening is offered to men with a life expectancy of at least 10 to 15 years. No consensus guidelines exist to direct physicians as to when to discontinue prostate cancer screening in older men, although the US Preventive Services Task Force has recommended discontinuing screening for those older than 75.[41–44] The Iowa Prostate Cancer Consensus has also published state consensus recommendations regarding screening men older than 7.[45] They suggest at least discussing the potential risks and benefits of screening, life expectancy, and the desire to pursue treatment if a patient is diagnosed with cancer. A recent longitudinal cohort study of men undergoing PSA screening revealed that no men between ages 75 and 80 with a PSA of less than 3.0 ng/mL died of prostate cancer, potentially identifying a subset of men in which PSA screening could be safely omitted.[46] Additional similar identifying variables would benefit this and younger age groups.

Most prostate cancers currently detected in the United States are clinically localized. Many older men have low or intermediate risk disease yet they seek treatment.[47] Older men who seek treatment for low-risk prostate cancer, however, are unlikely to die from their disease. Unfortunately, current risk stratification models cannot predict with 100% accuracy those who would benefit from treatment and those who can safely be followed. As demonstrated by Mohile and colleagues,[48] a patient's relative life expectancy needs to be factored into treatment decision analysis. Relative life estimation is of significant importance in this population given the approximately 10-year lead time to associated morbidity and mortality from screen-detected prostate cancers.[49] Counseling with regard to disease risk, life expectancy, and the likelihood of benefit with intervention allows elderly patients to make more informed treatment decisions.

Bladder Cancer

The risk of bladder cancer is significantly increased in individuals older than 65.[36] Bladder cancer mortality also seems higher in the elderly compared with that of younger individuals.[30] For nonmuscle invasive disease, endoscopic procedures, including transurethral resection, are generally well tolerated in this older age group. Intravesical immunotherapy and/or chemotherapy is often used to reduce disease recurrence and progression. Bacille Calmette-Guérin is the most common form of intravesical therapy used in the United States; however, the efficacy of intravesical bacille Calmette-Guérin in older patients has been questioned. Retrospective studies suggest a decreased response to bacille Calmette-Guérin therapy in patients older than 70 and may have an increased complication rate.[50,51]

The gold standard treatment for muscle-invasive bladder cancer is radical cystectomy (RC) and urinary diversion.[52] RC is a major operation and urinary diversion can have significant QOL implications. Systemic cisplatin-based chemotherapy is also often used for treatment, in combination with radical surgery.[53] With diminished functional reserve related to either advanced cancer or chronologic age, delivery of cytotoxic chemotherapy can prove particularly challenging in the geriatric population.[54] Surveillance, Epidemiology and End Results data have demonstrated that patients ages 80 and older are less likely to undergo RC; nevertheless, when RC is performed on this group, it is associated with a significant reduction in death from bladder cancer.[55] The exact nature of the bias for or against RC in the elderly is unknown, but possible reasons include delay in diagnosis, the use of less-aggressive therapy inappropriately, or the perception that older patients would not tolerate a major operative procedure.[30] Because RC has a proved benefit in the geriatric population, chronologic age alone should not be used to exclude patients from surgery. In patients who are unfit or unwilling to undergo RC, bladder-sparing protocols in the form of systemic chemotherapy, external beam radiation, and aggressive transurethral resection may present a viable option.[56] Bladder-sparing protocols, however, may be less likely to provide a cure, affect long-term QOL, have significant side effects, and only palliate in the short term.

Noncontinent diversion in the form of an ileal conduit is the most common urinary diversion used in elderly patients after RC.[57] Although continent neobladder diversion or orthotopic bladder substitution offers the advantage of continence without the need for an external appliance, complications have been noted to be higher in the geriatric population.[58,59] Both methods require intermittent catheterization. Also, continence rates with orthotopic urinary diversion have been shown to be lower in older patients.[60] Thus, the potential for improved QOL and body image with continent diversion must be balanced against the possibility of increased risk for perioperative complications and long-term continence problems in this age group.

Kidney Cancer

The gold standard treatment for renal cell carcinoma (RCC) remains surgical. Alternatives exist for patients unfit for or unwilling to undergo surgery, including percutaneous ablation and/or active surveillance. With the increased detection of small, localized renal masses due to the prevalent use of cross-sectional imaging, active surveillance has become an attractive option in the management of small renal masses (<4 cm) in highly selected individuals. Active surveillance may be a viable option for patients with small renal masses who are too debilitated to undergo active intervention or unwilling to accept the potential risks of such interventions. Several factors should be taken into consideration when assessing elderly patients for RCC treatment, including performance status, comorbidity, life expectancy, and contralateral renal function. Serum creatinine estimates in the elderly (discussed previously) can be incorrect and, therefore, glomerular filtration rate should be estimated using a standardized equation, such as the Modification of Diet in Renal Disease, or doing a 24-hour urine creatinine clearance.[61]

Several studies have demonstrated the importance of comorbidity assessment rather than absolute age when evaluating elderly patients for renal surgery. Surgical extirpation remains the gold standard treatment for patients with enhancing renal masses. Both laparoscopic and open renal surgery have proved safe, with acceptable complication rates in elderly patients.[33,62] Overall survival for elderly patients who undergo cytoreductive nephrectomy in the setting of metastatic RCC has been shown similar to that of younger patients, albeit in a small sample size. Cytoreductive nephrectomy, however, is associated with an increased risk of perioperative mortality in those ages 75 and older and, therefore, the risk of a major operation in the setting of metastatic disease must be balanced with that of potential benefit on an individual basis in this age group.[63,64] For elderly patients with advanced RCC, immunochemotherapy has been shown equally effective in this age group as in younger patients.[65] Unfortunately, these therapies are rarely curative in the setting of advanced disease but can provide improvement in progression-free survival, most commonly in patients with lower burdens of metastatic disease and a good performance status.[66] Systemic therapy can have significant side effects in this patient population and nomograms are currently under development to predict adverse events with these therapies.[65]

OTHER UROLOGIC CONDITIONS IN THE ELDERLY
Erectile Dysfunction

Erectile dysfunction (ED) is defined as the inability to acquire or maintain an erection for adequate sexual intercourse. ED should be differentiated from decreased libido, which generally results from androgen deficiency.[67] The prevalence of ED rises with age and can be as high as 70% by the seventh decade.[68] Vascular disease from hypercholesterolemia, hypertension, smoking, and diabetes is the most common cause of ED in the geriatric population. Neurologic disorders are also a significant cause of ED in the elderly.[67] Finally, medication-related ED is not uncommon in the elderly. ED can cause significant decrements in QOL in elderly men and, therefore, should be addressed and treated.

The initial history and physical examination can determine the most likely cause of ED and any reversible conditions. In a focused physical examination, signs of hypogonadism and longstanding chronic diseases, such as hypertension or diabetes, are looked for. Basic laboratory studies, including serum cholesterol, testosterone, and glucose, are helpful but not necessarily mandatory in the initial work-up.[67]

Initial treatment should eliminate any modifiable risk factors that may lead to ED (including smoking and medications). Consideration of the potential adverse medical consequences of changing a geriatric patient's medical regimen to improve ED is necessary to avoid unintended complications of medication changes. Phosphodiesterase inhibitors (sildenafil, vardenafil, and tadalafil) are now considered first-line therapy for ED. Sildenafil has been shown safe and effective in the elderly population, but efficacy decreases in men older than 80.[69] Also, dose reductions should be considered in elderly patients with hepatic or renal insufficiency.[68] For elderly patients in whom oral therapy fails or is contraindicated, vacuum erection devices are an option. The use of vacuum erection devices, however, requires some degree of manual dexterity in applying and operating the device. Other more invasive forms of ED management include intracavernosal injection, intraurethral administration of prostaglandin E_1 medications, and surgical implantation of a penile prosthesis. These are generally not contraindicated in the geriatric population but are less frequently used.[67]

Urinary Tract Infection

It is estimated that 20% of all women and 10% of all men 65 and older have bacteriuria.[70] These rates increase to 25% to 50% of women and 15% to 40% of men in institutionalized settings.[71] Most bacteriuria in the elderly is asymptomatic. The increased prevalence of bacteriuria in the elderly population is not entirely understood. Theories include a decline in cell-mediated immunity, worsening bladder function, increased perineal soiling, increased incidence of indwelling catheters and pH, and estrogenic changes in the vagina.[72] Although *Escherichia coli* remains the most common type of bacteria in the elderly population, Proteus, Klebsiella, Enterobacter, Pseudomonas, and Enterococcus species urinary tract infections are also common in the elderly.[73]

Studies have not demonstrated a benefit in treating asymptomatic bacteriuria with antibiotics in the elderly, and, therefore, it is currently not recommended.[72] This is an important management point because unnecessary use of antibiotics can lead to infection with resistant organisms or cause adverse side effects in the elderly. Pyuria can be present in the setting of asymptomatic bacteriuria in up to 90% of cases and, therefore, in itself does not merit treatment.[73] Patients with lower urinary tract symptoms and bacteriuria, however, should be treated with antibiotic therapy. Also, elderly patients with acute cognitive changes and bacteriuria should be treated, because mental status changes are often the initial presenting signs in this population.[74] A 7-day course of antibiotics is recommended; however, if a patient is febrile or has signs of systemic infection, a 14-day course should be instituted.[72] There is an increased incidence of antibiotic resistance in nursing home patients. Antibiotics should be administered according to local patterns of resistance, pending culture results. Worsening or deteriorating symptoms once treatment has started should lead to a high index of suspicion for antibiotic resistance.

SUMMARY

Elderly urologic patients require careful planning when developing a treament program for various urologic problems. Because of potential interference with poor renal function or crossover effects with central or peripheral nervous system, however, many urologic drugs must be titrated appropriately. In treating cancer, ED, incontinence or urinary infection, patient QOL, and life span become dominant factors in making therapeutic decisions, by behavioral change, medication, or surgical intervention.

REFERENCES

1. He W, Sengupta M, Velkoff VA, et al. 65+ in the United States: 2005. United States Census Bureau, Current Population Reports. U.S. Census Bureau and National Institute on Aging; 2005. p. 23–209. Available at: http://www.census.gov/prod/2006pubs/p23-209.pdf. Accessed August 24, 2010.
2. Population Division, DESA, United Nations. World Population Aging 1950–2050. Executive Summary. Available at: http://www.un.org/esa/population/publications/worldageing19502050/Pdf/62executivesummary.english.pdf. Accessed February 2010. Accessed February 15, 2010.
3. Surveillance Epidemiology and End Results (SEER). SEER data for 200–2004. Available at: www.cancer.gov. Accessed February 15, 2010.
4. Barnett SR. Polypharmacy and perioperative medications in the elderly. Anesthesiol Clin 2009;27(3):377–89.
5. Fried LP, Tangen CM, Walston J, et al. Frailty in older adults: evidence for a phenotype. J Gerontol A Biol Sci Med Sci 2001;56:M146–57.
6. Trueman P, Hood SC, Nayak US, et al. Prevalence of lower urinary tract symptoms and self-reported diagnosed benign prostatic hyperplasia, and their effect on quality of life in community-based survey of men in the UK. BJU Int 1999;83:410–5.
7. Haidinger G, Temml C, Schatzl, et al. Risk factors for lower urinary tract symptoms in elderly men. For the Prostate Study Group of the Austrian Society of Urology. Eur Urol 2000;37:413–20.
8. Nix JW, Carson CC. Medical management of benign prostatic hypertrophy. Can J Urol 2007;14(Suppl 1):53–7.

9. Reohrborn CG, Rosen RC. Medical therapy options for aging men with benign prostatic hyperplasia: focus on alfuzosin 10 mg once daily. Clin Interv Aging 2008;3(3):511–24.

10. McConnell JD, Roehrborn CG, Bautista OM, et al. The long-term effect of doxazosin, finasteride, and combination therapy on the clinical progression of benign prostatic hyperplasia. N Engl J Med 2003;349(25):2387–98.

11. Malhotra V. Transurethral resection of the prostate. Anesthesiol Clin North Am 2000;18(4):883–97.

12. Berger J, Robert G, Descazeaud A. Laser treatment of benign hyperplasia in patients on oral anticoagulant therapy. Curr Urol Rep 2010;11(4):236–41.

13. Mebust WK, Holtgrewe HL, Cockett AT, et al. Transurethral prostatectomy: immediate and postoperative complications. A cooperative study of 13 participating institutions evaluating 3,885 patients. J Urol 1989;141:243–7.

14. Donnell RF. Minimally invasive therapy of lower urinary tract symptoms. Urol Clin North Am 2009;36(4):497–509.

15. Appell RA, Sand PK. Nocturia: etiology, diagnosis and treatment. Neurourol Urodyn 2008;27(1):34–9.

16. Stewart RB, Moore MT, May FE, et al. Nocturia: a risk factor for falls in the elderly. J Am Geriatr Soc 1992;40:1217–20.

17. Benca RM, Peterson MJ. Insomnia and depression. Sleep Med 2008;9(Suppl 1):S3–9.

18. Rembratt A, Riis A, Norgaard JP. Desmopressin treatment in nocturia; an analysis of risk factors for hyponatremia. Neurourol Urodyn 2006;25:105–9.

19. Kay GG, Granville LJ. Antimuscarinic agents: implications and concerns in the management of overactive bladder in the elderly. Clin Ther 2005;27(1):127–38.

20. McGrother C. Epidemiology and etiology of urinary incontinence in the elderly. World J Urol 1998;16:S3–9.

21. Hu TW, Wagner TH, Bentkover JD, et al. Costs of urinary incontinence and overactive bladder in the United States: a comparative study. Urology 2004;63:461–5.

22. Gibbs CF, Johnson TM 2nd, Ouslander JG. Office management of geriatric urinary incontinence. Am J Med 2007;120(3):211–20.

23. Carr LK, Walsh PJ, Abraham VE, et al. Favorable outcome of pubovaginal slings for geriatric women with stress incontinence. J Urol 1997;157(1):125–8.

24. Yakovlev AE, Resch BE. Treatment of urinary voiding dysfunction syndromes with spinal cord stimulation. Clin Med Res 2010;8(1):22–4.

25. da Silva CM, Cruz F. Has botulinum toxin therapy come of age: what do we know, what do we need to know, and should we use it? Curr Opin Urol 2009;19(4):347–52.

26. Moore KN, Fader M, Getliffe K. Long-term bladder management by intermittent catheterization in adults and children. Cochrane Database Syst Rev 2007;4:CD006008.

27. Etzioni DA, Liu JH, Maggard MA, et al. The aging population and its impact on the surgery workforce. Ann Surg 2003;238:170–7.

28. Pasetto LM, Lise M, Monfardini S. Preoperative assessment of elderly cancer patients. Crit Rev Oncol Hematol 2007;64(1):10–8.

29. Shariat SF, Milowsky M, Droller MJ. Bladder cancer and the elderly. Urol Oncol 2009;27(6):653–67.

30. Extermann M, Overcash J, Lyman GH, et al. Comorbidity and functional status are independent in older cancer patients. J Clin Oncol 1998;16:1582–7.

31. Conwell Y, Forbes NT, Cox C, et al. Validation of a measure of physical illness burden at autopsy: the cumulative illness rating scale. J Am Geriatr Soc 1993;41:38–41.

32. Sanchez-Salas R, Prapotnich D, Rozet F, et al. Laparoscopic radical prostatectomy is feasible and effective in "fit" senior men with localized prostate cancer. BJU Int 2010. [Epub ahead of print].

33. Guzzo TJ, Allaf ME, Pierorazio PM, et al. Perioperative outcomes of elderly patients undergoing laparoscopic renal procedures. Urology 2009;73(3):572–6.

34. Rubenstein LZ, Stuck AE, Siu AL, et al. Impacts of geriatric evaluation and management programs on defined outcomes: overview of the evidence. J Am Geriatr Soc 1991;39:8–16.

35. Edwards BK, Eisner MP, Kosary CL. SEER cancer statistics review, 1975–2002. Available at: http://seer.cancer.gov/csr/1975_2002/. Accessed February 15, 2010.

36. Pal SK, Katheria V, Hurria A. Evaluating the older patient with cancer: understanding frailty and the geriatric assessment. CA Cancer J Clin 2010;60(2):120–32.

37. Gronberg H. Prostate cancer epidemiology. Lancet 2003;361:859–64.

38. Walter LC, Bertenthal D, Lindquist K, et al. PSA screening among elderly men with limited life expectancies. JAMA 2006;296(19):2336–42.

39. Andriole GL, Crawford ED, Grubb RL, et al. Mortality results from a randomized prostate cancer screening trial. N Engl J Med 2009;360(13):1310–9.

40. Schroder FH, Hugosson J, Roobol MJ, et al. Screening and prostate cancer mortality in a randomized European study. N Engl J Med 2009;360(13):1320–8.

41. Heidenreich A, Aus G, Bolla M, et al. EAU guideline on prostate cancer. Eur Urol 2008;53:68–80.

42. Smith RA, Cokkinides V, Brooks D, et al. Cancer screening in the United States, 2010: a review of current American Cancer Society guidelines and issues in cancer screening. CA Cancer J Clin 2010;60(2):99–119.

43. Carroll P, Albertsen P, Greene K, et al. Prostate-specific antigen best practice statement. Available at: http://www.auanet.org/content/media/psa09.pdf? CFID=1550596&CFTOKEN=18680908&jsessionid=84306ef13330b74de9953 e52462942505420. Accessed April, 2010.

44. Screening for Prostate Cancer, Topic Page. August 2008. U.S. Preventive Services Task Force. Rockville (MD): Agency for Healthcare Research and Quality; 2008. Available at: http://www.ahrq.gov/clinic/uspstf/uspsprca.htm. Accessed April, 2010.

45. Konety BR, Sharp VJ, Raut H, et al. Screening and management of prostate cancer in elderly men: the Iowa prostate cancer consensus. Urology 2008;71(3):511–4.

46. Schaeffer EM, Carter HB, Kettermann A, et al. Prostate specific antigen testing among the elderly-when to stop? J Urol 2009;181(4):1606–14.

47. Cooperberg MR, Lubeck DP, Meng MV, et al. The changing face of low-risk prostate cancer: trends in clinical presentation and primary management. J Clin Oncol 2004;22:2141–9.

48. Mohile SG, Lachs M, Dale W. Management of prostate cancer in the older man. Semin Oncol 2008;35(6):597–617.

49. Draisma G, Boer R, Otto SJ, et al. Lead times and overdetection due to prostate specific antigen screening: estimates from the European randomized study of screening for prostate cancer. J Natl Cancer Inst 2003;95:868–78.

50. Herr HW. Age and outcome of superficial bladder cancer treated with bacilli Calmeete-Guerin therapy. Urology 2007;70:65–8.

51. Joudi FN, Smith BJ, O'Donnell MA, et al. The impact of age on the response of patients with superficial bladder cancer to intravesical immunotherapy. J Urol 2006;175:1634–9.

52. Huang GJ, Stein JP. Open radical cystectomy with lymphadenectomy remains the treatment of choice for invasive bladder cancer. Curr Opin Urol 2007;17(5): 369–75.

53. Clark PE. Neoadjuvant versus adjuvant chemotherapy for muscle-invasive bladder cancer. Expert Rev Anticancer Ther 2009;9(6):821–30.

54. Carreca I, Balducci L. Cancer chemotherapy in the older patient. Urol Oncol 2009;27(6):633–42.

55. Hollenbeck BK, Miller DC, Taub D, et al. Aggressive treatment for bladder cancer is associated with improved overall survival among patients 80 years or older. Urology 2004;64:292–7.

56. Tran E, Souhami L, Tanguay S, et al. Bladder conservation treatment in the elderly population: results and prognostic factors of muscle-invasive bladder cancer. Am J Clin Oncol 2009;32(4):333–7.

57. Gore JL, Litwin MS. Quality of care in bladder cancer: trends in urinary diversion following radical cystectomy. World J Urol 2009;27(1):45–50.

58. Sogni F, Brausi M, Frea B, et al. Morbidity and quality of life in elderly patients receiving ileal conduit or orthotopic neobladder after radical cystectomy for invasive bladder cancer. Urology 2008;71:919–23.

59. Froehner M, Brausi M, Herr HW, et al. Complications following radical cystectomy for bladder cancer in the elderly. Eur Urol 2009;56(3):443–54.

60. Hautmann RE, Miller K, Steiner U, et al. The ileal neobladder: six years of experience with more than 200 patients. J Urol 1993;150:40–5.

61. Carnevale V, Pastore L, Camaioni M, et al. Estimate of renal function in oldest old inpatients by MDRD study equation, Mayo Clinic equation and creatinine clearance. J Nephrol 2010;23(3):306–13.

62. Berdjis N, Hakenberg OW, Novotny V, et al. Treating renal cell cancer in the elderly. BJU Int 2006;97:703–5.

63. Kader AK, Tamboli P, Luongo T, et al. Cytoreducttive nephrectomy in the elderly patient: the M.D. Anderson Cancer Center experience. J Urol 2007;177(3):855–60.

64. Atzpodien J, Wandert T, Reitz M. Age does not impair the efficacy of immunochemotherapy in patients with metastatic renal carcinoma. Crit Rev Oncol Hematol 2005;55:193–9.

65. Pond GR, Siu LL, Moore M, et al. Nomograms to predict serious adverse events in phase II clinical trials of molecularly targeted agents. J Clin Oncol 2008;26:1324–30.

66. Bellmunt J, Negrier S, Escudier B, et al. The medical treatment of metastatic renal cell cancer in the elderly: position paper of a SIOG Taskforce. Crit Rev Oncol Hematol 2009;69(1):64–72.

67. Mulligan T, Reddy S, Gulur P, et al. Disorders of male sexual function. Clin Geriatr Med 2003;19:473–81.

68. Heidelbaugh JJ. Management of erectile dysfunction. Am Fam Physician 2010;81(3):305–12.

69. Muller A, Smith L, Parker M, et al. Analysis of the efficacy and safety of sildenafil citrate in the geriatric population. BJU Int 2007;100(1):117–21.

70. Boscia JA, Kaye D. Asymptomatic bacteriuria in the elderly. Infect Dis Clin North Am 1987;1:893–905.

71. Nicolle LE. Urinary infections in the elderly: symptomatic or asymptomatic? Int J Antimicrob Agents 1999;11:265–8.

72. Schaeffer AJ, Schaeffer EM. Infections of the urinary tract. Campbells Urology. 9th edition. Maryland Heights (MO): Saunders; 2006. Chapter 8.

73. Boscia JA, Abrutyn E, Levison ME, et al. Pyuria and asymptomatic bacteriuria in elderly ambulatory women. Ann Intern Med 1989;110:404–5.

74. Woodford HJ, George J. Diagnosis and management of urinary tract infections in hospitalized older people. J Am Geriatr Soc 2009;57(1):107–14.

Index

Note: Page numbers of article titles are in **boldface** type.

A

Abdominal trauma, 245–246
Abscess
    kidney, 45–46
    perinephric, 45–46
Acyclovir, for herpes simplex virus infections, 53
Adenomatoid tumors, paratesticular, 239
Age-adjusted prostate-specific antigen test, 195
Age-specific factors, in urinary tract infections, 29–30
AIDS. *See* HIV infection.
Alfuzosin
    for lower urinary tract symptoms, 94
    for prostatitis, 80
Alpha agonists, for incontinence, 107
Alpha blockers
    for lower urinary tract symptoms, 94
    for prostatitis, 80
    for stones, 136–137, 173
ALTESS (Alfuzosin Long Term Efficacy and Safety
    Study), 94
Amitriptyline, for bladder pain syndrome, 68
Amoxicillin, for hydronephrosis, 5
Antibiotics. *See specific antibiotics.*
Anticholinergic drugs
    for incontinence, 256
    for nocturia, 255
Antidepressants
    for bladder pain syndrome, 68
    for prostatitis, 81
Antiinflammatory agents, for prostatitis, 80
Antimicrobial Resistance Epidemiology in Females with Cystitis
    study, 37
Antimuscarinics
    for incontinence, 108
    for lower urinary tract symptoms, 95
Apomorphine, for erectile dysfunction, 209–210
Autonomic dysreflexia, in spinal cord injury, 117–118
Azithromycin
    for chancroid, 52
    for *Chlamydia* infections, 51
    for urethritis, 132–133
Azoospermia, 225, 227

Med Clin N Am 95 (2011) 265–287
doi:10.1016/S0025-7125(10)00197-5
0025-7125/11/$ – see front matter © 2011 Elsevier Inc. All rights reserved.

medical.theclinics.com

B

Bacille Calmette-Guérin, for bladder cancer, 258
Baclofen, for prostatitis, 80
Bacteriuria
    in elderly persons, 260–261
    in nursing homes, 30
    in pregnancy, 30–31
    in prostatitis, 78
    unresolved, 34
Bedwetting, 6
Behavioral therapy, for incontinence, 106, 256
Benign prostatic hyperplasia. See also Lower urinary tract symptoms, male.
    in elderly persons, 254
    kidney failure in, 164
Biofeedback, for incontinence, 106
Biopsy
    for bladder pain syndrome, 61
    for renal cell carcinoma, 185
Bladder
    augmentation of, for incontinence, 108–109
    cancer of
        in elderly persons, 258–259
        irritative voiding symptoms after, 123, 125
    dysfunction of, 6, 20–23
    fistulae of, in HIV infection, 143
    infections of. See Cystitis.
    injury of, 248
    neurogenic. See Neurogenic bladder.
    outlet obstruction of. See Lower urinary tract symptoms, male.
    poor compliance of, in neurologic disorders, 115
    posterior urethral valves and, 20–21
Bladder pain syndrome, **55–73**
    classic form of, 62–64
    classification of, 62–64
    comorbidity with, 57
    definition of, 56–57
    differential diagnosis of, 60
    etiology of, 57–59
    evaluation of, 59, 61, 64–66
    natural history of, 57
    nomenclature of, 55–56
    nonulcer form of, 62–64
    phenotyping of, 66
    prevalence of, 57
    refractory, 69–70
    taxonomy issues in, 61–64
    treatment of, 66–70
Bladder training, for incontinence, 106
Botulinum toxin
    for detrusor-sphincter dyssynergia, 116

for incontinence, 108
Bowen disease, in HIV infection, 142
Bradycardia, in autonomic dysreflexia, 117–118
Burch suspension, for incontinence, 107–108
Burns
    penile, 249
    scrotal, 250

C

Calcium stones, 170, 174
Calculi. *See* Stone disease.
Cancer
    bladder, 123, 125, 258–259
    epididymis, 239–240
    in elderly persons, 256–260
    in HIV infection, 141–143
    kidney, **179–189,** 259–260
    prostate. *See* Prostate, cancer of.
    scrotal wall, 238–239
    testicular, 240–241
Carcinoma
    renal cell, **179–189**
    scrotal skin, 238–239
Carcinoma in situ, penile, in HIV infection, 142
Cardiovascular disease, erectile dysfunction in, 214–216
Catheterization
    indwelling
        for bladder injury, 248
        for neurogenic bladder, 116–117
    intermittent
        for detrusor-sphincter dyssynergia, 115–116
        for incontinence, 256
        for neurogenic bladder, 116–117
    urinary tract infections in, 30, 50
Cavernous nerves, in penile erection, 202, 204
Cefixime
    for *Chlamydia* infections, 51
    for gonorrhea, 51
    for urethritis, 132–133
    for urinary tract infections, 1–2
Ceftriaxone
    for chancroid, 52
    for *Chlamydia* infections, 51
    for gonorrhea, 51
Cellulitis, 133
Cerniliton, for prostatitis, 81
Chancroid, 51–52
Chelating agents, for stone disease, 174
Chemotherapy
    for bladder cancer, 259

Chemotherapy (*continued*)
  irritative voiding symptoms after, 123, 125
Chlamydia trachomatis
  in lymphogranuloma venereum, 52
  in urethritis, 33, 51, 132–133
Chlorthalidone, for stone disease, 174
Chordee, 19
Chronic Kidney Disease Epidemiology Collaboration equation, 162
Chronic pelvic pain syndrome
  definition of, 76
  etiology of, 76
  evaluation of, 77–79
  phenotypes of, 81–84
  treatment of, 79–81
Chronic Prostatitis Symptom Index, 78
Ciprofloxacin
  for chancroid, 52
  for prostatitis, 79–80
  for urethritis, 132–133
  for urinary tract infections, 37
Circumcision
  HIV infection and, 143–144
  injury in, 11
Citrate, deficiency of, stone formation in, 171, 174
Clean intermittent self-catheterization, for neurogenic bladder, 116–117
Cockcroft-Gault equation, 162
Cocktail solutions, for bladder pain syndrome, 68
Colic, renal, 171–173
Cologne Male Survey, of erectile dysfunction, 217
CombAT (Combination of Avodart and Tamsulosin) study, 95–96
Computed tomography
  for bladder injury, 248
  for hematuria, 157
  for kidney failure, 163
  for pyelonephritis, 47
  for renal abscess, 45
  for renal cell carcinoma, 182–183
  for renal injury, 246
  for stone disease, 172
  for testicular tumors, 240
  for trauma, 246
  for ureteral injury, 247
  for urinary tract infections, 33, 44
Condyloma acuminata, 53, 133
Condyloma lata, 52
Constipation, irritative voiding in, 126
Contusions, renal, 246–247
Coronary artery disease, erectile dysfunction in, 214–215
Corticosteroids, for prostatitis, 80
Creatinine, in kidney failure, 162
Cryotherapy

for human papilloma virus infections, 53
    for molluscum contagiosum, 53
Cryptococcus neoformans, in prostatitis, 132
Cryptorchidism, 10
Culture, urine. *See* Urine culture.
Cyclic adenosine monophosphate, in penile erection, 202, 204
Cyclic guanosine monophosphate, in penile erection, 202, 204
Cyclobenzaprine, for prostatitis, 80
Cyclophosphamide, irritative voiding symptoms after, 123, 125
Cyst(s)
    epididymis, 239
    scrotal wall, 238
Cystadenomas, papillary, paratesticular, 239
Cystectomy
    for bladder cancer, 259
    for bladder pain syndrome, 68–69
Cystic fibrosis, infertility in, 227
Cystinuria, stone formation in, 174–175
Cystitis, 48–50
    approach to, 33
    evaluation of, 32–33
    in HIV infection, 130
    in pediatric patients, 1–4
    interstitial. *See* Bladder pain syndrome.
    pathogenesis of, 31
    prophylaxis for, 38
    red flags in, 35
    treatment of, 35–37
Cystography
    for bladder injury, 248
    for trauma, 246
Cystometry, in urodynamic studies, 112–113
Cystoscopy
    for bladder pain syndrome, 61, 64–66
    for hematuria, 157–158
Cystourethropexy, retropubic, for incontinence, 107–108
Cytology, for hematuria, 157–158

D

Darifenacin, for irritative voiding symptoms, 126
Desmopressin
    for enuresis, 6
    for nocturia, 255
Detrusor contractions, involuntary, 112–113
Detrusor-sphincter dyssynergia, 113, 115–116
Diabetes mellitus, erectile dysfunction in, 214–216
DiaPat urine test, for prostate cancer, 197
DIAPPERS mnemonic, for incontinence, 102
Diazepam, for prostatitis, 80
Diet

Diet (*continued*)
  for bladder pain syndrome, 68
  for incontinence, 105
  for prostatitis, 79
  for stone disease, 137
Digital rectal examination
  for lower urinary tract symptoms, 91
  for prostatitis, 78
Dimercaptosuccinic acid renal scan, for urinary tract infections, 4
Dimethylsulfoxide, for bladder pain syndrome, 68
Dipstick test
  for hematuria, 154
  for kidney failure, 162
  for urinary tract infections, 32
Diuresis, in obstructive uropathy, 163–164
Diuretics, for stone disease, 174
DNA integrity, of sperm, 227
Doppler imaging
  for scrotal injury, 250
  for stone disease, 172
Doxazosin
  for lower urinary tract symptoms, 94
  for prostatitis, 80
Doxycycline
  for bladder pain syndrome, 66, 68
  for *Chlamydia* infections, 51
  for lymphogranuloma venereum, 52
  for urethritis, 132–133
Drainage, of perinephric abscess, 46
Duloxetine, for incontinence, 107
Dutasteride
  for lower urinary tract symptoms, 94–95
  for prostatitis, 80
Dysuria, 5–6

E

ED. *See* Erectile dysfunction.
Elderly persons, **253–264**
  benign prostatic hyperplasia in, 254
  bladder cancer in, 258–259
  cancer in, 256–260
  demographics of, 253
  erectile dysfunction in, 260
  incontinence in, 102, 255–256
  kidney cancer in, 259–260
  nocturia in, 254–255
  prostate cancer in, 258
  surgical considerations in, 256–258
  urinary tract infections in, 30, 260–261
  voiding dysfunction in, 254–256

Electromyography, in urodynamic studies, 112–113
Emphysematous pyelonephritis, 46–47
Endothelial dysfunction, in erectile dysfunction, 215–217
Enterobacter, in cystitis, 130
Enuresis, 6
Epididymis, masses of, 239–240
Epididymo-orchitis, 9, 50–51, 132, 240
Erectile dysfunction, **201–221**
  assessment of, 203, 205–207
  definition of, 201, 213
  in cardiovascular disease, 214–216
  in elderly persons, 260
  in HIV infection, 137–140
  in lower urinary tract symptoms, 216–217
  in testosterone deficiency, 217–218
  pathophysiology of, 203, 214–217
  physiology of, 202–204
  referral in, 206–207
  treatment of, 137–140, 207–211
ERSPC (European Randomized Study of Screening for Prostate Cancer), 194, 196–197
Erythromycin
  for chancroid, 52
  for lymphogranuloma venereum, 52
Escherichia coli
  in cystitis, 130
  in urinary tract infections, 31, 47, 260–261
Estrogen status
  in irritative voiding, 126
  in urinary tract infections, 29–30
European Association of Urology, bladder pain syndrome taxonomy of, 62
European Randomized Study of Screening for Prostate Cancer, 194, 196–197
European Society for the Study of Interstitial Cystitis, bladder pain syndrome definition of, 56, 66
Exercise
  for prostatitis, 79
  pelvic floor, for incontinence, 105–106

F

Famciclovir, for herpes simplex virus infections, 53
Fertility. *See also* Infertility.
  HIV infection and, 140–141
Fesoterodine
  for irritative voiding symptoms, 126
  for lower urinary tract symptoms, 95
Fetus, hydronephrosis in, 4–5
Finasteride
  for lower urinary tract symptoms, 94–95
  for prostatitis, 80
Fistulae, urinary tract, in HIV infection, 143
Fluid intake, irritative voiding and, 126

Fluid restriction, with neurogenic bladder, 117
Fluoroquinolones
    for gonorrhea, 51
    for prostatitis, 79, 131–132
    for urinary tract infections, 37, 49
Foley catheter, for neurogenic bladder, 116–117
Follicle-stimulating hormone, infertility and, 230–231
Foreskin, disorders of, 11
Fosfomycin, for urinary tract infections, 36–37
Fournier gangrene, 133
Fractional excretion of sodium test, for kidney failure, 162
Free prostate-specific antigen test, 195
Frequency, urinary, in irritative voiding symptoms, 121–127
Frequency volume charts, for lower urinary tract symptoms, 91, 93
Fungi, in cystitis, 130

    G

Gabentinoids, for prostatitis, 81
Genetic factors
    in prostate cancer, 196
    in urinary tract infections, 29
Genital warts, 53, 133
Genitalia, disorders of
    female, 11–12
    male, 8–11
Germ cell tumors, testicular, 142, 240–241
Glomerular filtration rate
    in kidney failure, 161–164
    in renal cell carcinoma, 182
Gubernaculum, masses of, 239–240

    H

Haemophilus ducreyi, in urinary tract infections, 51–52
Hematuria, **153–159**
    causes of, 153–154
    evaluation of, 154–158
    follow-up in, 158
    in bladder injury, 248
    in HIV infection, 134
    in irritative voiding, 122–123
    in kidney injury, 246
    in pediatric patients, 7–8
    in renal cell carcinoma, 181
    in urethral injury, 248
    in urinary tract infections, 35
    prevalence of, 153
Henoch-Schönlein purpura, of scrotal wall, 239
Hernia, 242
    inguinal, 9

Herpes simplex virus
    genital, 133
    in urethritis, 33
    in urinary tract infection, 52–53
HIV infection, **129–151**
    cancer in, 141–143
    circumcision and, 143–144
    hematuria in, 134
    infertility in, 140–141
    kidney failure in, 143
    sexual dysfunction in, 137–140
    skin infections in, 133
    urinary fistulae in, 143
    urinary tract infections in, 129–133
    urolithiasis in, 135–137
    voiding dysfunction in, 134–135
Human immunodeficiency virus infection. *See* HIV infection.
Human leukocyte antigens, in urinary tract infections, 29
Human papilloma virus infections, 53, 133
Hydrocele, 9–10, 242
Hydronephrosis
    antenatal, 4–5
    in cancer, 141
    in urinary tract infections, 47–48
Hydroxyzine, for bladder pain syndrome, 68
Hypercalciuria, stone formation in, 170, 174
Hyperlipidemia, erectile dysfunction in, 214–216
Hyperoxaluria, stone formation in, 171, 174
Hyperparathyroidism, hypercalciuria in, stone formation in, 170
Hypertension
    erectile dysfunction in, 214–216
    in autonomic dysreflexia, 117–118
    in renal injury, 247
    in scarred kidneys, 16–17
Hyperuricosuria, stone formation in, 170, 174
Hypocitraturia, stone formation in, 171, 174
Hypogonadism
    erectile dysfunction in, 217–218
    evaluation of, 203, 205–207
    in HIV infection, 138, 140–141
Hypospadias, 10–11, 19–20

I

Imipramine, for incontinence, 107
Immune modulators, for prostatitis, 80
Immunotherapy, for kidney cancer, 260
In vitro fertilization, for HIV patients, 140–141
Incontinence
    in elderly persons, 255–256
    in pediatric patients, 5–6

Incontinence (*continued*)
    in posterior urethral valves, 21
    in women, **101–109**
        classification of, 101–102
        definition of, 101–102
        evaluation of, 102, 104–105
        mixed, 102
        prevalence of, 102
        risk factors for, 102–103
        stress, 101, 105–108
        treatment of, 105–109
        types of, 101–102
        urge, 101–102, 108–109
    urinary tract infections in, 30
Indinavir, urolithiasis due to, 136
Infections, urinary tract. *See* Urinary tract infections.
Infertility, **223–234**
    causes of, 228–230
    definitions of, 223–224
    epidemiology of, 223–224
    evaluation for
        initial, 227–230
        laboratory, 230–231
        radiologic, 230–231
    follow-up for, 231
    in HIV infection, 140–141
    pathophysiology of, 223–224
    semen analysis in, 224–227
Inguinal hernia, 9
Intercavernous therapy, for erectile dysfunction, 210
International Children's Continence Society, recommendations of, 5–6
International Continence Society, bladder pain syndrome taxonomy of, 62
International Index of Erectile Function, 203, 215
International Prostate Symptoms Score, 88, 92, 217
Interstitial cystitis. *See* Bladder pain syndrome.
Intestine, reconstruction of, 21–23
Intraurethral therapy, for erectile dysfunction, 210
Intravenous pyelography, for trauma, 246
Intravenous urography, for hematuria, 157
Iowa Prostate Cancer Consensus, 258
Irritative voiding symptoms, **121–127**

K

Kaposi sarcoma, in HIV infection, 141
Karyotype testing, for infertility, 227
Kegel exercises, for incontinence, 105–106
Kidney
    abscess of, 45–46
    cancer of, **179–189**, 259–260
    congenital anomalies of, 4–5

damage of, with neurogenic bladder, 115–116
failure of, **161–168**
    assessment of, 161–162
    causes of, 162–163
    in HIV infection, 143
    in pediatric patients, 16–17
    in posterior urethral valves, 20–21
infections of, 43–48. *See also* Pyelonephritis.
    in HIV infection, 130–131
injury of, 246–247
lymphoma of, 142
renal cell carcinoma of, **179–189**
resection of, 185–187, 259–260
scarring of, 16–17
stone disease of. *See* Stone disease.
ultrasonography of, 162–163
Klebsiella, in cystitis, 130
Kruger classification, of sperm morphology, 226

L

Labial adhesions, 11
Lacerations, renal, 246–247
Lactobacilli, reduction of, urinary tract infections in, 29–30
Laser lithotripsy, for stone disease, 173
Laser therapy, for human papilloma virus infections, 53
Leiomyomas, paratesticular, 239
Leukocyte esterase test, for urinary tract infections, 32
Levofloxacin
    for prostatitis, 80
    for urinary tract infections, 37
Lewis blood group antigen, in urinary tract infections, 29
Leydig cell tumors, 241
Lifestyle changes
    for erectile dysfunction, 207
    for incontinence, 105–107
Lipomas, of spermatic cord, 242
Lipomatosis, pelvic, obstructive uropathy in, 166–167
Lithotripsy, for stone disease, 173
Lomefloxacin, for prostatitis, 79
Lower urinary tract symptoms
    comorbidities with, 122
    differential diagnosis of, 122, 124
    erectile dysfunction in, 216–217
    in HIV infection, 134–135
    irritative voiding symptoms in, **121–127**
    male, **87–100**
        assessment of, 89–92
        definitions of, 87–88
        epidemiology of, 88–89
        natural history of, 88–89

Lower (*continued*)
    treatment of, 93–96
    watchful waiting in, 93
  pathophysiology of, 217
  treatment of, 135
Lymphogranuloma venereum, 52
Lymphomas, non-Hodgkin's, in HIV infection, 141–142

M

Magnetic resonance imaging
  for hematuria, 157
  for penile injury, 249
  for renal cell carcinoma, 182–183
  for trauma, 246
  for urinary tract infections, 33
Massage, for prostatitis, 81
Meatal stenosis, 11
Medical Therapy of Prostatic Symptoms (MTOPS), 94
Medicated urethral system for erection (MUSE), 210
Menopause, urinary tract infections and, 29–30
α-Mercaptopropionylglycine, for stone disease, 174
Metastasis
  from renal cell carcinoma, 187
  ureteral, kidney failure in, 166
Midurethral slings, for incontinence, 107–108
Modification of Diet in Renal Disease equation, 162, 259
Molluscum contagiosum, 53, 133
Motility, of sperm, 225–226
MTOPS (Medical Therapy of Prostatic Symptoms), 94
Multicystic dysplastic kidney disease, 5
Muscle relaxants, for prostatitis, 80
Mycobacterium, in kidney infections, 131

N

National Health and Social Life Survey, 216–217
National Institutes of Health, prostatitis classification of, 75–76
Neisseria gonorrhoeae, in urethritis, 33, 51, 132–133
Nephrectomy
  for kidney cancer, 259–260
  for renal cell carcinoma, 185–187
Nephrocalcinosis, 171
Nephrolithotomy, for stone disease, 173
Nephropathy, in HIV infection, 143
Nephrostomy tubes, for tumor obstruction, 166
Neurogenic bladder, **111–120**
  definition of, 112
  detrusor-sphincter dyssynergia in, 115–116
  in injury of micturition center, 113–114

in pediatric patients, 6
in suprasacral spinal cord injury, 114–115
irritative voiding symptoms in, 125
kidney damage in, 115–116, 165–166
management of, 116–118
micturition reflex and, 111–112
urodynamic testing for, 112–113
Neuromodulation, for incontinence, 108
Nitric oxide
in erectile dysfunction, 215
in penile erection, 202, 204
Nitrite test, for urinary tract infections, 32
Nitrofurantoin, for urinary tract infections, 36–37
Nocturia
in elderly persons, 254–255
in irritative voiding symptoms, 121–127
Nonsteroidal antiinflammatory drugs
for prostatitis, 80
for stone disease, 173
Norfloxacin, for prostatitis, 79
Nuclear scan, for kidney failure, 163
Nursing homes, urinary tract infections in, 30

O

Obesity, erectile dysfunction in, 214–216
Obstructive uropathy, 47–48
bilateral versus unilateral, 163
in cancer, 141
kidney failure in, 163–167
at tumor, 166
at ureteropelvic junction, 165
in benign prostatic hyperplasia, 164
in neurogenic bladder, 165–166
in stone disease, 164–165
in stricture, 165
physiologic changes with, 163–164
Ofloxacin
for prostatitis, 79
for urethritis, 132–133
Oligoasthenospermia, 231
Olmsted County Study, of erectile dysfunction, 214–215
ONTARGET trial, 215
Orchiectomy, for testicular tumors, 240
Orchitis, 50–51
Oxalate stones, 171
stone formation in, 174
Oxybutinin
for irritative voiding symptoms, 126
for lower urinary tract symptoms, 95

P

Pain
  in bladder pain syndrome, **55–73**
  in irritative voiding symptoms, 121–127
  in stone disease, 171–173
Painful bladder syndrome. *See* Bladder pain syndrome.
Papaverine, for erectile dysfunction, 210
Papillary cystadenomas, paratesticular, 239
Paraphimosis, 11
Parasites, in cystitis, 130
PCA 3 test, for prostate cancer, 197
Pediatric patients, **1–13, 15–25**
  antenatal hydronephrosis in, 4–5
  bladder dysfunction in, 21–23
  circumcision injury in, 11
  hematuria in, 7–8
  hypospadias in, 10–11, 19–20
  incontinence in, 5–6
  intestinal reconstruction in, 21–23
  labial disorder in, 11
  lower urinary tract dysfunction in, 5–6
  paraphimosis and phimosis in, 11
  posterior urethral valves in, 20–21
  pyeloplasty in, 18–19
  scrotal swelling in, 8–10
  testicular torsion in, 8–9
  undescended testicle in, 10, 240
  ureteral implantation in, 15–18
  ureteropelvic junction obstruction in, 18–19
  urinary tract infections in, 1–4, 15–18
  vesicoureteral reflux in, 15–18
  vulvitis in, 11–12
Pelvic floor dysfunction, irritative voiding symptoms in, 125–126
Pelvic floor exercises, for incontinence, 105–106
Pelvic fluid, in bladder injury, 248
D-Penicillamine, for stone disease, 174–175
Penicillin G, for syphilis, 52
Penis
  cancer of, 142
  congenital defects of, 10–11, 19–20
  erection of
    dysfunctional. *See* Erectile dysfunction.
    physiology of, 202–203
  injury of, 249
  prosthesis for, for erectile dysfunction, 210
Pentosanpolysulfate, for bladder pain syndrome, 68
Perinephric abscess, 45–46
Phentolamine, for erectile dysfunction, 210
Phenylpropranolamine, for incontinence, 107
Phimosis, 11

Phosphodiesterase inhibitors, for erectile dysfunction, 138–140, 208–209
Physical therapy
    for bladder pain syndrome, 68
    for prostatitis, 81
Phytotherapy
    for prostatitis, 81
    in lower urinary tract symptoms, 93
PLCO (Prostate, Lung, Colorectal, and Ovarian) Cancer Screening Trial, 194–197
Pneumaturia, in HIV infection, 143
Pneumocystis carinii, in kidney infections, 131
Podofilox, for human papilloma virus infections, 53
Podophyllin, for human papilloma virus infections, 53
Pokyuria, in lower urinary tract symptoms, 93
Polyps, scrotal wall, 237
Polyuria, in lower urinary tract symptoms, 93
Positron emission tomography, for renal cell carcinoma, 182–183
Posterior urethral valves, 20–21
Postvoid residual
    for incontinence, 104–105
    for irritative voiding symptoms, 122–123
PREDICT study, of lower urinary tract symptom treatment, 95–96
Pregnancy, urinary tract infections in, 30–31
Prolactinomas, infertility due to, 230
Prostaglandin E1, for erectile dysfunction, 210
Prostate
    benign hyperplasia of. *See also* Lower urinary tract symptoms, male.
        in elderly persons, 254
        kidney failure in, 164
    cancer of
        in elderly persons, 258
        in HIV infection, 142–143
        markers for, 197
        natural history of, 193
        prostate-specific antigen in, **191–200**
        risk factors for, 196
        screening for, 194, 258
        survival in, 193–194
        treatment of, 193–194
        watchful waiting for, 193
    massage of, 78, 81
Prostate, Lung, Colorectal, and Ovarian Cancer Screening Trial, 194–197
Prostate Cancer Prevention Trial, 195, 214
Prostatectomy
    for benign prostatic hyperplasia, 254
    for prostate cancer, 258
    for prostatitis, 81
Prostate-specific antigen
    for lower urinary tract symptoms, 88–89, 91
    for prostate cancer, 142–143, **191–200**
        current recommendations for, 197–198
        history of, 192

Prostate-specific (*continued*)
    limitations of, 196–197
    manipulations of, 195
    screening with, 192–194
    versus other markers, 197
  for prostatitis, 78–79
Prostate-specific antigen density test, 195
Prostate-specific antigen velocity test, 195
Prostatitis syndromes, **75–86**
  approach to, 82–84
  classification of, 75–76, 81–84
  epidemiology of, 75
  etiology of, 76
  evaluation of, 77–79
  in HIV infection, 131–132
  phenotypes of, 81–84
  treatment of, 79–81
Prosthesis, penile, for erectile dysfunction, 210
Proteus, in cystitis, 130
Pseudoephedrine, for incontinence, 107
Psychological support, for prostatitis, 81
Pyelitis, 46–47
Pyelography
  intravenous, for trauma, 246
  retrograde, for hematuria, 157
Pyelonephritis, 43–45
  abscess development in, 45–46
  approach to, 33–34
  complicated versus uncomplicated, 44–45
  emphysematous, 46–47
  evaluation of, 32–33
  in HIV infection, 130–131
  in pediatric patients, 1–4
  pathogenesis of, 31
  treatment of, 37–38
  xanthogranulomatous, 47–48
Pyeloplasty, 18–19
Pyonephrosis, 47–48
Pyuria, 49
  in elderly persons, 261
  red flags in, 35

Q

Quercetin, for prostatitis, 81

R

Racial factors, in prostate cancer, 195–196
Radiofrequency ablation, for renal cell carcinoma, 186
Radiography

for hematuria, 157
for kidney injury, 246
for renal cell carcinoma, 183
for urinary tract infections, 32–33, 44
Rand Corporation study, of bladder pain syndrome, 57
5-α-Reductase inhibitors, for lower urinary tract symptoms, 94–95
Renal cell carcinoma, **179–189**
  clinical presentation of, 180–181
  evaluation of, 181–185
  gross appearance of, 184
  in elderly persons, 259–260
  incidence of, 180–181
  subtypes of, 187–188
  treatment of, 185–188
  watchful waiting for, 186–187
Renovascular injuries, 246–247
Retrograde pyelography, for hematuria, 157
Retrograde urography
  for kidney failure, 163
  for trauma, 246
  for urethral injury, 248–249
Retroperitoneal adenopathy, in HIV infection, 141
Retroperitoneal fibrosis, obstructive uropathy in, 166
Retropubic cystourethropexy, for incontinence, 107–108
Rhabdomyosarcomas, 239, 242
RH-PET test, for erectile definition, 216

S

Sacral root, neuromodulation of, for incontinence, 108
Salmonella
  in cystitis, 130
  in epididymo-orchitis, 132
Sarcomas, Kaposi, in HIV infection, 141
Saw palmetto
  for lower urinary tract symptoms, 93
  for prostatitis, 81
Scarring, kidney, 16–17
Schistosomiasis, irritative voiding symptoms in, 123
Scrotum. *See also* Testis.
  injury of, 249–250
  masses in, **235–244**
    examination of, 235–236
    germ cell tumors, 142
    history of, 235
    imaging for, 237
    lymphoma, 142
    paratesticular, 239–240
    spermatic cord, 242
    testicular, 240–242
    types of, 238

Scrotum (*continued*)
    wall, 237–239
    swelling of, 8–10
Semen analysis, 224–227
  reference values for, 224
  sperm characteristics in
    concentration, 225
    DNA integrity, 227
    morphology, 226
    motility, 225–226
    number, 225
    vitality, 225
  volume, 224
Seminomas, 240–241
Sertoli cell tumors, 241
Sexual activity. *See also* Erectile dysfunction.
  penile injury during, 249
  urinary tract infections in, 28–29
Sexual dysfunction
  in HIV infection, 137–140
  in hypospadias, 19–20
Sexually transmitted diseases
  in HIV infection, 133
  in men, 51–53
  scrotal skin involvement in, 238
Shock wave lithotripsy, for stone disease, 173
Sildenafil, for erectile dysfunction, 138–140, 208–209, 260
Silodosin, for lower urinary tract symptoms, 94
Skin infections
  in HIV infection, 133
  scrotal, 238
Slings, midurethral, for incontinence, 107–108, 256
Sodium bicarbonate, for stone disease, 174
Solifenacin
  for irritative voiding symptoms, 126
  for lower urinary tract symptoms, 95
Sperm abnormalities, in HIV infection, 140–141
Sperm characteristics, evaluation of, for infertility, 225–227
Spermatic cord
  examination of, in infertility, 229
  masses of, 242
Spermatoceles, 239
Spermicides, urinary tract infections and, 28–29
Sphincterotomy, for detrusor-sphincter dyssynergia, 116
Spinal cord injury, suprasacral, neurogenic bladder in, 114–115
Staghorn calculi, 173
Staphylococcus aureus, in perineal cellulitis, 133
Staphylococcus saphrophyticus, in urinary tract infections, 31
Stents
  ureteral
    for stricture, 165

for tumor obstruction, 166
    urethral, for detrusor-sphincter dyssynergia, 116
Stone disease, **168–177**
    clinical manifestations of, 171–172
    diagnosis of, 171–172
    epidemiology of, 169–170
    in HIV infection, 135–137
    kidney failure in, 171
    morbidity in, 171
    obstruction in, kidney failure in, 164–165
    pathogenesis of, 170–171
    recurrent, 173–174
    treatment of, 172–175
Stranguria, in irritative voiding symptoms, 121–127
Stress, in bladder pain syndrome, 59
Stress incontinence
    in elderly persons, 255–256
    in women, 101, 105–108
Stricture, ureteral, kidney failure in, 165
Stroke, neurogenic bladder in, 113–114
Syphilis, 52, 133

T

Tadalafil, for erectile dysfunction, 208–209
Tamulosin
    for lower urinary tract symptoms, 94
    for prostatitis, 80
    for stone disease, 173
Teratomas, 241
Teratozoospermia, 226
Terazosin
    for lower urinary tract symptoms, 94
    for prostatitis, 80
Testis
    cancer of, 142, 240–241
    examination of, 229
    fracture of, 250
    germ cell tumors of, 142, 240–241
    infections of, 50–51, 132
    injury of, 249–250
    lymphoma of, 142
    masses of, 240–242
    rupture of, 9
    torsion of, 8–9, 241–242
    undescended, 10, 240
Testosterone deficiency
    erectile dysfunction in, 217–218
    in HIV infection, 138
    infertility in, 229–230
Tetracyclines, for irritative voiding symptoms, 123

Thermotherapy, for prostatitis, 81
Timed voiding, for incontinence, 106
TIMES study, of lower urinary tract symptom treatment, 96
Tolterodine, for irritative voiding symptoms, 126
Torsion, testicular, 8–9, 241–242
TRANSCEND trial, 215
Transillumination, of scrotum, 237
Trauma, **245–251**
    bladder, 248
    blunt, 245–246
    penetrating, 246
    penile, 249
    renal, 246–247
    scrotal, 249–250
    testicular, 249–250
    ureteral, 247
    urethral, 248–249
Treponema pallidum infections, 52
Trichloroacetic acid, for human papilloma virus infections, 53
Trimethoprim-sulfamethoxazole
    for prostatitis, 79
    for urinary tract infections, 2, 36, 49
Trospium, for lower urinary tract symptoms, 95
Tuberculosis
    cystitis in, 130
    irritative voiding symptoms in, 123
    pyelonephritis in, 131
Tumor(s)
    kidney, **179–189**
    scrotal, 9–10
        paratesticular, 239–240
        testicular, 240–242
        wall, 237–239
    ureteral, 166
Tygerberg morphology, of sperm, 226

U

Ulcers
    genital, 51–52, 133
    in bladder pain syndrome, 62–64
Ultrasonography
    for hematuria, 157
    for kidney failure, 162–163
    for penile injury, 249
    for renal abscess, 45
    for renal cell carcinoma, 183
    for scrotal injury, 250
    for scrotal masses, 237
    for stone disease, 172
    for trauma, 246
    for urinary tract infections, 2–3

UPOINT (Urinary, Psychosocial, Organ specific, Infection, Neurologic/systemic and Tenderness) classification, 64, 81–84
Ureter
    hydronephrosis in, 4–5
    implantation of, 15–18
    injury of, 247
    obstruction of, in cancer, 141
    reconstruction of, in stricture, 165
    stones in. *See* Stone disease.
    stricture of, 165
    tumor of, kidney failure in, 166
Ureteropelvic junction obstruction, 18–19, 165
Urethra
    bulking procedures for, 107
    devices for, in incontinence, 106–107
    injury of, 248–249
    slings for, for incontinence, 107–108
    stent for, for detrusor-sphincter dyssynergia, 116
Urethritis
    approach to, 33
    in HIV infection, 132–133
Urge incontinence
    in elderly persons, 255–256
    in women, 101–102, 108–109
Urgency, urinary, in irritative voiding symptoms, 121–127
Uric acid stones, 136–137, 170, 174
Urinalysis
    for hematuria, 154–156
    for incontinence, 104
    for kidney failure, 162–163
    for lower urinary tract symptoms, 91
    for urinary tract infections, 32
Urinary diversion, 21–23
    for bladder cancer, 259
    for bladder pain syndrome, 68–69
Urinary tract, obstruction of. *See* Obstructive uropathy.
Urinary tract infections
    hematuria in, 155–156
    in elderly persons, 260–261
    in HIV infection, 129–133
    in men, **43–54**
        bladder, 48–50
        epididymitis, 50–51
        kidney, 43–48
        orchitis, 50–51
        recurrent, 49–50
        sexually transmitted, 51–53
        with obstruction, 47–48
    in neurogenic bladder, 117
    in pediatric patients, 1–4, 15–18
    in women, **27–41**

Urinary tract infections (*continued*)
 age-specific factors in, 29–30
 behavioral factors in, 28–29
 economic burden of, 27
 epidemiology of, 27–28
 evaluation of, 32–33
 genetic factors in, 29
 in pregnancy, 30–31
 in urinary catheterization, 30
 pathogenesis of, 31
 prophylaxis for, 38
 recurrent, 34–35
 red flags in, 35
 susceptibility factors in, 28
 treatment of, 35–37
 types of, 33–35
 unresolved, 34
 irritative voiding in, 123
 stone disease in, 171
Urine
 involuntary loss of. *See* Incontinence.
 sample collection of, 32
Urine culture
 for epididymo-orchitis, 132
 for incontinence, 104
 for irritative voiding symptoms, 122–123
 for prostatitis, 78
 for pyelonephritis, 131
 for urinary tract infections, 32, 34
Urodynamic studies
 for bladder pain syndrome, 61
 for neurogenic bladder, 112–113
Urodynamic testing, for incontinence, 105
Urography
 computed tomography, for kidney failure, 163
 for hematuria, 157
 retrograde. *See* Retrograde urography.
Urolithiasis. *See* Stone disease.
Urologic disorders
 bladder pain syndrome, **55–73**
 erectile dysfunction. *See* Erectile dysfunction.
 hematuria. *See* Hematuria.
 in elderly persons. *See* Elderly persons.
 in HIV infection, **129–151**
 incontinence. *See* Incontinence.
 infections. *See* Urinary tract infections.
 infertility, **223–234**
 irritative voiding symptoms, **121–127**
 lower tract symptoms. *See* Lower urinary tract symptoms.
 neurogenic bladder. *See* Neurogenic bladder.
 pediatric. *See* Pediatric patients.

pelvic pain syndrome, **75–86**
prostate cancer. *See* Prostate, cancer of.
prostatitis, **75–86,** 131–132
renal failure. *See* Kidney, failure of.
renal masses, **179–189**
scrotal masses, **235–244**
stone disease, **169–177**
trauma, **245–251**

V

VA COOP study, of lower urinary tract symptom treatment, 95–96
Vacuum constriction devices, for erectile dysfunction, 210, 260
Vaginal prolapse, irritative voiding symptoms in, 125–126
Vaginitis, versus urinary tract infections, 33
Valacyclovir, for herpes simplex virus infections, 53
Vardenafil, for erectile dysfunction, 208–209
Varicocele, 9–10, 229–230, 242
Vas deferens
    congenital absence of, 227
    examination of, in infertility, 229
    masses of, 242
Vascular pedicle, of testis, 242
Vasectomy, 230
Vasoactive intestinal peptide, for erectile dysfunction, 210
Vesicoenteric fistula, in HIV infection, 143
Vesicoureteral reflux, 3–4, 15–18
Vitality, of sperm, 225
Voiding
    dysfunctional, in elderly persons, 254–256
    irritative symptoms in, **121–127**
Voiding cystourethrography
    for hydronephrosis, 5
    for urinary tract infections, 2–3
Vulvitis, 11–12

W

Warts, genital, 53, 133
Weight loss, for incontinence, 105
World Health Organization, semen analysis reference values of, 224

X

Xanthogranulomatous pyelonephritis, 47–48

Y

Y chromosome microdeletions, infertility and, 227
Yohimbine, for erectile dysfunction, 210
Yolk sac tumors, 241